Acupuncture Therapeutics

Companion volumes

Diagnostics of Traditional Chinese Medicine
Edited by Zhu Bing and Wang Hongcai
ISBN 978 1 84819 036 8
International Acupuncture Textbooks

Basic Theories of Traditional Chinese Medicine
Edited by Zhu Bing and Wang Hongcai
ISBN 978 1 84819 038 2
International Acupuncture Textbooks

Meridians and Acupoints
Edited by Zhu Bing and Wang Hongcai
ISBN 978 1 84819 037 5
International Acupuncture Textbooks

Case Studies from the Medical Records of Leading Chinese Acupuncture Experts
Edited by Zhu Bing and Wang Hongcai
ISBN 978 1 84819 046 7
International Acupuncture Textbooks

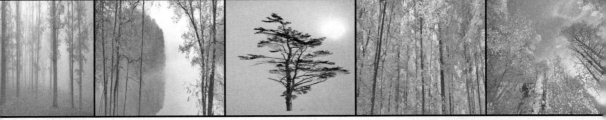

International
Acupuncture
Textbooks

Acupuncture Therapeutics

Chief Editors: Zhu Bing and Wang Hongcai

Advisor: Cheng Xinnong

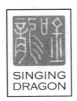

SINGING
DRAGON

LONDON AND PHILADELPHIA

China Beijing International Acupuncture Training Center
Institute of Acupuncture and Moxibustion
China Academy of Chinese Medical Sciences
Advisor: Cheng Xinnong
Chief Editors: Zhu Bing, Wang Hongcai
Deputy Editors: Hu Xuehua, Huang Hui, Yu Min, Wang Huizhu
Members of the Editorial Board: Huang Hui, Hong Tao, Hu Xuehua, Liu Xuan, Liu Yuting,
Wang Fang, Wang Hongcai, Wang Huizhu, Wang Yue, Wu Mozheng, Yu Min, Zhu Bing,
Zhang Nan, Zhang Yi

First published in 2011
by Singing Dragon (an imprint of Jessica Kingsley Publishers)
in co-operation with People's Military Medical Press
116 Pentonville Road
London N1 9JB, UK
and
400 Market Street, Suite 400
Philadelphia, PA 19106, USA

Library of Congress Cataloging in Publication Data
A CIP catalog record for this book is available from the Library of Congress

British Library Cataloguing in Publication Data
A CIP catalogue record for this book is available from the British Library

ISBN 978 1 84819 039 9

Printed and bound in Great Britain
by MPG Books Group

CHINA BEIJING INTERNATIONAL ACUPUNCTURE TRAINING CENTER

China Beijing International Acupuncture Training Center (CBIATC) was set up in 1975 at the request of the World Health Organization (WHO) and with the approval of the State Council of the People's Republic of China. Since its foundation, it has been supported and administered by WHO, the Chinese government, the State Administration of Traditional Chinese Medicine (SATCM) and the China Academy of Chinese Medical Sciences (CACMS). Now it has developed into a world-famous, authoritative training organization.

Since 1975, aiming to popularize acupuncture to the world, CBIATC has been working actively to accomplish the task, 'to perfect ways of acupuncture training and provide more opportunities for foreign doctors', assigned by WHO. More than 30 years' experience has created an excellent teaching team led by the academician, Professor Cheng Xinnong, and a group of professors. The multiple courses here are offered in different languages, including English, German, Spanish and Japanese. According to statistics, so far CBIATC has provided training in acupuncture, Tuina Massage, Traditional Chinese Medicine, Qigong, and so on for over 10,000 medical doctors and students from 106 countries and regions.

The teaching programmes of CBIATC include three-month and various short courses, are carefully and rationally worked out based on the individual needs of participants. Characterized by the organic combination of theory with practice, there are more than ten cooperating hospitals for the students to practice in. With professional teaching and advanced services, CBIATC will lead you to the profound and wonderful world of acupuncture.

Official website: www.cbiatc.com
Training support: www.tcmoo.com

PREFACE

More than 2000 years ago, a Chinese doctor named Bianque saved the life of a crown prince simply with an acupuncture needle. The story became one of the earliest acupuncture medical cases and went down in history. It is perhaps since then that people have been fascinated by the mystery of acupuncture and kept on studying it. In 1975, at the request of the World Health Organization, an acupuncture school was founded in Beijing, China, namely the China Beijing International Acupuncture Training Center. As one of the sponsor institutions, the Center compiled a textbook of Chinese Acupuncture and Moxibustion for foreign learners, published in 1980 and reprinted repeatedly afterwards, which has been of profound, far-reaching influence. It has been adopted as a 'model book' for acupuncture education and examination in many countries, and has played a significant role in the global dissemination of acupuncture.

Today, with the purpose of extending this 'authentic and professional' knowledge, we have compiled a series of books entitled *International Acupuncture Textbooks* to introduce incisively the basic theories of Traditional Chinese Medicine (TCM) and acupuncture–moxibustion techniques, by building on and developing the characteristics of the original textbook of Chinese Acupuncture and Moxibustion; and presenting authoritatively the systematic teaching materials with concise explanation based on a core syllabus for TCM professional education in China.

In addition, just as the same plant might have its unique properties when growing in different geographical environments, this set of books may reflect, in its particular style, our experience accumulated over 30 years of international acupuncture training.

Zhu Bing and Wang Hongcai

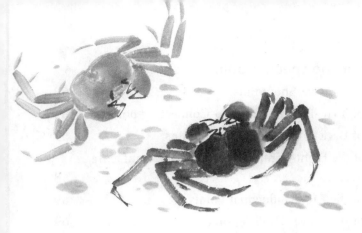

CONTENTS

GENERAL INTRODUCTION

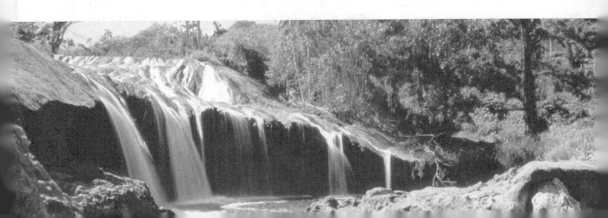

I. FUNCTIONS OF ACUPUNCTURE

1. TO UNBLOCK THE MERIDIANS AND COLLATERALS

Acupuncture is a therapy in which points are stimulated by needles or moxibustion in order to activate circulation, regulate Qi and Blood to remove pathogenic factors and treat diseases, on the basis that meridians, collaterals and the Zang Fu organs are physiologically related and pathologically influenced. So, unblocking the meridians and collaterals is the main and most direct effect of acupuncture in the treatment of disease. Obstruction in the meridians and collaterals can be removed and circulation activated through the use of the appropriate acupuncture manipulation techniques.

Meridians and collaterals are pathways through which Qi and Blood circulate and where the exterior of the body connects with the interior. They are closely related to the Zang Fu organs. When a disease occurs, the meridians and collaterals can be affected first, and then Zang Fu organs involved, or vice versa. Acupuncture can promote Qi and Blood circulation, remove pathogenic factors, regulate Qi activities, adjust the functions of the Zang Fu organs, and treat both deficient and excess syndromes of Qi and Blood in the meridians and collaterals.

2. TO STRENGTHEN BODY RESISTANCE AND ELIMINATE PATHOGENIC FACTORS

Strengthening body resistance and eliminating pathogenic factors are fundamental principles underlying the use of acupuncture in the treatment of disease. To strengthen the body resistance is to reinforce the anti-pathogenic Qi, and enhance the body's resistance.

Once the anti-pathogenic Qi is strengthened, pathogenic factors will be eliminated. To eliminate pathogenic factors is to remove the causative factors of disease. When the pathogenic factors are removed, the injury to the anti-pathogenic Qi can be alleviated. The course of a disease, including its occurrence, development and transmission, is actually the process of the conflict between the anti-pathogenic Qi and pathogenic factors. When anti-pathogenic Qi defeats pathogenic Qi, pathogenic factors are removed, and a disease is cured; when anti-pathogenic Qi fails to fight against the pathogenic Qi, a disease becomes worse. So the function of acupuncture in the treatment of disease is one of engagement in the conflict between anti-pathogenic Qi and pathogenic Qi. The effect of acupuncture in strengthening the anti-pathogenic Qi and eliminating pathogenic factors is achieved by different needling techniques and combinations of acupoints:

1. **Methods of treatment**: Moxibustion has the function of strengthening the anti-pathogenic Qi; while Blood-letting puncturing therapy is effective in removing the pathogenic factors.

2. **Acupuncture techniques**: Reinforcing and reducing techniques of acupuncture are applied in order to strengthen the anti-pathogenic Qi and eliminate pathogenic factors respectively.

3. **Points with reinforcing and reducing effects**: Gaohuang (BL43), Qihai (CV6), Guanyuan (CV4), Mingmen (GV4), etc. are often used to strengthen the anti-pathogenic Qi; the twelve Jing-Well points, Shixuan (EX-UE11), Renzhong (GV26), etc. are frequently selected to eliminate the pathogenic Qi.

4. **Order of treatment**: The order in which to strengthen the anti-pathogenic Qi and eliminate pathogenic Qi depends on the conditions of increasing, decreasing and transformation of anti-pathogenic Qi and pathogenic Qi, whether the condition is the primary and secondary, and whether the syndrome is acute or chronic. In treating a disease, either the pathogenic factors can be eliminated first, and then anti-pathogenic Qi strengthened; or anti-pathogenic Qi strengthened first, then pathogenic Qi removed; or, alternatively, anti-pathogenic Qi can be strengthened and pathogenic Qi eliminated simultaneously. Generally speaking, there is a principle 'to strengthen the anti-pathogenic Qi but leave no pathogenic Qi; to eliminate pathogenic Qi but not to hurt anti-pathogenic Qi'.

3. TO REGULATE YIN AND YANG

The key purpose of acupuncture in treating diseases is to regulate the excess and deficiency conditions of Yin and Yang, keep the body in a state of 'balance of Yin and Yang', and restore the normal physiological functions for the recovery of health. The occurrence of a disease results from a relative imbalance of Yin and Yang, namely excess and deficiency of Yin and Yang, leading to pathological changes such as 'a Yang syndrome due to Yin excess, or Yin syndrome due to excess of Yang'. The regulation of Yin and Yang by acupuncture is fulfilled through the reinforcing and reducing needling techniques and combination of acupuncture points. For instance, in treating chronic diarrhoea caused by Spleen Yang deficiency, Yinlingquan (SP9) is punctured with the reinforcing technique combined with moxibustion based on the principle of warming Yang and dispelling Cold. In treating toothache due to excessive Stomach Fire in which Yang Heat is excessive, Neiting (ST44) is punctured with the reducing technique. During regulation of Yin and Yang, Front-Mu and Back-Shu points are often used clinically to regulate and replenish Yin and Yang of the Zang Fu organs according to the principle 'to gain Yang from Yin, and gain Yin from Yang'.

II. PRINCIPLES OF TREATMENT

1. TO CLEAR HEAT AND DISPEL COLD

Cold syndromes: Syndromes caused by pathogenic Cold or Yang deficiency.

Heat syndromes: Syndromes caused by pathogenic Heat or Yin deficiency in the interior.

These two types of syndromes can be treated by applying the principle 'short retention of the needles for Heat syndromes and longer retention of needles for Cold syndromes'.

1.1 Short retention of the needles for Heat syndromes

To clear Heat: The clearing method is used in acupuncture to treat Heat syndromes by dispelling and reducing Heat; namely, Heat is treated by Cold.

Application

1. Shallow insertion with quick removal of the needle, or pricking to cause bleeding with gentle and quick needling techniques, with short retention or without retention of the needles to clear Heat through use of reducing acupuncture techniques.

2. Apply three-edged needle, cutaneous needle, or filiform needles to cause bleeding to clear Heat.

3. Select Ying-Spring points to clear Heat. For example, Laogong (PC8) is punctured to clear Heart Fire. Bleeding at Dazhui (GV14), Quchi (LI11), and twelve Jing-Well points can clear Heat.

4. When pathogenic Heat moves into the interior, needling techniques of deep insertion with retention of the needles combined with a comprehensive 'Penetrating-heaven coolness' method should be applied.

1.2 Longer retention of needles for Cold syndromes

To warm Cold: The warming method is used in acupuncture to treat Cold syndromes by warming up Yang Qi and dispelling Cold, and to restore Yang from collapse; namely, Cold is treated by warmth.

Application

1. Deep insertion with longer retention of the needles, or combined with moxibustion to warm the meridians and dispel Cold.

2. Dispel Cold by applying moxibustion, cupping, and Fire needling therapies.

3. Apply moxibustion at Mingmen (GV4), Guanyuan (CV4).

4. For retention of Cold in the interior Zang Fu organs, deep insertion with longer retention of the needles should be applied combined with a comprehensive 'Setting the mountain on Fire' method or warming needle therapy. When there is Cold in the Blood, moxibustion will be effective for warming up the Blood vessels. But for a complicated syndrome of Cold and Heat, both clearing and warming methods should be applied at the same time.

2. TO REINFORCE DEFICIENCY AND REDUCE EXCESS

Deficiency syndromes: Syndromes in which the anti-pathogenic Qi is deficient.

Excess syndromes: Syndromes in which pathogenic Qi is excessive.

For deficiency and excess syndromes, the principles of acupuncture treatment are 'reinforcing deficiency and reducing excess'. For a condition that involves neither a deficiency nor an excess syndrome, points of the affected meridians are selected.

2.1 To reinforce deficiency

Reinforcing deficiency means strengthening the anti-pathogenic Qi, promoting the functions of the Zang Fu organs and tissues, replenishing Yin, Yang, Qi and Blood of the body to improve the body resistance against diseases.

Application

Acupuncture using reinforcing needling techniques or moxibustion, which pertains to the reinforcing method, can be used to treat deficiency syndromes. Yang and Qi deficiency syndromes can be treated by the acupuncture reinforcing method combined with moxibustion. Qihai (CV6) is punctured for Qi deficiency, Mingmen (GV4) for Yang deficiency. For Yin or Blood deficiency syndromes, either acupuncture reinforcing or uniform reinforcing and the reducing methods can be applied. Moxibustion is applicable for Blood deficiency. When Yin and Yang are both deficient, Guanyuan (CV4), Qihai (CV6), Mingmen (GV4), Zusanli (ST36), Back-Shu points of the related organs, and the Yuan-Primary points can be punctured with the reinforcing technique, or moxibustion therapy be applied for tonification.

MOXIBUSTION FOR SYNDROMES OF SINKING

Syndromes of sinking: Those syndromes in which the Qi in the Middle Burner is deficient and fails to control, resulting in hypofunction or prolapse of the Zang Fu organs; syndromes with empty vessels, syndromes with a deep and weak pulse; or a dangerous syndrome of collapse of Yang with a feeble and fading pulse.

Moxibustion for syndromes of sinking: This method pertains to reinforcing for deficiency. For syndromes of hypofunctions or prolapse of the Zang Fu organs due to Qi deficiency in the Middle Burner, moxibustion can be applied at Baihui (GV20), Shenqu (CV8), Qihai (CV6), Guanyuan (CV4), Zhongwan (CV12), Pishu (BL20), Weishu (BL21), Shenshu (BL23), Zusanli (ST36), etc. to tonify Qi in the Middle Burner, lift Yang Qi to keep the internal organs in their normal position. For syndromes with too much loss of Blood, or collapse of Yang with decreased blood pressure, heavy moxibustion can be applied at the above mentioned points to promote Yang for consolidation, and restore Yang from collapse.

2.2 To reduce excess

Reducing excess means to eliminate the pathogenic factors so as to support the recovery of anti-pathogenic Qi.

Application

Excess syndromes are treated with the reducing methods. Blood-letting puncturing is a type of reducing technique. In treating excess Heat syndromes such as high fever, sunstroke, loss of consciousness, convulsions, and severe pain when the anti-pathogenic Qi has not been weakened, Dazhui (GV14), Hegu (LI4), Taichong (LR3), Weizhong (BL40), Shuigou (GV26), Shixuan (EX-UE11), and twelve Jing-Well points are punctured with the reducing or bleeding techniques but without moxibustion, to clear excessive Heat; but if the root cause of the disease is deficient with excess symptoms and signs, and the anti-pathogenic Qi has been weakened already, reinforcing and reducing techniques can be applied simultaneously, or the deficiency reinforced first, then the excess reduced.

REMOVAL OF STAGNATION

Stagnation: This refers to pathological changes of obstruction in the meridians and collaterals.

Removal of stagnation: Blood-letting puncturing, one of the reducing techniques, is used to remove Blood stagnation. For syndromes caused by obstruction of the meridians and collaterals, a three-edged needle is used to prick and cause bleeding; in severe cases, cupping can be added after bleeding to get rid of more Blood stasis. Other diseases such as thecal cyst, or infantile retention of food can also be treated using the pricking technique.

2.3 To select points from the affected meridian for treating a condition that involves neither a deficiency nor an excess syndrome

Cases without obvious manifestations of deficiency and excess, or complicated by both deficiency and excess syndromes of the Zang Fu organs or meridians and collaterals are understood to be temporary conditions of derangement of Qi and Blood, in which the other organs, meridians and collaterals are not involved, and the affected organ is only related to its relevant meridian. So, to treat such a syndrome, points from the affected meridian are selected. The Yuan-Primary points and Five-Shu points will be the best ones to be punctured. Once the Qi has arrived, a uniform reinforcing and the reducing method (using even movement) is applied by lifting and thrusting the needle to regulate Qi of the affected meridian and restore the normal functions of the affected organ.

Application

Reinforcing and reducing techniques are applied simultaneously to treat a complicated syndrome of deficiency and excess. The order and intensity of the treatment depend on the severity, the primary and secondary conditions of the syndrome, or following the order either reinforcing first, then reducing; or reducing first, then reinforcing; or reinforcing the upper, reducing the lower, or vice versa; or reinforcing the left and reducing the right, or vice versa.

3. MIND CONCENTRATION AND RESPONSE TO QI ACTIVITIES

3.1 Mind concentration

Mind concentration runs through the whole process of treating disease through acupuncture. Before and after the treatment, the patient's mental state should be observed and regulated; during the treatment, the doctor should concentrate his Mind.

Application

Before acupuncture treatment, especially for a patient having treatment for the first time, the doctor should tell him about the precautions taken for his safety, give him a general idea about acupuncture treatment, and ask him to calm the Mind and not to be nervous. If the patient is extremely nervous, or is in a state of severe fright, fear, or grief, avoid giving the treatment for the time being and prevent the Mind and Qi from being distracted and dispersed. When treating intractable, chronic and mental diseases, doctors should also give psychological treatment and explain to the patients how their body is changing, because the psychological condition of the patient affects greatly the state of the disease. Ask the patient to be confident that they can conquer the disease and should cooperate with the doctor to receive treatment for the recovery of health.

3.2 Response to Qi activities

Qi here refers to meridian Qi, which is a general term for the forms of movement and functional activities of the meridian system. Meridian Qi is manifested by the arrival of Qi, flow of Qi, and Qi running to the affected area of the disease, etc. The doctor's concentration of his Mind on needling, and the patient's concentration of his Mind on feeling the needling sensation will all be significant in stimulating meridian Qi, speeding up the arrival of Qi, and promoting Qi flow and Qi running to the affected area of the disease.

Application

When with the patient, the doctor should be serious and kind. During acupuncture treatment, he should concentrate his Mind completely on needling. He should select the points carefully and locate the points precisely. When puncturing the points, he must notice what happens below the point and observe the patient's response and expression, and ask how the patient feels about the needling sensation. If Qi doesn't arrive, use the proper manipulation techniques to promote the arrival of Qi, such as palpation, percussion, massage along the meridian and pressing methods. The patient should be calm, not nervous. When receiving the treatment, he should keep quiet and relax his muscles, and concentrate his Mind on feeling the needling sensation and on the area affected by the disease.

III. PRINCIPLES OF SYNDROME DIFFERENTIATION

1. TREATMENT OF DISEASES BASED ON SYNDROME DIFFERENTIATION ACCORDING TO THE EIGHT PRINCIPLES

The Eight Principles are the principles of Yin and Yang, exterior and interior, Cold and Heat, deficiency and excess.

Treatment based on syndrome differentiation according to the Eight Principles is a method of treatment, by which the location and nature of the diseases, and the relations between the anti-pathogenic Qi and pathogenic factors are generalized and analyzed based on the information obtained clinically from the four diagnostic methods of inspection, auscultation and olfaction, inquiring and palpation, according to the Eight Principles, the general principles for syndrome differentiation and treatment of diseases, including Yin and Yang, exterior and interior, Cold and Heat, deficiency and excess.

1.1 Treatment of diseases based on syndrome differentiation according to Yin and Yang principles

Yin and Yang are basic and general principles.

	Yin syndromes	Yang syndromes
Syndrome differentiation	Declined and weakened Yang Qi, or retention of Cold	Hyperactivity of Yang Qi, accumulation of excessive Heat
Manifestations	Hypofunction, declining, inhibition, and Cold. The interior, Cold and deficiency are Yin syndromes; deficiency Cold syndrome is a Yin syndrome	Hyperfunction, excitement, excessive, restlessness and Heat. The exterior, Heat, excess are Yang syndromes, excess Heat syndrome is a Yang syndrome
Principles of treatment	Warm up Yang, benefit Qi, and dispel Cold	Relieve the exterior symptoms, clear Heat, and reduce the excess
Meridians treated	Yin meridians are treated primarily, Yang meridians secondarily	Yang meridians are treated primarily and Yin meridians secondarily
Methods of treatment	Moxibustion, cupping	Needling, Blood-letting puncturing
Manipulation	Reinforcing method, deep insertion with longer retention of the needles	Reducing method, shallow insertion with quick removal of the needles
Prognosis	A Yang syndrome turning into a Yin syndrome suggests that the disease is getting worse; a Yin syndrome transforming into a Yang syndrome indicates that the disease has made a turn for the better	

1.2 Treatment of diseases based on syndrome differentiation according to exterior and interior principles

Exterior and interior are principles which determine the depth of the diseases.

	Exterior syndromes	Interior syndromes
Definition	Syndromes resulting from the invasion of the superficial portion of the body (body surface) by exogenous pathogenic factors, marked by fever, chills, headache, and superficial pulse	Syndromes resulting from the transmission of exogenous pathogenic factors to the interior of the body to affect the Zang Fu organs, or from the dysfunctions of the Zang Fu organs
Characteristics	Sudden onset, shallow depth, mild disease, short duration. Chills and fever, no obvious changes of the tongue coating, normal tongue, superficial pulse	Slow onset, deep depth, severe disease, long duration. Fever without chills, or chills without fever, various changes of the tongue coating, deep pulse
Principles of treatment	Unblock the meridians and collaterals, dispel Wind and relieve the exterior symptoms	Regulate Zang Fu organs, promote Qi and activate Blood circulation
Commonly used points	Dazhui (GV14), Hegu (LI4), Quchi (LI11), Waiguan (TE5), Lieque (LU7), Fengchi (GB20), Fengmen (BL12), Feishu (BL13), etc.	Zhongwan (CV12), Tianshu (ST25), Daheng (SP15), Zhigou (TE6), Fenglong (ST40), Qihai (CV6), Guanyuan (CV4), Zusanli (ST36), Sanyinjiao (SP6), Shangjuxu (ST37), Xiajuxu (ST39), etc.
Methods of treatment	Exterior Heat and excess syndromes are treated only by acupuncture without moxibustion with the reducing method, shallow insertion and quick removal of the needles; exterior Cold and deficiency syndromes are treated by acupuncture and moxibustion with the reinforcing and reducing methods; for exterior Cold syndromes, needles are retained, exterior deficiency syndrome, moxibustion is applied	Interior excess and Heat syndromes are treated only by acupuncture without moxibustion, with the deep insertion and reducing method; interior deficiency and Cold syndromes are treated by both acupuncture and moxibustion; for interior deficiency syndromes, gentle needling with the reinforcing method combined with moxibustion; for interior Cold syndromes, deep insertion of the needles with longer retention, with the reinforcing and reducing methods, combined with warming needling technique
Prognosis	An exterior syndrome tuning into an interior syndrome indicates an aggravation of the disease; an interior syndrome turning into an exterior one suggests an alleviation of the disease	

1.3 Treatment of diseases based on syndrome differentiation according to Cold and Heat principles

Cold and Heat are two principles to determine the nature of the diseases.

	Cold syndromes	**Heat syndromes**
Definition	Syndromes caused by exogenous pathogenic Cold, or hypofunctions of the body	Syndromes caused by exogenous pathogenic Heat, or hyperfunctions of the body
Classification	Excess Cold, deficiency Cold	Excess Heat, deficiency Heat
Manifestations	Symptoms of Cold: aversion to Cold, preference for warmth and warm drinks, loose stools, clear urine, Cold limbs, slow, or deep, thready pulse, pale tongue, white moist, sticky coating	Symptoms of Heat: fever, preference for Cold and Cold drinks, constipation and deep-yellow urine; rapid, or surging rapid pulse, red tongue, yellow and dry coating
Principles of treatment	A Cold syndrome is treated by Heat with retention of the needles, warming therapies and moxibustion	A Heat syndrome is treated by acupuncture with quick needling therapies
Methods of treatment	Moxibustion, cupping, warming method, longer retention of the needles, or warming and reinforcing needling techniques can be applied, Back-Shu points, Front-Mu points, Yuan-Primary points and points of tonification can be selected	Shallow insertion with quick removal of the needles, or Blood-letting puncturing, cooling, reducing methods can be applied, Jing-Well points, Ying-Spring points can be selected

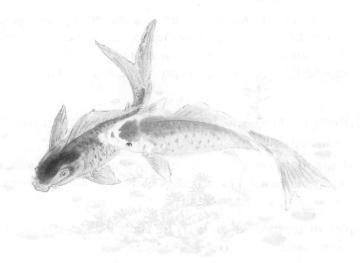

1.4 Treatment of diseases based on syndrome differentiation according to deficiency and excess principles

Deficiency and excess are principles used to distinguish the relative strength of the anti-pathogenic Qi and pathogenic factors.

	Deficiency syndromes	Excess syndromes
Definition	Syndromes in which the anti-pathogenic Qi is deficient	Syndromes in which the pathogenic Qi is excessive
Characteristics	Slow onset, long duration, marked by hypofunctions, present in chronic diseases. Weak pulse, pale tongue with no coating	Sudden onset, short duration, marked by hyperfunctions, present in acute diseases. Forceful pulse, red tongue with thick and sticky coating
Principles of treatment	"Reinforcing deficiency", "moxibustion for sinking"	"Reducing excess", "removal stagnation"
Methods of treatment	Reinforcing method, heavy moxibustion, selection of tonifying points (Yuan-Primary points, Back-Shu points and Front-Mu points), etc.	Reducing method, acupuncture without moxibustion, Blood-letting puncturing, selection of Jing-Well and Ying-Spring points to remove pathogenic factors

2. TREATMENT OF DISEASES BASED ON SYNDROME DIFFERENTIATION ACCORDING TO THE THEORY OF THE ZANG FU ORGANS

This is a method of treatment to generalize and analyze the symptoms and signs obtained from the four diagnostic methods so as to determine the affected Zang Fu organs, the nature of the disease and the relative strength of the anti-pathogenic Qi and pathogenic Qi based on the Theory of the Zang Fu Organs.

2.1 Differentiation and treatment of the Lung syndromes

2.1.1 Invasion of the Lungs by Wind Cold

Clinical manifestations: Severe chills, slight fever, headache, general aching, absence of sweat, nasal discharge, cough with clear thin sputum, thin, white tongue coating, superficial, and tense pulse.

Principles of treatment: Dispel Wind and Cold, improve the Lung function in dispersing, and relieve the exterior symptoms.

Methods of treatment: Points are selected from the Lung, Large Intestine, and Bladder Meridians and punctured with the reducing method or combined with moxibustion.

2.1.2 Accumulation of Heat in the Lungs

Clinical manifestations: High fever, slight chills, sweating, thirst, dry nose, or yellow nasal discharge, epistaxis, sore throat, cough with yellow and sticky sputum, constipation, deep yellow urine, red tongue with yellow coating, superficial and rapid pulse.

Principles of treatment: Dispel Wind and clear Heat, improve the Lung function in dispersing, and relieve the exterior symptoms.

Methods of treatment: Points are mainly selected from the Lung, Large Intestine and Stomach Meridians and punctured with the reducing method or Blood-letting puncturing method.

2.1.3 Retention of Phlegm Damp in the Lungs

Clinical manifestations: Cough with shortness of breath, fullness and stuffiness in the chest, orthopnoea in severe cases, cough with white and sticky sputum, sticky tongue coating, and a rolling pulse.

Principles of treatment: Promote the Lung function in descending, eliminate Damp and resolve Phlegm.

Methods of treatment: Points from the Lung, Spleen and Stomach Meridians and relevant Back-Shu points are selected. For Heat Phlegm, points are selected and punctured with the reducing method; for Cold Phlegm, points are punctured with uniform reinforcing and the reducing method, and combined with moxibustion.

2.1.4 Lung Qi deficiency

Clinical manifestations: Feeble cough, shortness of breath, dislike of speaking, weak voice, pale complexion, general lassitude, spontaneous sweating, a pale tongue and a thready pulse.

Principles of treatment: Tonify the Lungs and regulate Qi, strengthen the Spleen and benefit Qi, warm the Kidneys and improve their function in receiving Qi.

Methods of treatment: Points from the Lung, Spleen, and Kidney Meridians, Conception Vessel and Back-Shu points are selected and punctured combined with moxibustion.

2.1.5 Lung Yin deficiency

Clinical manifestations: Dry cough without sputum, or with little, sticky sputum, or with bloody sputum, dry throat, hoarse voice, emaciation, feverish sensation in the palms and soles, tidal fever, flushed cheeks, a red tongue with lack of fluid, and a thready, rapid pulse.

Principles of treatment: Nourish Lung and Kidney Yin, clear and reduce Heat caused by deficiency.

Methods of treatment: Points of the Lung and Kidney Meridians, and Back-Shu points are selected and treated by acupuncture mainly with reinforcing method. (For Yin deficiency with Fire, a uniform reinforcing and the reducing method is applied.)

2.2 Differentiation and treatment of the Large Intestine syndromes

2.2.1 Excess syndrome of the Large Intestine

Clinical manifestations: Abdominal pain worse on pressure, constipation; yellow and sticky tongue coating; deep, excess and forceful pulse. The syndrome is often caused by overeating, resulting in retention of Heat in the intestine.

Principles of treatment: Improve digestion, remove retained food, promote and regulate Qi in the Fu organs.

Methods of treatment: Points from the Large Intestine and Stomach Meridians are punctured with the reducing method and with no moxibustion.

2.2.2 Damp Heat in the Large Intestine

Clinical manifestations: Abdominal pain, tenesmus, diarrhoea with Blood and mucus in the stools, or, yellow stools of offensive smell; a burning sensation of the anus; thirst, deep yellow urine; yellow, sticky tongue coating, and a rolling and rapid pulse.

Principles of treatment: Clear Heat and dry Dampness, regulate the intestine and remove obstruction.

Methods of treatment: Points from the Large Intestine and Stomach Meridians, Front-Mu and Lower He-Sea points of the affected meridian are selected and punctured with the reducing method, with no moxibustion.

2.2.3 Deficiency syndrome of the Large Intestine

Clinical manifestations: Incontinence of stools, frequent diarrhoea, prolapse of the rectum, dull pain of the abdomen alleviated by pressure and warmth, Cold limbs; pale tongue with white and sticky coating, a thready and weak pulse.

Principles of treatment: Tonify and lift Yang Qi, stop diarrhoea, and promote consolidation.

Methods of treatment: Points from the Spleen and Stomach Meridians, and the Conception Vessel are selected and punctured with the reinforcing method combined with moxibustion.

2.2.4 Cold syndrome of the Large Intestine

Clinical manifestations: Abdominal pain, borborygmus, diarrhoea, white, sticky tongue coating, and a deep and slow pulse.

Principles of treatment: Warm the interior, dispel Cold. Relieve pain and stop diarrhoea.

Methods of treatment: Front-Mu and Lower He-Sea points of the affected meridian are punctured with the reinforcing method combined with moxibustion.

2.2.5 Consumption of the fluid of the Large Intestine

Clinical manifestations: Dry stools, constipation, dry mouth and throat; red tongue lack of fluid, a thready and hesitant pulse.

Principles of treatment: Nourish Yin and generate fluid, moisten the intestine and promote bowel movement.

Methods of treatment: Points of the Spleen, Large Intestine and Stomach Meridians, Back-Shu, and Front-Mu points of the affected organ are selected and punctured with the reinforcing or uniform reinforcing and the reducing methods, but with less moxibustion.

2.3 Differentiation and treatment of the Spleen syndromes

2.3.1 Spleen Qi deficiency

Clinical manifestations: Reduced appetite, abdominal distension, borborygmus, loose stools or diarrhoea, pale or sallow complexion, general lassitude, dislike of speaking, pale tongue with white coating, weak forceless pulse.

Principles of treatment: Tonify Qi in the Middle Burner.

Methods of treatment: Points of the Spleen and Stomach Meridians and relevant Back-Shu points are punctured with the reinforcing method combined with moxibustion.

2.3.2 Spleen Yang deficiency

Clinical manifestations: Dull pain of the abdomen alleviated on pressure and warmth, dysuria, watery thin discharge of leucorrhoea, Cold limbs or oedema, pale tongue with white coating, deep, slow and forceless pulse.

Principles of treatment: Warm up Yang and strengthen the Spleen

Methods of treatment: Points of the Spleen and Stomach Meridians and relevant Back-Shu points are selected and punctured with the reinforcing method combined with moxibustion.

2.3.3 Damp Heat in the Spleen

Clinical manifestations: Abdominal distension, poor appetite, dislike of oily food, nausea, vomiting, thirst with no desire to drink, general lassitude, heavy sensation of the head, loose stools, dysuria, jaundice, deep yellow urine, yellow, sticky tongue coating, soft and rapid pulses.

Principles of treatment: Clear Heat and eliminate Damp.

Methods of treatment: Points of the Spleen and Liver Meridians are punctured with the reducing method without moxibustion.

2.4 Differentiation and treatment of the Stomach syndromes
2.4.1 Retention of food in the Stomach

Clinical manifestations: Epigastric and abdominal fullness and distension, pain worse upon pressure, nausea, vomiting, regurgitation, diarrhoea, a thick and sticky tongue coating, and a rolling pulse.

Principles of treatment: Improve digestion, remove retained food, and regulate the Stomach and intestine.

Methods of treatment: Points of the Stomach Meridian, the Front-Mu point of the Stomach, and points of the Conception Vessel are selected and punctured with the reducing method without moxibustion.

2.4.2 Excess Cold in the Stomach

Clinical manifestations: Epigastric and abdominal pain with Cold sensation, alleviated on pressure and warmth, vomiting of clear and thin fluid; a white and slippery tongue coating, and a deep, string-taut, and tense pulse.

Principles of treatment: Warm the Middle Burner, and dispel Cold.

Methods of treatment: Points of the Stomach and Spleen Meridians and their relevant Back-Shu and Front-Mu points are punctured with a uniform reinforcing and reducing method combined with moxibustion.

2.4.3 Hyperactivity of Fire in the Stomach

Clinical manifestations: Burning sensation and pain in the epigastric region, acid regurgitation and an empty and uncomfortable feeling in the Stomach; thirst with preference for Cold drinks, foul breath, constipation, swelling and pain or ulceration and bleeding of the gums; a red tongue with lack of fluid, with little coating or with no coating, a surging, rolling and rapid pulse.

Principles of treatment: Clear and reduce Stomach Fire.

Methods of treatment: Points of the Stomach and Large Intestine Meridians are punctured with the reducing method without moxibustion.

2.4.4 Stomach Yin deficiency

Clinical manifestations: Pain and an empty and uncomfortable sensation in the Stomach, dry vomiting, hiccups, dry mouth and throat, dry stools and scanty urine; a red tongue lack of fluid, with little coating or no coating; a thready, and rapid pulse.

Principles of treatment: Nourish the Stomach and generate fluid.

Methods of treatment: Points of the Stomach and Large Intestine Meridians, and Front-Mu point of the Stomach are punctured with the reinforcing method but less moxibustion. (For Yin deficiency with Fire, a uniform reinforcing and reducing technique is applied.)

2.5 Differentiation and treatment of the Heart (Pericardium) syndromes

2.5.1 Heart Qi deficiency

Clinical manifestations: Pale complexion, palpitations, spontaneous sweating, lassitude worse on exertion; a pale tongue with white coating; a weak and forceless pulse, and sometimes there is a knotted and intermittent pulse. In severe cases, there are symptoms of extreme Cold limbs, and loss of consciousness.

Principles of treatment: Warm up Heart Yang, regulate Qi and Blood.

Methods of treatment: Points of the Heart and Pericardium Meridians and Back-Shu points are punctured with the reinforcing method combined with moxibustion.

2.5.2 Heart Blood deficiency

Clinical manifestations: Pale complexion, palpitations, easily frightened, poor memory, dream-disturbed sleep, feverish sensation in the palms and soles, night sweating, pale tongue or red tongue with lack of fluid; a thready, weak pulse, or a knotted and intermittent pulse.

Principles of treatment: Benefit Qi, nourish Blood and calm the Mind.

Methods of treatment: Points of the Heart and Pericardium Meridians and Back-Shu and Front-Mu points are punctured with the reinforcing method combined with moxibustion. (For Yin deficiency with Fire, a uniform reinforcing and reducing technique is applied.)

2.5.3 Hyperactivity of the Heart Fire

Clinical manifestations: Restlessness, insomnia, thirst, ulceration of the tongue, haematemesis, epistaxis, deep yellow urine with hesitant urination, or bloody urine, skin diseases, a red tongue, and rapid pulse.

Principles of treatment: Clear Heat, and reduce Fire; calm the Heart and relieve restlessness.

Methods of treatment: Points of the Heart, Kidney and Pericardium Meridians are punctured with the reducing method.

2.5.4 Phlegm misting the Heart

Clinical manifestations: Restlessness, insomnia, mental derangement, unconsciousness, dullness, incoherent speech, weeping and laughing without an apparent reason, or sudden collapse, coma and gurgling with sputum in the throat; a red tongue with sticky coating, and a string-taut and rolling pulse.

Principles of treatment: Resolve Phlegm, bring back consciousness, and tranquillize the Mind.

Methods of treatment: Points of the Heart and Pericardium Meridians and Governor Vessel are punctured with filiform needles or a three-edged needle for bleeding with the reducing method.

2.5.5 Stagnation of Heart Blood

Clinical manifestations: Chest fullness, palpitations, angina pectoris referring to the shoulder and arm. In severe cases, profuse sweating may occur, Cold limbs, cyanosis of the lips. A purplish dark tongue with purplish spots, and a hesitant pulse or a knotted and intermittent pulse.

Principles of treatment: Activate Blood, remove stagnation, unblock the meridian, and relieve pain.

Methods of treatment: Points of the Heart and Pericardium Meridians, and relevant Back-Shu and front-Mu points are punctured with the reducing method.

2.6 Differentiation and treatment of the Small Intestine syndromes

2.6.1 Deficiency Cold of the Small Intestine

Clinical manifestations: Dull lower abdominal pain alleviated by pressure and warmth, borborygmus, diarrhoea, frequent urination, pale tongue with white coating, a thready, weak or deep, slow and tense pulse.

Principles of treatment: Warm the intestine, and dispel Cold; regulate Qi and relieve pain.

Methods of treatment: The Back-Shu, Front-Mu points and Lower He-Sea points of the Small Intestine are selected and punctured mainly with the reinforcing method combined with moxibustion.

2.6.2 Excess Heat of the Small Intestine

Clinical manifestations: Restlessness, thirst, ulceration of the mouth and tongue, deep yellow and scanty urine, or hesitant and painful urination with bloody urine, lower abdominal distension and pain alleviated by intestinal flatus; a red tongue with yellow coating, and a rolling and rapid pulse.

Principles of treatment: Clear Heat, reduce Fire, promote urination.

Methods of treatment: Points of the Heart, Small Intestine, and Gallbladder Meridians are punctured with the reducing method without moxibustion.

2.6.3 Qi stagnation of the Small Intestine

Clinical manifestations: Protrusion around the umbilicus or a bearing-down colicky pain and distension in the lower abdomen relating to the scrotum; a white and slippery tongue coating, and a deep, string-taut, and tense pulse.

Principles of treatment: Warm the meridian, dispel Cold, regulate Qi and relieve pain.

Methods of treatment: Points of the Conception Vessel, Stomach, and Liver Meridians are punctured with the reducing method combined with moxibustion.

2.7 Differentiation and treatment of the Kidney syndromes

2.7.1 Kidney Yang deficiency

Clinical manifestations: Pallor, Cold limbs, seminal emission, spermatorrhoea, premature ejaculation, impotence; or irregular menstruation, loose stools, enuresis, clear urine, weakness and soreness of the lower back and knees; when the Kidneys fail to dominate the function of Water metabolism, there will be scanty urine and oedema; or once the Kidneys fail to receive Qi, there are symptoms of shortness of breath and wheezing (exhalation more than inhalation and worse on exertion); the tongue is pale with white coating; the pulse is deep, slow, and weak.

Principles of treatment: Warm and tonify Kidney Yang, improve the Kidney functions for Water metabolism and receiving Qi.

Methods of treatment: Points of the Kidney Meridian and Conception Vessel, and relevant Back-Shu points are selected and punctured with the reinforcing method combined with moxibustion.

2.7.2 Kidney Yin deficiency

Clinical manifestations: Emaciation, dizziness and tinnitus, poor sleeping and memory, dry throat and tongue, seminal emission, loose teeth, feverish sensation of the palms and soles of the feet, tidal fever and night sweating, soreness and weakness of the lower back and knees; a red tongue with little coating, and a thready, rapid pulse.

Principles of treatment: Nourish the Kidney, and replenish Essence, strengthen the Water to control Fire.

Methods of treatment: Points of the Kidney and Liver Meridians and relevant Back-Shu points are punctured with the reinforcing method but less moxibustion.

(For Yin deficiency with Fire, a uniform reinforcing and reducing technique is applied.)

2.8 Differentiation and treatment of the Bladder syndromes

2.8.1 Deficiency Cold of the Bladder

Clinical manifestations: Frequent urination with clear urine, incontinence of urine, dribbling urination, or dysuria, oedema; a pale tongue with moist coating, and a deep and thready pulse.

Principles of treatment: Warm up Yang and promote Qi, activate the functions of the Bladder.

Methods of treatment: Points of the Conception Vessel and Bladder Meridian are punctured with the reinforcing method combined with moxibustion.

2.8.2 Damp Heat in the Bladder

Clinical manifestations: Frequent and urgent urination with scanty deep yellow and turbid urine, or with haematuria, burning pain in the urethra; a red tongue with yellow coating, and a rapid pulse.

Principles of treatment: Clear Heat, eliminate Damp, regulate the functions in the Lower Burner.

Methods of treatment: Points of the Conception Vessel, Bladder, and Spleen Meridians are mainly selected and punctured by needles with the reducing method without moxibustion.

2.9 Differentiation and treatment of the Triple Burner syndromes

2.9.1 Deficiency Cold of the Triple Burner

Clinical manifestations: Oedema, abdominal distension, dysuria, or enuresis, incontinence of urine; a white and slippery tongue coating, and a deep, thready and weak pulse.

Principles of treatment: Warm and regulate the Triple Burner, promote functional activity of Qi.

Methods of treatment: Points of the Conception Vessel, and relevant Back-Shu points are punctured with the reinforcing method combined with moxibustion.

2.9.2 Excess Heat of the Triple Burner

Clinical manifestations: Feverish sensation of the body, thirst, wheezing, oedema, dry stools, dysuria; a yellow tongue coating, and a rolling, rapid pulse.

Principles of treatment: Regulate and activate the functions of the Triple Burner, eliminate Damp and promote water flow.

Methods of treatment: Points of the Conception Vessel and the Triple Burner Meridians are mainly selected and punctured only by needles with the reducing method.

2.10 Differentiation and treatment of the Liver syndromes

2.10.1 Liver Qi stagnation

Clinical manifestations: Emotional depression, sighing, chest and hypochondriac fullness and distension, belching, stomach ache with poor appetite, irregular menstruation, dysmenorrhoea, breast distension and pain; a thin yellow tongue coating, and a string-taut pulse.

Principles of treatment: Pacify the Liver and regulate Qi.

Methods of treatment: Points of the Liver Meridian are mainly selected and punctured only by needles with the reducing method without moxibustion.

2.10.2 Hyperactivity of Liver Yang

Clinical manifestations: Headache, dizziness, distension of the eyes, hypochondriac distension and pain, irritability; a red tongue, and a string-taut pulse.

Principles of treatment: Soothe the Liver and subdue Yang.

Methods of treatment: Points of the Liver and Kidney Meridians and relevant Back-Shu points are mainly selected and punctured only with the reducing method without moxibustion.

2.10.3 Flare-up of the Liver Fire

Clinical manifestations: Red complexion, headache, dizziness, redness, swelling and pain of the eyes, bitter taste, dry throat, irritability, insomnia, deep yellow urine, or epistaxis; a red tongue with yellow coating, and a string-taut pulse.

Principles of treatment: Reduce Liver Fire.

Methods of treatment: Points of the Liver Meridian are mainly selected and punctured by needles or by Blood-letting puncturing technique with the reducing method without moxibustion.

2.10.4 Stirring of Liver Wind in the interior

Clinical manifestations: Dizziness, vertigo, numbness of the hand and foot, tremor of the limbs, high fever, delirium, convulsions, stiffness of the neck and back; a red and deviated tongue, and string-taut pulse.

Principles of treatment: Dispel Wind, relieve convulsions.

Methods of treatment: Points of the Liver Meridian and Governor Vessel are mainly selected and punctured only with the reducing method.

2.10.5 Retention of Cold in the Liver meridian

Clinical manifestations: Lower abdominal distension, fullness, and pain referring to the testes with a bearing-down sensation, Cold sensation and contracted scrotum; white and slippery tongue coating, deep and string-taut pulse.

Principles of treatment: Warm the meridian and dispel Cold.

Methods of treatment: Points of the Liver Meridian are mainly selected and punctured with reinforcing method combined with moxibustion.

2.10.6 Liver Blood deficiency

Clinical manifestations: Pallor, dizziness and vertigo, Dryness and distension of the eyes, blurred vision, or night blindness, tinnitus, numbness of the fingers, reduced menstrual flow or amenorrhoea; pale tongue with scanty coating, and string-taut, and thready pulse.

Principles of treatment: Nourish Liver Blood.

Methods of treatment: Points of the three Yin meridians of foot and the relevant Back-Shu points are mainly selected and punctured with the reinforcing method combined with moxibustion.

2.10.7 Damp Heat in the Liver and Gallbladder

Clinical manifestations: Chest and hypochondriac distension and pain, yellow sclera, deep yellow urine, itching of genitalia, swelling, burning pain of the testes; and for female, yellow, foul discharge of leucorrhoea; yellow, sticky tongue coating, and string-taut, rapid pulse.

Principles of treatment: Pacify the Liver and Gallbladder, clear Heat and eliminate Damp.

Methods of treatment: Points of the Gallbladder, Liver and Spleen Meridians and the relevant Back-Shu points are punctured only by needles with the reducing method.

2.10.8 Hyperactivity of Gallbladder Fire

Clinical manifestations: Migraine, tinnitus, deafness, bitter taste, dry throat, vomiting of bitter fluid, hypochondriac pain; red tongue, and string-taut, rapid pulse.

Principles of treatment: Clear Heat and reduce Fire of the Gallbladder.

Methods of treatment: Points of the Gallbladder and Liver Meridians are mainly selected and punctured only with the reducing method.

2.11 Meridians related to the syndromes of the five Zang Fu organs

2.11.1 Meridians related to the Lung syndromes

The Lung Meridian is externally and internally related with the Large Intestine Meridian; the Heart Meridian ascends and connects with the Lungs; the Kidney Meridian enters the Lungs; the Major Collateral of the Stomach links with the Lungs; the Lung Meridian originates in the Middle Burner, communicating with the Spleen Meridian at Zhongfu (LU1).

2.11.2 Meridians related to the Heart syndromes

The Heart Meridian is externally and internally related with the Small Intestine Meridian; the Spleen Meridian flows into the Heart; the Kidney Meridian joins the Heart; the Liver Meridian distributes at Tanzhong (CV17); the Divergent Meridians of the three Yang meridians of foot communicate with the Heart; the Governor Vessel runs through the Heart and communicates with the brain; the Heart Meridian ascends and connects with the Lungs.

2.11.3 Meridians related to the Kidney syndromes

The Bladder Meridian is externally and internally related with the Kidney Meridian; the Kidney Meridian enters the Lungs, connects with the Heart, runs through the diaphragm, linking with the Heart, Lung, Liver and Spleen Meridians; the Kidneys connect with the Conception, Governor, Thoroughfare and Belt Vessels; the Yin Heel, and Yin Link Vessels are supported by Qi of the Kidney Meridian.

2.11.4 Meridians related to the Liver syndromes

The Kidney Meridian runs through the Liver. The Kidneys and Liver share the same source; the Liver Meridian curves around the Stomach, connects with the Gallbladder, flows into the Lungs in the upper Burner, linking with the Lungs and Stomach; the Gallbladder Meridian connects with the Liver, and its Divergent Meridian communicates with the Heart; the Liver Meridian is externally and internally related with the Gallbladder Meridian.

3. DIFFERENTIATION AND TREATMENT OF QI AND BLOOD SYNDROMES

This is a method of syndrome differentiation and treatment based on analysis of the pathological changes of Qi and Blood. Qi and Blood are the material basis for vital activities of the body; they are important in nourishing the Zang Fu organs, meridians and collaterals; unblocking the circulation of the meridian, and regulating the functions of balance. Disorders of the Zang Fu organs will affect circulation of Qi and Blood, and equally, changes of Qi and Blood will affect the functional activities of the Zang Fu organs, too.

3.1 Differentiation and treatment of Qi syndromes

Qi syndromes are generally divided into deficiency and excess types. 'Deficiency' refers to insufficiency of Qi, marked by hypofunctions or declining of Qi, such as deficiency of Qi and sinking of Qi; 'excess' means surplus of Qi, manifested by hyperfunctions or over activities, such as stagnation of Qi, adverse flow of Qi.

3.1.1 Syndromes of Qi deficiency

Manifestations: General lassitude, dizziness and vertigo, dislike of speaking, spontaneous sweating, shortness of breath that is worse on exertion, a pale, flabby tongue with teeth marks, and a thready, weak, and forceless pulse.

Principles of treatment: Tonify and replenish Qi. Acupuncture is applied with the combination of moxibustion.

Selection of points: Includes Qihai (CV6), Guanyuan (CV4), Tanzhong (CV17), Feishu (BL13), Pishu (BL20), Shenshu (BL23), Zusanli (ST36), etc.

3.1.2 Syndromes of sinking of Qi

Manifestations: Chronic diarrhoea, enuresis, uterine bleeding, abdominal bearing-down sensation, prolapse of uterus or rectum; a pale tongue with white coating, and a deep, weak and forceless pulse.

Principles of treatment: According to the principle 'Moxibustion for sinking of Qi', this syndrome is treated by both acupuncture and moxibustion with reinforcing method to tonify and benefit Qi in the Middle Burner so as to lift Yang Qi to relieve Qi sinking.

Selection of points: Baihui (GV20), Shenque (CV8), Qihai (CV6), Guanyuan (CV4), Zhongwan (CV12), Pishu (BL20), Weishu (BL21), Shenshu (BL23), Zusanli (ST36), etc.

3.1.3 Syndromes of Qi stagnation

Manifestations: Local distension and pain (distension is greater than pain), unfixed pain, belching and hiccups, tendency to sigh; for females, breast distension and pain, irregular menstruation; a thin, yellow tongue coating, and a string-taut or hesitant pulse.

Principles of treatment: Aim to activate the meridian circulation, regulating Qi and relieving pain. Acupuncture treatment is given with the reducing method without moxibustion.

Selection of points: Zhongwan (CV12), Tanzhong (CV17), Hegu (LI4), Taichong (LR3), Qimen (LR14), Zhigou (TE6), Yanglingquan (GB34), Zusanli (ST36), Shangjuxu (ST37), Xiajuxu (ST39), etc.

3.1.4 Syndromes of adverse flow of Qi

1. **Upward flow of Lung Qi**

   Manifestations: Cough, and asthma.

   Principles of treatment: To promote the Lung functions in dispersing and descending of Qi, regulate Qi, relieve cough, and arrest asthma. Acupuncture therapy is applied with the reducing method with no moxibustion.

2. **Upward flow of Stomach Qi**

   Manifestation: Nausea, vomiting, belching, hiccups.

Principles of treatment: To regulate Qi, harmonize the Stomach, promote Qi activities for descending. Acupuncture therapy is applied with the reducing method with no moxibustion.

Selection of points: Zhongwan (CV12), Liangmen (ST21), Neiguan (PC6), Tanzhong (CV17), Zusanli (ST36), Weishu (BL21), and Qichong (ST30), etc.

3.2 Differentiation and treatment of Blood syndromes

3.2.1 Syndromes of Blood deficiency

Manifestations: Sallow or pale complexion, pale conjunctivae, lips, and nails; dizziness, vertigo, palpitations, insomnia, numbness of foot and hand, delayed menstruation, scanty menstrual flow with light red colour; a pale tongue, and a thready, forceless pulse.

Principles of treatment: To tonify and nourish Blood, benefit Qi and produce Blood. Acupuncture therapy is applied with reinforcing method and combined with moxibustion.

Selection of points: Xuehai (SP10), Qihai (CV6), Tanzhong (CV17), Xuanzhong (GB39), Sanyinjiao (SP6), Zusanli (ST36), Xinshu (BL15), Geshu (BL17), Pishu (BL20), Ganshu (BL18), Gaohuang (BL43), etc.

3.2.2 Syndromes of Blood stasis

Manifestations: Local swelling, distending and stabbing pain which is fixed, and aggravated on pressure, subcutaneous bleeding, cyanosis, or scattered stagnated spots; lower abdominal pain before or during menstruation, with either profuse or scanty menstrual flow with purplish colour or with clots. In severe cases, there are symptoms of Blood stasis in general, such as dark complexion, squamous and dry skin, subcutaneous bleeding; a purple, dark tongue with purplish spots, a hesitant pulse.

Principles of treatment: To activate Blood, remove stagnation, relieve swelling, and stop pain. At the early stage, acupuncture treatment is given with the reducing method, or by Blood-letting puncturing therapy combined with cupping; at the late period of treatment, acupuncture is combined with moxibustion with uniform reinforcing and the reducing method for removing Blood stasis.

Selection of points: Xuehai (SP10), Geshu (BL17), Qihai (CV6), Tanzhong (CV17), Hegu (LI4), Taichong (LR3), Ashi points, etc.

3.2.3 Syndromes of bleeding

1. **Qi fails to control Blood**

   Manifestations: Various bleeding syndromes (haematemesis, haematochezia, subcutaneous bleeding, profuse menstrual flow, uterine bleeding with light red colour, etc.); general lassitude, shortness of breath, dislike of speaking, pale complexion; a pale tongue, and thready, weak and forceless pulse.

   Principles of treatment: To tonify Qi and control Blood. Acupuncture therapy is applied with reinforcing method and combined with moxibustion.

2. **Heat in Blood**

   Manifestations: Epistaxis, haemoptysis, haematemesis, haematuria, haematochezia, profuse menstrual flow, uterine bleeding with fresh red colour; accompanied by fever, restlessness, thirst, dry stools, deep yellow scanty urine; a deep red tongue, and a thready rapid pulse.

   Principles of treatment: To clear Heat and cool Blood, and stop bleeding. Acupuncture is applied simply with the reducing method, without moxibustion.

   Selection of points: For epistaxis: Yingxiang (LI20), Shangxing (GV23), Yintang (EX-HN 3), Fengchi (GB20), Hegu (LI4); for haemoptysis: Zhongfu (LU1), Chize (LU5), Yuji (LU10), Kongzui (LU6), Geshu (BL17); for haematemesis: Zhongwan (CV12), Liangmen (ST21), Neiguan (PC6), Geshu (BL17), Neiting (ST44), Zusanli (ST36); for haematuria: Zhongji (CV3), Sanyinjiao (SP6), Yanglingquan (GB34), Xiajuxu (ST39), Shenshu (BL23), Pangguangshu (BL28), Xiaochangshu (BL27); for haematochezia, Changqiang (GV1), Zhongwan (CV12), Liangmen (ST21), Kongzui (LU6), and Chengshan (BL57); for profuse menstrual flow and uterine bleeding: Hegu (LI4), Taichong (LR3), Dadun (LR1), Xingjian (LR2), Geshu (BL17), Sanyinjiao (SP6), etc.

3. **Yin deficiency with excessive Fire**

   Manifestations: Bleeding syndromes of the Lungs, such as haemoptysis, cough with Blood, or bloody sputum, usually with a small amount of Blood, accompanied by dry throat, feverish sensation of the palms and soles, afternoon fever, flushed cheeks, insomnia, dream-disturbed sleep; a red tongue with lack of fluid, and a thready, rapid pulse.

   Principles of treatment: Nourish Yin, clear Heat, and stop bleeding. Acupuncture treatment is given with uniform reinforcing and the reducing method.

Selection of points: Zhongfu (LU1), Yuji (LU10), Chize (LU5), Taixi (KI3), Feishu (BL13), Gaohuang (BL43), etc.

4. **Blood stagnation in the interior**

Manifestation: Lower abdominal pain which is stabbing and fixed before or during menstruation, purple dark menstrual flow with clots; a purple tongue with spots, a hesitant pulse.

Principles of treatment: To activate Blood and remove stagnation. Acupuncture is applied with the reducing method combined with moxibustion.

Selection of points: The same as those for treating the 'syndromes of Blood stasis'.

3.3 Differentiation and treatment of both Qi and Blood syndromes

Qi pertains to Yang, and Blood to Yin. Being the Commander of Blood, Qi can produce Blood, and controls Blood. When Qi is freely circulating, Blood flows freely, too. So, stagnation of Qi leads to stagnation of Blood. Blood is the mother of Qi, it carries Qi. Non substantial Qi in the body depends on substantial Blood for nourishment. Physiologically, Qi and Blood are related; and pathologically, they influence each other, resulting in both Qi and Blood disorders.

3.3.1 Qi and Blood deficiency

Manifestations: Common symptoms and signs of Qi and Blood deficiency.

Principles of treatment: To tonify both Qi and Blood. Both acupuncture and moxibustion are applied with reinforcing method.

Selection of points: Qihai (CV6), Xuehai (SP10), Tanzhong (CV17), Pishu (BL20), Weishu (BL21), Ganshu (BL18), Geshu (BL17), Xuanzhong (GB39), Zusanli (ST36), etc.

3.3.2 Qi deficiency due to loss of Blood

Manifestations: Common symptoms and signs of Qi deficiency and bleeding syndromes.

Principles of treatment: To benefit Qi and control Blood. Acupuncture is applied with reinforcing method combined with moxibustion.

Selection of points: Qihai (CV6), Zusanli (ST36), Pishu (BL20), Weishu (BL21).

3.3.3 Loss of Qi combined with loss of Blood

Manifestations: Considerable loss of Blood, suddenly reduced blood pressure, pallor, extreme Cold limbs, profuse sweating, feeble breathing, or even coma, loss of consciousness; a pale tongue, and an extremely weak, fading or hollow and large pulse.

Principles of treatment: To tonify Qi and Blood forcefully, and restore Yang from collapse. Acupuncture is applied with reinforcing method, and heavy moxibustion is recommended.

Selection of points: Apply moxibustion immediately on Shenque (CV8), Qihai (CV6), Guanyuan (CV4), Baihui (GV20), Zusanli (ST36); or puncture Suliao (GV25), Neiguan (PC6), Zusanli (ST36), and Sanyinjiao (SP6), etc.

3.3.4 Qi deficiency combined with Blood stagnation

Manifestations: Common symptoms and signs of Qi deficiency and Blood stagnation.

Principles of treatment: To tonify and regulate Qi, activate Blood and remove Blood stasis. Acupuncture can be combined with moxibustion with a uniform reinforcing and the reducing method, or cutaneous needling therapy for bleeding.

Selection of points: Qihai (CV6), Tanzhong (CV17), Zusanli (ST36), Hegu (LI4), Pishu (BL20), Weishu (BL21), Geshu (BL17), and Ashi points, etc.

3.3.5 Blood stagnation with Blood deficiency

Manifestations: Local redness, swelling and stabbing pain worse on pressure, pale complexion, dizziness and vertigo, palpitations, insomnia; a pale tongue with stagnated spots, and a thready, hesitant pulse.

Principles of treatment: To activate Blood and remove Blood stasis. Acupuncture can be combined with moxibustion with uniform reinforcing and the reducing method.

Selection of points: Xuehai (SP10), Geshu (BL17), Hegu (LI4), Taichong (LR3), Zusanli (ST36), Pishu (BL20), Ganshu (BL18), Sanyinjiao (SP6), and Ashi points, etc.

3.3.6 Qi and Blood stagnation

Manifestations: Common symptoms and signs of both Qi and Blood stagnation syndromes.

Principles of treatment: To promote Qi flow and activate Blood, regulate Qi and remove stagnation. Acupuncture of the reducing method is applied combined with Blood-letting puncturing technique with a three-edged needle for bleeding, or followed by cupping.

Selection of points: Tanzhong (CV17), Hegu (LI4), Taichong (LR3), Weizhong (BL40), Qimen (LR14), Geshu (BL17), and Ashi Points, etc.

4. DIFFERENTIATION AND TREATMENT OF MERIDIAN SYNDROMES

This is a method to determine the affected and involved meridians of a disease in order to select the points for treatment from the relevant meridians based on the theory of meridians and collaterals, including the running courses, distribution of the meridians and collaterals, the physiological functions of their pertaining organs, and characteristics of the related syndromes of diseases.

In a broad sense, meridian syndromes include syndromes of the pertaining organs of the meridians, termed as 'Zang Fu and meridian syndromes'; in a narrow sense, they refer to the syndromes of muscles, skin and hair, tendons, vessels, bone, five sense organs and nine orifices. Excess syndromes are marked by local swelling, Heat and pain, and convulsions; deficiency syndromes are manifested by Cold limbs, numbness, flaccidity, and paralysis.

4.1 Identification of the affected meridians

This method identifies the affected meridians according to the clinical manifestations on the basis of Chapter 10 of *Miraculous Pivot* (concerning 'a disease, the pathological changes', and 'the affected meridians of the pertaining Zang Fu organs').

For example:

- symptoms of fullness and distension of the Lungs, accompanied by cough and asthma, pain in the clavicular fossa, or referring to the arm in severe cases, are differentiated as a syndrome of the Lung Meridian of Hand-Taiyin

- stiffness and pain of the tongue, a syndrome of the Spleen Meridian of Foot-Taiyin

- dry tongue and throat, a syndrome of the Kidney Meridian of Foot-Shaoyin.

4.2 Identification of the affected meridians according to the location of the diseases

The affected meridians are identified based on the location of the pathological changes, and the running courses and distribution of the meridians. For example:

Headache
- Frontal: Yangming Meridian
- Temporal: Shaoyang Meridian
- Occipital: Taiyang Meridian
- Parietal: Jueyin Meridian

Toothache
- Toothache in the upper gum: the Stomach Meridian of Foot-Yangming Meridian enters the upper gum
- Toothache in the lower gum: the Large Intestine Meridian of Hand-Yangming Meridian enters the lower gum

If a disease area covers several meridians, then the involved meridians should be differentiated according to the symptoms.

Hypochondria pain referring to
- Foot-Shaoyang: accompanied by bitter taste, yellow sclera
- Foot-Jueyin: accompanied by restlessness, irritability, hiccups
- Foot-Taiyin: accompanied by epigastric and abdominal distension and fullness

Pathological tongue changes referring to
- Hand-Shaoyin: accompanied by ulcer of the mouth and tongue, deep yellow urine
- Foot-Shaoyin: accompanied by weakness and soreness of the lower back and knees, tinnitus
- Foot-Taiyin: accompanied by stiffness and pain of the tongue, abdominal pain, poor appetite

4.3 Meridian diagnosis

Diseases can be diagnosed according to the theories of the meridians and collaterals in the following ways.

4.3.1 Inspection of the meridians

This is a method of analyzing the pathological changes by observing the colour, surface conditions, and the shape of the tissues of the affected areas on the running courses of the meridians so as to determine the affected meridians.

Clinical significance:

1. To reflect the pathological changes of the Zang Fu organs and meridians, and improve the accuracy of the diagnosis.

2. Changes of colour can distinguish a deficiency syndrome from an excess syndrome; a Cold from a Heat syndrome; and improve the accuracy of diagnosis and therapeutic effect.

3. Helpful in predicting the prognosis. Examples:

   • 'Red line' on the anterior border of the medial aspect of the upper limb; pertaining to the Lung Meridian, indicating respiratory diseases.

   • 'Loss of hair' on the posterior border of the medial aspect of the lower limb; pertaining to the Kidney Meridian, indicating urinary, genital dysfunctions.

   • Infantile superficial venule of index finger. Observation of three crease-regions indicates the severity of a disease, whether it is a mild or a severe case; the depth, superficial or deep, determines an exterior or interior syndrome; the colour, red or purple distinguishes the nature of the disease, a Cold or a Heat syndrome; the stagnated or pale condition indicates a deficiency or an excess syndrome.

4.3.2 Palpation of the meridian points

Palpation of the meridian points is also known as 'meridian point-pressure', or 'meridian point-diagnosis'. It is a method to identify the affected meridians of the disease by palpating and pressing the relevant meridian points on certain parts of the running courses of the meridians in order to discover the pathological reaction areas or spots. This works because diseases of the internal organs may have their outward manifestations on the body surface through the transmission functions of the meridians and collaterals, which can be investigated by palpation along the running course of the meridians and palpation of points.

Positive reactant:

1. Substances such as round, diamond, oval, cord-like, or vesical nodules and tumours.

2. Morphological changes of the meridian points: protrusion, depression, loose, and hard changes or changes of colour and temperature.

3. Abnormal sensation of the points and along the meridians: pain, sensitive feeling, numbness, Cold, Heat, or delayed response.

Methods:

1. Sliding (finding a superficial reactant), pressing and kneading (finding a deeper reactant), moving (finding a deepest reactant), pushing (on the lower back and back regions), pinching and other methods.

2. Palpation with even pressure, comparison of the left and right.

3. The order of examination: lower back and back first, then the chest, abdomen, and the four limbs.

4.3.3 Examination of the meridians and acupoints using an electric device

This is a diagnostic method of identifying the pathological changes of the Zang Fu organs and meridians by analyzing the changes of electric resistance and conductivity of the meridians and points by an electric device. The acupoints chosen for the test can be Yuan-Primary points and Jing-Well points. For patients with a deformity of the fingers or toes or loss of limbs, Back-Shu points can be selected instead.

Clinical significance: To determine the deficiency and excess conditions of Qi and Blood of the affected Zang Fu organs and their meridians, and select the best acupoints for treatment of the disease.

Result of examination:

1. If the electric conductivity of an acupoint is one third higher than the average conductivity, that meridian exhibits an excess syndrome.

2. If the electric conductivity of an acupoint is one third lower than the average conductivity, that meridian exhibits a deficiency syndrome.

3. If the electric conductivity of an acupoint on both sides of the same meridian differs greatly, that meridian must be out of order; there is imbalance between the left and right.

4. The examination of the meridians and points for identifying the affected meridians also depends on a general analysis based on syndrome differentiation.

4.3.4 Perception examination with Heat or heating device

This is a diagnostic method which involves placing an ignited incense or spot-shaped heating device close to the Jing-Well points on both sides or on the Back-Shu points to examine the perception, and to compare the difference on the left and right in order to analyze the conditions of imbalance or deficiency and excess of the meridians. (The first choice will be Jing-Well points, or Back-Shu points if that is inconvenient.) For convenience, Zhiyin (BL67, medial aspect of the nail of the small toe) can be examined instead of Yongquan (KI1); Geshu (BL17) is in correspondence with Zhongze (on the ulnar side of the nail of the middle finger); Weiguanxiashu (EX-B3) with Lidui (ST45, lateral side of the nail of the middle toe).

Clinical significance: To examine the differences in the temperature of acupoints (Jing-Well points), so as to identify the changes of balance, deficiency and excess of the Zang Fu organs and meridians.

Result of examination:

1. Similar or the same temperature suggests that there is no disease of that meridian.

2. Temperature difference twice or several times higher than that of the average (sometimes, on one side, there is no warm sensation, but on the other side, there is very sensitive sensation) indicates that the meridian is in disorder.

3. Comparison of the left and right: Higher temperature difference indicates a deficiency syndrome, while lower temperature difference, an excess syndrome.

4. Comparison of the meridians: Temperature difference higher than that of the average suggests a deficiency syndrome, lower than that of the average, an excess syndrome.

4.4 Differentiation and treatment of syndromes according to the theory of meridians and collaterals

4.4.1 Syndromes of the Lung Meridian of Hand-Taiyin

Manifestations: Cough, asthma, shortness of breath, chest fullness, nasal obstruction, sore throat, chills and fever, sweating, aversion to Wind, frequent urination with scanty urine, soreness, pain and numbness of the anterior border of the medial aspect of the upper limb along the running course of the Lung Meridian.

Principles of treatment: Promote and regulate Lung Qi, activate the circulation of the meridian and collaterals.

Treatment: Main points are selected from the affected Lung Meridian, combined with points from the Large Intestine and Stomach Meridians, and are punctured with reinforcing method for a deficiency syndrome, and the reducing method for an excess syndrome. Moxibustion is added for treating a Cold syndrome.

4.4.2 Syndromes of the Large Intestine Meridian of Hand-Yangming

Manifestations: Soreness, pain and numbness of the anterior border of the lateral aspect of the upper limb along the running course of the Large Intestine Meridian, weakness and soreness of the upper limb with limitation of movement, muscular atrophy, paralysis, swelling of the neck, shoulder pain, nasal discharge, epistaxis, toothache of the lower gum, sore throat, facial pain, facial paralysis, facial spasm, abdominal pain, borborygmus, diarrhoea, dysentery, haemorrhoid, and constipation.

Principles of treatment: Unblock the meridian and activate the collaterals, promote and regulate the functions of the intestine.

Treatment: Points are mainly selected from the affected meridian and combined with points of the Lung and Stomach Meridians, and are punctured with reinforcing method for a deficiency syndrome, and the reducing method for an excess syndrome. Moxibustion is added for treating a Cold syndrome.

4.4.3 Syndromes of the Stomach Meridian of Foot-Yangming

Manifestations: Epigastric pain, reduced appetite, vomiting, abdominal pain, borborygmus, dysentery, constipation, fever; soreness, pain and numbness of the anterior border of the lateral aspect of the lower limb, weakness and soreness of the lower limbs with limited movement, muscular atrophy, paralysis, swelling of the neck, sore throat, toothache of the upper gum, nasal and eye disorders; facial pain, paralysis, and spasm; and frontal headache.

Principles of treatment: Regulate the Stomach and intestine, activate the circulation of the meridians and collaterals.

Treatment: Points are mainly selected from the affected meridian and combined with points of the Spleen Meridian and the Back-Shu and Front-Mu points of the Stomach, and are punctured with reinforcing method for a deficiency syndrome, and the reducing method for an excess syndrome. Moxibustion is added for treating a Cold syndrome.

4.4.4 Syndromes of the Spleen Meridian of Foot-Taiyin

Manifestations: Epigastric and abdominal distension and fullness, diarrhoea, poor appetite, jaundice, oedema, heaviness of the body, lassitude, irregular menstruation, uterine bleeding, soreness, pain and numbness of the anterior border of the medial aspect of the lower limbs, rigidity of the root of the tongue.

Principles of treatment: Build up the Spleen and harmonize the Stomach; activate the circulation of the meridians and collaterals.

Treatment: Points are mainly selected from the affected meridian and combined with points of the Stomach Meridian and the Back-Shu and Front-Mu points of the Spleen, and are punctured with reinforcing method for a deficiency syndrome, and the reducing method for an excess syndrome. Moxibustion is added for treating a Cold syndrome.

4.4.5 Syndromes of the Heart Meridian of Hand-Shaoyin

Manifestations: Chest pain, palpitations, cardiac pain, restlessness, insomnia, mental disorder, dry throat, ulcers of the mouth and tongue, soreness, pain and numbness of the posterior border of the medial aspect of the upper limbs, pain and feverish sensation of the palms.

Principles of treatment: Regulate the Heart and Mind, activate the circulation of the meridians and collaterals.

Treatment: Points are mainly selected from the affected meridian and combined with the points of the Pericardium Meridian and the Front-Mu and Back-Shu points of the affected organ, and are punctured with reinforcing method for a deficiency syndrome, and the reducing method for an excess syndrome. Moxibustion is added for treating a Cold syndrome.

4.4.6 Syndromes of the Small Intestine Meridian of Hand-Taiyang

Manifestations: Soreness, pain and numbness of the posterior border of the lateral aspect of the upper limbs, pain in the scapula and shoulder, sore throat, swelling of the cheek, yellow sclera, tinnitus, deafness, lower abdominal pain, borborygmus, diarrhoea, deep yellow scanty urine.

Principles of treatment: Activate the circulation of the meridians and collaterals, regulate the functions of the intestines.

Treatment: Points are mainly selected from the affected meridian and combined with the points of the Stomach Meridian and the Front-Mu and Back-Shu points of the affected organ, and are punctured with reinforcing method for a deficiency syndrome, and the reducing method for an excess syndrome. Moxibustion is added for treating a Cold syndrome.

4.4.7 Syndromes of the Bladder Meridian of Foot-Taiyang

Manifestations: Enuresis, dysuria, lower abdominal distension, mental disorder, various Zang Fu, and five sense organ disorders, soreness, pain, numbness of the posterior aspect of the lower limbs along the running course of the meridian, neck, back, lower back, lumbar and sacral pain, chills and fever, occipital headache.

Principles of treatment: Regulate the functions of the Bladder, unblock the meridians and activate the collaterals.

Treatment: Points are mainly selected from the affected meridian and combined with the Front-Mu point of the affected organ, and are punctured with reinforcing method for a deficiency syndrome, and the reducing method for an excess syndrome. Moxibustion is added for treating a Cold syndrome.

4.4.8 Syndromes of the Kidney Meridian of Foot-Shaoyin

Manifestations: Enuresis, dysuria, seminal emission, impotence, irregular menstruation, sterility, infertility, wheezing, haemoptysis insomnia, dream-disturbed sleep, soreness, pain and numbness of the posterior border of the medial aspect of the lower limbs, lumbago, feverish sensation of the soles, dry throat, myopia, blurred vision, tinnitus, and deafness.

Principles of treatment: Tonify the Kidney and replenish the primary Qi, activate the circulation of the meridians and collaterals.

Treatment: Points are mainly selected from the affected meridian, combined with the points of the Conception Vessel, and Bladder Meridian, and are treated by both acupuncture and moxibustion with reinforcing method.

4.4.9 Syndromes of the Pericardium Meridian of Hand-Jueyin

Manifestations: Chest pain, palpitations, cardiac pain, restlessness, insomnia, mental disorder, dry throat, ulcers of the mouth and tongue, soreness, pain and numbness of the midline of the medial aspect of the upper limbs along the running course of the meridian.

Principles of treatment: Regulate the Heart and calm the Mind, activate the meridians and collaterals.

Treatment: Points are mainly selected from the affected meridian and combined with points of the Back-Shu and Front-Mu points of the affected organ, and are punctured with reinforcing method for a deficiency syndrome, and the reducing method for an excess syndrome. Moxibustion is added for treating a Cold syndrome.

4.4.10 Syndromes of the Triple Burner Meridian of Hand-Shaoyang

Manifestations: Soreness, pain and numbness of the midline of the lateral aspect of the upper limbs along the running course of the meridian, shoulder, neck and retroauricular pain, tinnitus and deafness, migraine, sore throat, abdominal distension, oedema, dysuria.

Principles of treatment: Activate the circulation of the meridians and collaterals, unblock and regulate the functions of the Triple Burner.

Treatment: Points are mainly selected from the affected meridian and combined with points of the Gallbladder and Bladder Meridians, Back-Shu, Front-Mu and Lower He-Sea points of the affected organ, and are punctured with reinforcing method for a deficiency syndrome, and the reducing method for an excess syndrome. Moxibustion is added for treating a Cold syndrome.

4.4.11 Syndromes of the Gallbladder Meridian of Foot-Shaoyang

Manifestations: Jaundice, bitter taste, yellow sclera, yellow skin of the body, fright and fear, insomnia, soreness, pain and numbness of the midline of the lateral aspect of the lower limbs along the running course of the meridian, migraine, eye diseases, tinnitus, deafness.

Principles of treatment: Pacify the Liver and promote the functions of the Gallbladder; unblock the meridians and collaterals.

Treatment: Points are mainly selected from the affected meridian and combined with points of the Triple Burner and Liver Meridians, and are punctured with reinforcing method for a deficiency syndrome, and the reducing method for an excess syndrome. Moxibustion is added for treating a Cold syndrome.

4.4.12 Syndromes of the Liver Meridian of Foot-Jueyin

Manifestations: Hypochondriac distension and pain, jaundice, bitter taste, reduced appetite, belching, hiccups, restlessness, irritability, soreness, pain and numbness of the midline of the medial aspect of the lower limbs along the running course of the meridian, hernia, facial paralysis, dizziness and vertigo, parietal headache, myopia, night blindness, blurred vision, redness, swelling and pain of the eye.

Principles of treatment: Pacify the Liver, regulate Qi and activate the circulation of the meridians and collaterals.

Treatment: Points are mainly selected from the affected meridian and combined with points of the Gallbladder and Kidney Meridians, and are punctured with reinforcing method for a deficiency syndrome, and the reducing method for an excess syndrome. Moxibustion is added for treating a Cold syndrome.

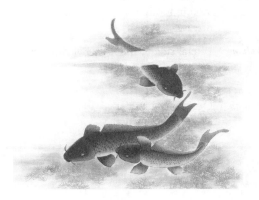

IV. ACUPUNCTURE PRESCRIPTION

1. GENERAL INTRODUCTION

Acupuncture prescription is a therapeutic plan consisting of the treatment of appropriately selected acupoints, needling techniques, reinforcing and the reducing methods and a combination of points based on the principles of treatment for the individual cases of disease according to differentiation of syndromes.

1.1 General indications of the meridians

Three Yin meridians of the hand

Name of the meridians	Indications		
	Diseases of the affected meridian	*Diseases of the two meridians*	*Diseases of the three meridians*
The Lung Meridian of Hand-Taiyin	Lung, throat diseases		Chest diseases
The Pericardium Meridian of Hand-Jueyin	Heart, Stomach diseases	Mental diseases	
The Heart Meridian of Hand-Shaoyin	Heart diseases		

Three Yang meridians of the hand

Name of the meridians	Indications		
	Diseases of the affected meridian	*Diseases of the two meridians*	*Diseases of the three meridians*
The Large Intestine Meridian of Hand-Yangming	Frontal head, nose, mouth, tooth diseases		Eye, throat, febrile diseases
The Triple Burner Meridian of Hand-Shaoyang	Lateral side of the head, hypochondriac diseases	Ear diseases	
The Small Intestine Meridian of Hand-Taiyang	Occipital, shoulder and scapula, mental diseases		

Three Yang meridians of the foot

Name of the meridians	Indications		
	Diseases of the affected meridian	*Diseases of the two meridians*	*Diseases of the three meridians*
The Stomach Meridian of Foot-Yangming	Frontal head, mouth, tooth, throat, gastrointestinal diseases		Mental, febrile diseases
The Gallbladder Meridian of Foot-Shaoyang	Lateral side of the head, ear, hypochondriac diseases	Ear diseases	
The Bladder Meridian of Foot-Taiyang	Occipital, lumbar, back diseases; Back-Shu points are indicated for Zang Fu diseases		

Three Yin meridians of the foot

Name of the meridians	Indications	
	Diseases of the affected meridian	*Diseases of the three meridians*
The Spleen Meridian of Foot-Taiyin	Spleen and Stomach diseases	Menstruation and urination disorders
The Liver Meridian of Foot-Jueyin	Liver and genital disorders	
The Kidney Meridian of Foot-Shaoyin	Kidney, Lung, throat diseases	

The Conception and Governor Vessel

Name of the meridians	Indications	
	Diseases of the affected meridian	*Diseases of the two meridians*
The Governor Vessel	Wind Stroke, coma, febrile disease, headache	Mental disorder, mouth, tooth, throat, chest, Lungs, Spleen, intestines, Kidneys, Bladder, and menstruation disorders
The Conception Vessel	Restore Yang from collapse	

1.2 Basic principles for prescription and selection of acupoints

The basic principles involve the selection of points along the running course of the meridians. The running course of the meridians, the distribution and indications of points are the basis for acupuncture prescription.

1.3 Symbols commonly used in a prescription

Reinforcing	⊤
Reducing	⊥
Uniform reinforcing and reducing	|
Three-edged needle for bleeding	↓
Cutaneous needle	※
Embedding needle	○-
Moxibustion with moxa sticks	×
Moxibustion with moxa cones (3 cones)	△3
Warming needle	△
Cupping	○
Electroacupuncture	IN
Point injection	IM

In an acupuncture prescription, these symbols should be marked after the point. For example, reinforcing Zusanli (ST36) ⊤, bleeding by puncturing Shaoshang (LU11) ↓

1.4 The form of a prescription

1. **Names of points**: 4 points are written on each line according to their importance as primary or secondary.

2. **Note of selection of points for puncturing**: Unilateral or bilateral puncturing.

3. **Note of needling techniques**: Specific needling or moxibustion techniques.

4. **Note of reinforcing and the reducing methods**: Reinforcing, reducing or uniform reinforcing and the reducing methods.

5. **Note of period of retention of the needles and courses of treatment.**

1.5 Frequency of treatment

1.5.1 Frequency of treatment in general

Acute syndromes: Short course of treatment for a few days or weeks, such as acute sprain, 1–2 treatments; common cold, 2–3 treatments.

Chronic syndromes: Longer course of treatment for several weeks, months or years, such as haemiplegia after Wind Stroke, 2–3 months, 6 months or one year

For cases without a clear diagnosis, 5–10 treatments are given at first to observe the result.

1.5.2 Course and interval

One course usually consists of 7–10 treatments. Between courses, there is an interval of 3–4 days.

1.5.3 Frequency of treatment

Generally speaking the treatment can be given once or twice daily. For treating chronic diseases, treatment can be given once every day or once every other day.

1.5.4 Retention of needles

Retention of the needles depends on the individual cases. Usually the needles are retained for 20–30 minutes, or if necessary, for one to several hours.

1.5.5 Optimal time for treatment

Choosing an optimal time for treatment can improve the therapeutic effect. For example, for treatment of irregular menstruation or dysmenorrhoea, start to give daily treatment 5–7 days before menstruation for 7–10 days; when treating insomnia, the optimal time for treatment is in the afternoon, or evening, especially 1–2 hours before sleep.

2. PRINCIPLES FOR SELECTION OF POINTS

Selection of points along the running course of the meridians is the basic principle in acupuncture treatment, which is a prerequisite of combination of points.

2.1 Selection of local points

This means selection of the points around the affected areas, Zang Fu organs, sense organs and tissues of the disease. Each acupoint has its local effect for treatment of diseases. For example, Baihui (GV20), Taiyang (EX-HN5) are selected for headache; Suliao (GV25), Yingxiang (LI20) for nose diseases; Jiache (ST6), Dicang (ST4) for facial paralysis; Huiyin (CV1), Changqiang (GV1) for prolapse of rectum.

2.2 Selection of adjacent points

Adjacent refers to the location close to the diseased Zang Fu organs, five sense organs, or limbs. Each acupoint has its local and nearby effect for treatment of diseases. For example, Fengchi (GB20) is selected for eye, ear diseases; Taiyang (EX-HN5) or Shangguan (GB3) for toothache; Shangxing (GV23) or Tongtian (BL7) for nose diseases.

2.3 Selection of distant points

Here, points far from the diseased areas are selected. Points along the running course of each meridian can be selected to treat diseases of the relevant organ. They can be divided as follows:

1. **Selection of the points from the affected meridian**: Points far from the diseased area, but on the running course of the affected meridian are selected. For instance, points distal to the ends of the upper or lower limbs are selected for diseases of the head, while points proximal are selected for diseases of the chest and abdomen.

2. **Selection of the points from the related meridians**: Points can be selected from the related meridians, such as the meridians which are externally and internally related, crossed, or connected. For example:

   - *From the meridians externally and internally related*: In treating a Lung disease, Taiyuan (LU9) is selected with the combination of Hegu (LI4); Liver disease, Taichong (LR3) is combined with Yanglingquan (GB34).

   - *From the crossing meridians*: Sanyinjiao (SP6) is selected for diseases of the Liver, Spleen and Kidney; Guanyuan (CV4), Zhongji (CV3), for diseases of the Conception Vessel and three Yin meridians of the foot.

   - *From the connected meridians*: Zhongwan (CV12), Zusanli (ST36), Taichong (LR3) are selected for disharmony between the Liver and Stomach, and stomach ache.

2.4 Selection of points according to the symptoms

Points are selected with the emphasis on relieving specific symptoms and signs. For example: Dazhui (GV14), Quchi (LI11) for fever; Renzhong (GV26), Shixuan

(EX-UE11) for loss of consciousness; Tianshu (ST25), Lanwei (EX-LE7) for appendicitis; Ashi points, for sprain and Bi syndrome.

2.5 Selection of points according to syndrome differentiation

Based on differentiation of syndromes, the prescription is guided by principles of treatment. For example, for a deficiency Cold syndrome of the Spleen and Stomach, the principles of the treatment should be warming the Middle Burner and dispelling Cold. Pishu (BL20), Weishu (BL21), Zhongwan (CV12), Zusanli (ST36) are selected and punctured with reinforcing method combined with moxibustion.

3. METHODS OF COMBINING POINTS

Based on the selection of points and the individual case of a disease, a prescription is made by combining those points with cooperative functions.

3.1 Combination of points according to the different parts of the body

This is a method to combine points according to their location in certain parts of the body.

3.1.1 Combination of points on the upper and lower parts of the body

This is a method of combining points located on the upper parts of the body (the upper limbs and region above the lower back) and on the lower parts of the body (the lower limbs and the region below the lower back). For example: Hegu (LI4) on the upper, and Neiting on the lower part of the body are selected for toothache; Neiguan (CV6), on the upper body combined with Gongsun (SP4) on the lower body for fullness of the chest and abdomen.

3.1.2 Combination of points in the front and on the back

This is a method of combining points located in the front part of the body and on the back. For example: the combination of Back-Shu and Front-Mu points: Weishu (BL21) combined with Zhongwan (CV12) for Stomach disorders; for regulating both the Spleen and the Liver functions, Pishu (BL20) with Zhangmen (LR13); Renzhong (GV26) combined with Fengfu (GV16) for loss of consciousness; Yamen (GV15) combined with Lianquan (CV23) for hoarse voice.

3.1.3 Combination of points on the left and right

This is a method of contralateral combination of points because the distribution of a meridian is symmetrical, and their running courses cross. For example: Hegu (LI4) on the right side is selected for treating facial paralysis on the left; Taiyang (EX-HN5) and Touwei (ST8) on the affected side are combined with Waiguan (TE5) and Zulinqi (GB41) on the healthy side for migraine on the right side; Jianliao (TE14) on the left is punctured to treat shoulder pain on the right.

3.1.4 Combination of distant and adjacent points

Based on the local and distal effects of the points, adjacent points are combined with distant points. For example, when treating eye diseases, Jingming (BL1) and Chengqi (ST1) are combined with Guangming (GB37) and Hegu (LI4); for Stomach disease, Weishu (BL21) and Zhongwan (CV12) are combined with Neiguan (PC6), Gongsun (SP4) and Zusanli (ST36).

3.2 Combination of points according to the meridians

This refers to a method of combination of points according to the theories and inter-relations of the meridians and collaterals.

3.2.1 Combination of points from the affected meridian

This is a method of point combination in which points are selected from the affected meridian only when a certain Zang or Fu organ and its meridian is in disorder, but the other Zang Fu organs and meridians are not involved. Following the principle that 'meridian points are selected to treat a syndrome neither excess nor deficient', Zhongfu (LU1), Lieque (LU7), Taiyuan (LU9) and Chize (LU5) are selected for a Lung disease.

3.2.2 Combination of points from the meridians externally and internally related

Here, points are selected from the Yin meridians for diseases of Yang meridians with which they are externally and internally related, or vice versa based on the externally–internally related relationship of the Zang Fu organs and meridians. For example:

- Yinxi (HT6), a point of the Heart Meridian, is combined with Houxi (SI3), a point of the Small Intestine Meridian for treatment of night sweating.

- Neiguan (PC6), a point of the Pericardium Meridian, is combined with Waiguan (TE5), a point of the Triple Burner Meridian for angina pectoris.

3.2.3 Combination of points from the meridians with the same names

Points of the hand and foot meridians that have the same names can be combined because 'Qi of their meridians communicates with each other'. For example:

- Hegu (LI4), a point of the Large Intestine Meridian of Hand-Yangming, is combined with Jiexi (ST41), a point of the Stomach Meridian of Foot-Yangming, to treat headache.

- Houxi (SI3), a point of the Small Intestine Meridian of Hand-Taiyang, is combined with Kunlun (BL60), a point of the Bladder Meridian of Foot-Taiyang, to treat torticollis, acute lumbar sprain, and occipital headache.

3.2.4 Combination of points from the mother and child meridians

According to the principle of 'reinforcing the mother for a deficiency syndrome and reducing the child for an excess syndrome', the child meridian is reduced for an excess syndrome of the Zang Fu organs; while the mother meridian is reinforced for a deficiency syndrome of the Zang Fu organs based on the theories of the Zang Fu organs, meridians and the Five Elements. For example, in the treatment of a deficiency type of cough, besides the points of the Lung Meridian of Hand-Taiyin, and its Back-Shu point, points from the Spleen Meridian of Foot-Taiyin and Stomach Meridian of Foot-Yangming are selected as a combination, such as Sanyinjiao (SP6), Zusanli (ST36), and Taibai (SP3) for strengthening the Earth (the Spleen and Stomach), so as to promote the Metal (the Lungs) according to the Theory of the Five Elements that the Earth produces Metal and the principle of reinforcing the mother for deficiency and reducing the child for excess.

3.2.5 Combination of points from the crossing meridians

This method is used when there are several meridians communicating at the affected area of the disease, or the disease is related with several crossing meridians. For example: Sanyinjiao (SP6) can be selected to treat diseases of the Liver, Spleen and Kidneys. Since the Stomach and Liver Meridians communicate at the frontal and temporal regions, so Touwei (ST8), Yangbai (GB14), Shuaigu (GB8) and Zulinqi (GB41) can be used to treat frontal headache referring to the lateral side of the head.

V. CLINICAL APPLICATION OF THE SPECIFIC POINTS

Various pathological changes of the diseases may be reflected in the specific points of the body. When these specific points are stimulated by needles, they can produce the effect that the ordinary meridian points may not reach.

1. CLINICAL APPLICATION OF THE FIVE-SHU POINTS

Five-Shu points refer to five specific points of Jing-Well, Ying-Spring, Shu-Stream, Jing-River and He-Sea points of the twelve regular meridians located below the elbows and knees.

Yin meridians	Five-Shu points				
	Jing-Well (Wood)	*Ying-Spring (Fire)*	*Shu-Stream (Earth)*	*Jing-River (Metal)*	*He-Sea (Water)*
The Lung Meridian of Hand-Taiyin (Metal)	Shaoshang (LU11)	Yuji (LU10)	Taiyuan (LU9)	Jingqu (LU8)	Chize (LU5)
The Pericardium Meridian of Hand-Jueyin (Fire)	Zhongchong (PC9)	Laogong (PC8)	Daling (PC7)	Jianshi (PC5)	Quze (PC3)
The Heart Meridian of Hand-Shaoyin (Fire)	Shaochong (HT9)	Shaofu (HT8)	Shenmen (HT7)	Lingdao (HT4)	Shaohai (HT3)
The Spleen Meridian of Foot-Taiyin (Earth)	Yinbai (SP1)	Dadu (SP2)	Taibai (SP3)	Shangqiu (SP5)	Yinlingquan (SP9)
The Liver Meridian of Foot-Jueyin (Wood)	Dadun (LR1)	Xingjian (LR2)	Taichong (LR3)	Zhongfeng (LR4)	Ququan (LR8)
The Kidney Meridian of Foot-Shaoyin (Water)	Yongquan (KI1)	Rangu (KI2)	Taixi (KI3)	Fuliu (KI7)	Yingu (KI10)

Yin meridians	Five-Shu points				
	Jing-Well (Metal)	*Ying-Spring (Water)*	*Shu-Stream (Wood)*	*Jing-River (Fire)*	*He-Sea (Earth)*
The Large Intestine Meridian of Hand-Yangming (Metal)	Shangyang (LI1)	Erjian (LI2)	Sanjian (LI3)	Yangxi (LI5)	Quchi (LI11)
The Triple Burner Meridian of Hand-Shaoyang (Fire)	Guanchong (TE1)	Yemen (TE2)	Zhongzhu (TE3)	Zhigou (TE6)	Tianjing (TE10)
The Small Intestine Meridian of Hand-Taiyang (Fire)	Shaoze (SI1)	Qiangu (SI2)	Houxi (SI3)	Yanggu (SI5)	Xiaohai (SI8)
The Stomach Meridian of Foot-Yangming (Earth)	Lidui (ST45)	Neiting (ST44)	Xiangu (ST43)	Jiexi (ST41)	Zusanli (ST36)
The Gallbladder Meridian of Foot-Shaoyang (Wood)	Zuqiaoyin (GB44)	Xiaxi (GB43)	Zulinqi (GB41)	Yangfu (GB38)	Yanglingquan (GB34)
The Bladder Meridian of Foot-Taiyang (Water)	Zhiyin (BL67)	Zutonggu (BL66)	Shugu (BL65)	Kunlun (BL60)	Weizhong (BL40)

1.1 The application of the Five-Shu points according to the seasonal changes

In spring and summer, Yang Qi tends to be up, and the Qi of the body remains at a superficial level, so points should be punctured shallowly.

In autumn and winter, Yang Qi tends to be down, Qi of the body moves inside, so points are punctured deeply.

According to the distribution of the Five-Shu points, Jing-Well and Ying-Spring points are located superficially at the region where the muscle is quite thin; while Jing-River and He-Sea points are located comparatively deeper at the place where the muscle is thick. Therefore, Jing-Well points are more often punctured in spring, Ying-Spring points in summer; Jing-River and He-Sea points in autumn and winter.

1.2 Main indications of Five-Shu points

- Jing-Well points are indicated for fullness of the chest.

- Ying-Spring points are indicated for febrile diseases.

- Shu-Stream points are indicated for heaviness of the body and joint pain.

- Jing-River points are indicated for cough and asthma.

- He-Sea points are indicated for disorders of reversed flow or diarrhoea.

1.3 Application of Five-Shu points according to the inter-promoting and inter-acting relationship of the Five Elements (mother and child relationship)

1.3.1 Reinforcing and the reducing method of the affected meridian

To select the mother and child points of the affected meridian.

- *Deficiency syndrome:* Reinforce the mother point of the affected meridian.

- *Excess syndrome:* Reduce the child point of the affected meridian.

- *Neither deficiency nor excess syndrome:* Select the mother and child points of the related or externally–internally related meridians.

1.3.2 Reinforcing and the reducing method for the related meridians

- *Deficiency syndrome:* Reinforce the mother point of the related or externally–internally related meridians.

- *Excess syndrome:* Reduce the child point of the related or externally–internally related meridians.

The mother and child reinforcing and reducing points

Meridians	Deficiency and excess	Point of the affected meridian	Points of the related meridian
The Lung Meridian of Hand-Taiyin	Deficiency	Taiyuan (LU9)	Taibai (SP3)
	Excess	Chize (LU5)	Yingu (KI10)
The Heart Meridian of Hand-Shaoyin	Deficiency	Shaochong (HT9)	Dadun (LR1)
	Excess	Shenmen (HT7)	Taibai (SP3)
The Pericardium Meridian of Hand-Jueyin	Deficiency	Zhongchong (PC9)	Dadun (LR1)
	Excess	Daling (PC7)	Taibai (SP3)
The Large Intestine Meridian of Hand-Yangming	Deficiency	Quchi (LI11)	Zusanli (ST36)
	Excess	Erjian (LI2)	Zutonggu (BL66)
The Small Intestine Meridian of Hand-Taiyang	Deficiency	Houxi (SI3)	Zulinqi (GB41)
	Excess	Xiaohai (SI8)	Zusanli (ST36)
The Triple Burner Meridian of Hand-Shaoyang	Deficiency	Zhongzhu (TE3)	Zulinqi (GB41)
	Excess	Tianjing (TE10)	Zusanli (ST36)
The Spleen Meridian of Foot-Taiyin	Deficiency	Dadu (SP2)	Shaofu (HT8)
	Excess	Shangqiu (SP5)	Jingqu (LU8)
The Kidney Meridian of Foot-Shaoyin	Deficiency	Fuliu (KI7)	Jingqu (LU8)
	Excess	Yongquan (KI1)	Dadun (LR1)
The Liver Meridian of Foot-Jueyin	Deficiency	Ququan (LR8)	Yingu (KI10)
	Excess	Xingjian (LR2)	Shaofu (HT8)
The Stomach Meridian of Foot-Yangming	Deficiency	Jiexi (ST41)	Yanggu (SI5)
	Excess	Lidui (ST45)	Shangyang (LI1)
The Bladder Meridian of Foot-Taiyang	Deficiency	Zhiyin (BL67)	Shangyang (LI1)
	Excess	Shugu (BL65)	Zulinqi (GB41)
The Gallbladder Meridian of Foot-Shaoyang	Deficiency	Xiaxi (GB43)	Zutonggu (BL66)
	Excess	Yangfu (GB38)	Yanggu (SI5)

2. CLINICAL APPLICATION OF YUAN-PRIMARY AND LUO-CONNECTING POINTS

Yuan-Primary points: Yuan means source and primary. Yuan-Primary points are located at the sites close to the wrist and ankle where the primary Qi of the Zang Fu organs is retained; there are twelve Yuan-Primary points.

Luo-Connecting points: Luo means connecting and linking. Luo-Connecting points connect the externally and internally related meridians. There are sixteen Luo-Connecting points (twelve Luo-Connecting points of the twelve regular meridians, one of the Governor Vessel, and one of the Conception Vessel, two of the major collaterals of the Spleen and Stomach)

The Yuan-Primary and Luo-Connecting points of the twelve regular meridians

Meridians	Yuan-Primary points	Luo-Connecting points
The Lung Meridian of Hand-Taiyin	Taiyuan (LU9)	Lieque (LU7)
The Pericardium Meridian of Hand-Jueyin	Daling (PC7)	Neiguan (PC6)
The Heart Meridian of Hand-Shaoyin	Shenmen (HT7)	Tongli (HT5)
The Spleen Meridian of Foot-Taiyin	Taibai (SP3)	Gongsun (SP4)
The Liver Meridian of Foot-Jueyin	Taichong (LR3)	Ligou (LR5)
The Kidney Meridian of Foot-Shaoyin	Taixi (KI3)	Dazhong (KI4)
The Large Intestine Meridian of Hand-Yangming	Hegu (LI4)	Pianli (LI6)
The Triple Burner Meridian of Hand-Shaoyang	Yangchi (TE4)	Waiguan (TE5)
The Small Intestine Meridian of Hand-Taiyang	Wangu (SI4)	Zhizheng (SI7)
The Stomach Meridian of Foot-Yangming	Chongyang (ST42)	Fenglong (ST40)
The Gallbladder Meridian of Foot-Shaoyang	Qiuxu (GB40)	Guangming (GB37)
The Bladder Meridian of Foot-Taiyang	Jinggu (BL64)	Feiyang (BL58)

Clinical application:

1. Yuan-Primary points can reflect diseases of the Zang Fu organs, which can be used for diagnosis as well as treatment of acute and chronic, deficiency and excess syndromes of the Zang Fu organs.

2. Luo-Connecting points are applied to treat diseases involving the two externally–internally related meridians.

3. Combination of Yuan-Primary and Luo-Connecting points: This combination is also known as the 'host and guest' combination, which is applied according to the occurring order of the diseases of the externally–internally related meridians. When a meridian is first affected, its Yuan-Primary point is used, while for second affected meridian, its Luo-Connecting point is selected.

3. CLINICAL APPLICATION OF BACK-SHU AND FRONT-MU POINTS

Back-Shu points: These are specific points on the back where Qi of the Zang Fu organs is infused, and termed according to the names of their relevant Zang Fu organs. There are twelve Back-Shu points.

Front-Mu points: They are specific points on the chest and abdomen where Qi of the Zang Fu organs is infused and converged, which are located close to their corresponding Zang Fu organs. There are twelve Front-Mu points.

Back-Shu and Front-Mu points of the Zang Fu organs

Zang Fu organs	Back-Shu points	Front-Mu points
Lung	Feishu (BL13)	Zhongfu (LU1)
Pericardium	Jueyinshu (BL14)	Tanzhong (CV17)
Heart	Xinshu (BL15)	Juque (CV14)
Spleen	Pishu (BL20)	Zhangmen (LR13)
Liver	Ganshu (BL18)	Qimen (LR14)
Kidney	Shenshu (BL23)	Jingmen (GB25)
Large Intestine	Dachangshu (BL25)	Tianshu (ST25)
Triple Burner	Sanjiaoshu (BL22)	Shimen (CV5)
Small Intestine	Xiaochangshu (BL27)	Guanyuan (CV4)
Stomach	Weishu (BL21)	Zhongwan (CV12)
Gallbladder	Danshu (BL19)	Riyue (GB24)
Bladder	Pangguangshu (BL28)	Zhongji (CV3)

Clinical application:

1. Both Back-Shu and Front-Mu points can reflect disorders of the internal organs. Tenderness or sensitive reaction may occur on the relevant Back-Shu and Front-Mu points when the Zang Fu organs are in disorder.

2. Both Back-Shu and Front-Mu points can regulate the functions of the Zang Fu organs, and treat diseases of the corresponding Zang Fu organ.

3. Combination of the Back-Shu and Front-Mu points follows the principle of 'treating a Yin syndrome from the Yang side; and treating a Yang syndrome from the Yin side'.

4. Back-Shu points of the five Zang organs are indicated for diseases of their relevant tissues and organs.

5. Front-Mu points are more often indicated for acute and pain syndromes of the relevant Zang Fu organs.

4. CLINICAL APPLICATION OF THE EIGHT CONFLUENT POINTS OF THE EIGHT EXTRA MERIDIANS

The Eight Confluent Points are eight points of the twelve regular meridians which connect with the eight extra meridians.

Combination and indications of the Eight Confluent Points

Confluent points	Regular meridians	Extra meridians	Indications
Lieque (LU7)	The Lung Meridian of Hand-Taiyin	Conception Vessel	Throat, chest, Lungs
Zhaohai (KI6)	The Kidney Meridian of Foot-Shaoyin	Yin Heel Vessel	
Houxi (SI3)	The Small Intestine Meridian of Hand-Taiyang	Governor Vessel	Ear, inner canthus, head and neck, shoulder and scapula, lower back
Shenmai (BL62)	The Bladder Meridian of Foot-Taiyang	Yang Heel Vessel	
Gongsun (SP4)	The Spleen Meridian of Foot-Taiyin	Thoroughfare Vessel	Heart, chest and Stomach
Neiguan (PC6)	The Pericardium Meridian of Hand-Jueyin	Yin Link Vessel	
Zulinqi (GB41)	The Gallbladder Meridian of Foot-Shaoyang	Belt Vessel	Ear, outer canthus, lateral side of the head, neck and shoulder, chest and hypochondrium
Waiguan (TE5)	The Triple Burner Meridian of Hand-Shaoyang	Yang Link Vessel	

Indications:

1. Diseases on the running course of the affected meridian.

2. Syndromes of the extra meridians with which the meridians of the relevant Zang Fu organs communicate.

3. Houxi (SI3) is indicated for syndromes of the Governor Vessel marked by pain and rigidity of the spine and opisthotonus; Gongsun (SP4) is indicated for syndromes of the Thoroughfare Vessel (Chong Meridian) marked by reversed flow of Qi in the chest and abdomen; Neiguan (PC6) and Gongsun (SP4) are indicated for diseases of the Heart, chest and Stomach.

5. CLINICAL APPLICATION OF THE EIGHT INFLUENTIAL POINTS

The Eight Influential Points refer to the eight specific points which have particular effects in the treatment of disorders relating to the Zang and Fu organs, Qi, Blood, tendon, pulse and vessels, bone and marrow.

The Eight Influential Points

Zang organs	Zhangmen (LR13)	Fu organs	Zhongwan (CV12)
Qi	Tanzhong (CV17)	*Blood*	Geshu (BL17)
Tendon	Yanglingquan (GB34)	*Pulse, vessel*	Taiyuan (LU9)
Bone	Dazhu (BL11)	*Marrow*	Xuanzhong (GB39)

Indications: Diseases of the Zang and Fu organs, Qi, Blood, tendon, vessels, bone and marrow respectively.

6. CLINICAL APPLICATION OF THE LOWER HE-SEA POINTS

'He' means convergence. Lower He-Sea points refer to the six points located in the lower limbs along the three Yang meridians of foot where Qi of the six Fu organs converges. So, they are called 'Lower He-Sea points of the six Fu organs'.

Lower He-Sea points

Hand
- Small Intestine: Xiajuxu (ST39)
- Triple Burner: Weiyang (BL39)
- Large Intestine: Shangjuxu (ST39)

Foot
- Bladder: Weizhong (BL40)
- Gallbladder: Yanglingquan (GB34)
- Stomach: Zusanli (ST36)

Indications: Diseases of the six Fu organs.

7. CLINICAL APPLICATION OF THE XI-CLEFT POINTS

'Xi' means cleft. Xi-Cleft points are those points located at the sites where Qi and Blood of the meridians is converged and accumulated. There are sixteen Xi-Cleft points in all.

The Xi-Cleft points

Meridians	Xi-Cleft points	Meridians	Xi-Cleft points
The Lung Meridian of Hand-Taiyin	Kongzui (LU6)	*The Large Intestine Meridian of Hand-Yangming*	Wenliu (LI7)
The Pericardium Meridian of Hand-Jueyin	Ximen (PC4)	*The Triple Burner Meridian of Hand-Shaoyang*	Huizong (TE7)
The Heart Meridian of Hand-Shaoyin	Yinxi (HT6)	*The Small Intestine Meridian of Hand-Taiyang*	Yanglao (SI6)
The Spleen Meridian of Foot-Taiyin	Diji (SP8)	*The Stomach Meridian of Foot-Yangming*	Liangqiu (ST34)
The Liver Meridian of Foot-Jueyin	Zhongdu (LR6)	*The Gallbladder Meridian of Foot-Shaoyang*	Waiqiu (GB36)
The Kidney Meridian of Foot-Shaoyin	Shuiquan (KI5)	*The Bladder Meridian of Foot-Taiyang*	Jinmen (BL63)
Yin Link Vessel	Zhubin (KI9)	*Yang Link Vessel*	Yangjiao (GB35)
Yin Heel Vessel	Jiaoxin (KI8)	*Yang Heel Vessel*	Fuyang (BL59)

Clinical application:

1. To reflect the diseases of the Zang Fu organs and meridians.

2. To treat the acute syndromes or acute attacks of diseases of the Zang Fu organs and meridians.

8. CLINICAL APPLICATION OF THE CROSSING POINTS

The Crossing points refer to those points located at the intersection of two or more meridians. There are about 100 Crossing points.

Indications: These are indicated to treat diseases of the meridians that cross each other, and disorders of their relevant Zang Fu organs.

TREATMENT OF DISEASES

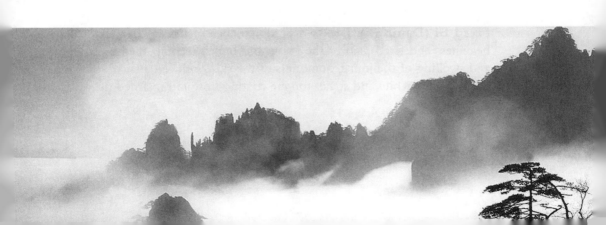

I. INTERNAL DISEASES

1. BI SYNDROMES
Brief introduction

Bi syndromes are syndromes caused by pathogenic Wind, Cold, Damp and Heat, marked by joint and muscular soreness, pain and numbness of the limbs, accompanied by limitation of movement or burning pain and swelling of the joints and limbs, which include rheumatic arthritis, acute rheumatic fever, rheumatoid arthritis, osteoarthritis, fibrositis, and neuralgia.

Aetiology and pathogenesis

When pathogenic Wind, Cold, Damp and Heat invade the body they may block the circulation of Qi and Blood in the meridians and collaterals, resulting in obstruction which causes Bi syndromes. Bi syndromes are generally classified into four types: wandering Bi caused by Wind; painful Bi caused by Cold; fixed Bi caused by Damp; and Heat Bi caused by either Heat, or constitutional Yang excess, or Yin deficiency with Fire, with further attacks of pathogenic Wind, Cold, or Damp that remain in the meridians for a long time, transforming into Heat.

Syndrome differentiation

Bi syndromes are characterized by muscular pain of the joints with limitation of movement.

1. **Wandering Bi (Wind Bi)**: Due to predominance of Wind manifested by migratory pain of the joints accompanied by limitation of movement, aversion to Wind, and fever, thin and white tongue coating and superficial pulse.

2. **Painful Bi (Cold Bi)**: Due to predominance of Cold marked by severe and fixed pain of the joints which is aggravated by Cold, and alleviated by warmth accompanied by limitation of movement. The local affected area is neither red nor hot. The tongue coating is thin and white, the pulse, string-taut and tense.

3. **Fixed Bi (Damp Bi)**: Due to a predominance of Damp characterized by heaviness and fixed pain of the joints and limbs, accompanied by soreness and swelling of the joints, numbness of the skin, induced attack on a Cold, or rainy day; white and sticky tongue coating, soft and retarded pulse.

4. **Heat Bi**: Due to accumulation of Heat that blocks the meridians, collaterals and joints, marked by joint pain with local burning sensation, redness and swelling, limitation of movement with a single or several joints involved; accompanied by aversion to Wind, fever, thirst, restlessness, yellow and dry tongue coating, rolling and rapid pulse.

Treatment
Body acupuncture

1. **Principles of treatment**

   Unblock the meridians and collaterals and relieve pain.

   - Dispel Wind and activate Blood for wandering Bi.
   - Dispel Cold and warm the meridians for painful Bi.
   - Eliminate Damp for fixed Bi.
   - Clear Heat and relieve swelling for Heat Bi.
   - Wandering, painful, and fixed Bi syndromes are treated by acupuncture with the reducing method, combined with moxibustion.
   - Heat Bi syndrome is treated by acupuncture only with the reducing method without moxibustion.

2. **Prescription**

   - *Wandering Bi*: Geshu (BL17), Xuehai (SP10).
   - *Painful Bi*: Shenshu (BL23), Guanyuan (CV4).
   - *Fixed Bi*: Yinlingquan (SP9), Zusanli (ST36).
   - *Heat Bi*: Dazhui (GV14), Quchi (LI11).

   Affected parts of the body:

   - *Shoulder*: Jianyu (LI15), Jianliao (TE14), Naoshu (SI10).
   - *Elbow*: Quchi (LI11), Tianjing (TE10), Chize (LU5), Shaohai (HT3), Xiaohai (SI8).
   - *Wrist*: Waiguan (TE5), Yangchi (TE4), Yangxi (LI5) Wangu (SI4).
   - *Back*: Shenzhu (GV12), Dazhui (GV14), Yaoyangguan (GV3), Jiaji points.
   - *Hip joint*: Huantiao (GB30), Juliao (GB29), Zhibian (BL54).
   - *Thigh*: Chengfu (BL36), Fengshi (GB31), Futu (ST32), Yanglingquan (GB34).

- *Knee joint*: Xiyan (EX-LE5), Liangqiu (ST34), Yanglingquan (GB34), Xiyangguan (GB33).
- *Ankle*: Qiuxu (GB40), Shenmai (BL62), Kunlun (BL60), Zhaohai (KI6).

3. **Explanation**

Selection of points on the local affected pain areas and along the running course of the meridians and collaterals can activate the circulation of Qi and Blood, regulate Ying (nutrient Blood) and Wei (defensive Qi) so the pathogenic Wind Cold can be dispelled, Damp eliminated and Heat cleared. When 'obstruction is removed, pain is alleviated', and Bi syndrome treated.

4. **Modification**

- *To activate and regulate Blood for wandering Bi syndrome*: + Geshu (BL17), Xuehai (SP10).
- *To tonify and warm up Yang Qi to dispel Cold*: + Shenshu (BL23), Guanyuan (CV4).
- *To strengthen the Spleen so as to eliminate Damp*: + Yinlingquan (SP9), Zusanli (ST36).
- *To clear Heat*: + Dazhui (GV14), Quchi (LI11).
- + Ashi points for each syndrome.

5. **Manipulation**

All points are punctured with routine needling techniques except for Dazhui (GV14), Quchi (LI11) which can be pricked to cause bleeding; Shenshu (BL23), Guanyuan (CV4) are treated with moxibustion or warming needle therapy.

Other therapies

1. **Electroacupuncture**

When Qi has arrived, connect the needle to an electroacupuncture stimulator; the point is stimulated by a continuous wave for 10–20 minutes.

2. **Cutaneous needle**

A plum blossom needle is used to tap heavily on both sides of the spine or on the affected joints until there is slight bleeding, and followed by cupping.

3. **Point injection**

To inject 0.5–1ml injection of Danggui (当归 *Radix Angelicae Sinensis*), Fangfeng (防风 *Radix Ledebouriellae*), Weilingxian (威灵仙 *Radix Clematidis*), etc. into the point of the local affected joint. This treatment is given once every other day or every 3 days.

Notes

1. Acupuncture is quite effective in treating Bi syndromes, especially in treating rheumatic arthritis. For rheumatoid arthritis with repeated attacks, it takes time.

2. Bone tuberculosis and tumour are excluded.

3. Patients should be advised to keep their joints warm and avoid being affected by Wind, Cold and Damp.

2. LOWER BACK PAIN

Brief introduction

Lower back pain is pain on one or both sides of the lumbar region, which is closely associated with the disorders of the Kidneys and their meridian, for the lumbus is the seat of the Kidneys. Lower back pain can be caused by many diseases, such as rheumatic diseases, Kidney diseases, bone injury, lumbar vertebra hyperplasia, and pelvic diseases.

Aetiology and pathogenesis

Invasion by exogenous Wind, Cold and Damp, or lumbar sprain or contusion may cause obstruction of the circulation of Qi and Blood in the meridians and collaterals, which causes pain; or a deficiency of the Kidneys fails to nourish the meridians of the lumbar region, so malnutrition results in pain. As far as the lower back pain is concerned, the meridians affected and involved are the Kidney and Bladder Meridians, Governor and Belt Vessels.

Lower back pain due to Cold Damp

Lower back pain usually occurs after exposure to Cold and Damp and is aggravated on rainy days. So, retained Cold Damp may block the meridians and collaterals and impair the circulation of Qi and Blood, resulting in pain.

Lower back pain due to Blood stasis

Over strain, sprain or contusion, traumatic injury, or inappropriate movement may cause Qi and Blood stagnation, which blocks the meridians and collaterals, resulting in lower back pain.

Lower back pain due to Kidney deficiency

Constitutional Kidney deficiency or deficiency of Kidney Essence and Blood due to the aging process, or consumption of Kidney Qi and Essence due to excessive sexual activity may all give rise to lower back pain.

Syndrome differentiation

If the pain is located on the mid-posterior line of the lumbar region, it is a syndrome of the Governor Vessel; if the pain is on both sides of the lower back, it is a syndrome of the Bladder Meridian.

1. **Lower back pain due to Cold Damp**: Lower back pain with a Cold and heavy sensation, accompanied by soreness and numbness, limitation of extension and flexion of the back, pain radiating downwards to the buttocks and lower limbs, repeated attacks aggravated on Cold, rainy days; white, sticky tongue coating, deep and slow pulse.

2. **Lower back pain due to Blood stagnation**: A history of traumatic injury, attack due to over strain, rigidity and pain fixed in a certain area, limitation of movement, purplish tongue, and hesitant pulse.

3. **Lower back pain due to Kidney deficiency**: Insidious onset of protracted pain and soreness, accompanied by lassitude and weakness of the lower back and knees, aggravated by fatigue and alleviated by pressure and rest.

Treatment

Body acupuncture

1. **Principles of treatment**

   Warm the meridians and dispel Cold for Cold Damp syndrome, activate Blood and remove Blood stasis for Blood stagnation syndrome, tonify and strengthen the Kidney for Kidney deficiency syndrome. The Cold Damp and stagnation syndromes are treated by both acupuncture and moxibustion with the reducing method; Kidney deficiency syndrome is treated by acupuncture and moxibustion with the reinforcing method.

2. **Prescription**

Weizhong (BL40), Shenshu (BL23), Dachangshu (BL25), Yaoyangguan (GV3) and Ashi points.

3. **Explanation**

Weizhong (BL40) is located at the intersection in the popliteal fossa, where the two branches of the Bladder Meridian converge; this is one of the Four General Points selected to activate and regulate the meridian Qi for 'treating disorders of the back and lower back'; Shenshu (BL23) is located at the site where the Kidney is located; it is selected to tonify and strengthen the Kidneys. Dachangshu (BL25), Yaoyangguan (GV3) and Ashi are local points used to promote circulation of Qi and Blood, and relieve pain.

4. **Modification**

- *To warm Yang and dispel Cold for Cold Damp syndrome:* + Dazhui (GV14).

- *To activate Blood and remove Blood stasis for Blood stagnation syndrome:* + Geshu (BL17).

- *To tonify and strengthen the Kidney:* + Mingmen (GV4) with moxa.

5. **Manipulation**

All points are punctured with routine needling techniques. Medicinal moxa, Fuzi (附子 *Radix Aconiti Lateralis Preparata*) of indirect moxibustion on Mingmen (GV4) is recommended to treat lower back pain due to Kidney deficiency.

Other therapies

1. **Auricular acupuncture**

Points: Lumbar and Sacral Vertebrae, Kidney, Ear-Shenmen on the affected side. Filiform needles are used to puncture the points, and at the same time, ask the patient to exercise his lower back; or Wangbuliuxing (王不留行 *Semen Vaccaria*) seeds are applied to the points.

2. **Cutaneous needle**

A plum blossom needle is used to tap on the lumbar region until there is slight bleeding, and followed by cupping. This therapy is used for treating lower back pain due to Cold Damp and Blood stagnation.

3. **Point injection**

Inject 0.5–1ml of a mixture of 5ml Dexamethasone and 2ml Procaine into an Ashi point after a strict disinfection procedure. The treatment is given once daily.

Notes

1. The therapeutic result differs because of different aetiological factors of the lower back pain. Acupuncture can effectively treat lower back pain due to rheumatic diseases, or muscular injury, relieve symptoms and signs of lower back pain due to disorders of the lumbar vertebrae and protrusion of lumbar vertebrae disc; however, it fails to have good results in treating lower back pain caused by a lacerated ligament of the small joints of the lumbar region. For lower back pain caused by diseases of the internal organs, the primary disease should be treated. Tuberculosis of the spinal column and tumour are beyond acupuncture indications.

2. Massage on the lumbar region with palms twice a day in the morning and in the evening can relieve and prevent lower back pain.

3. Massage (Tuina), and traction therapies can be combined with acupuncture to treat lower back pain caused by protrusion of the lumbar vertebrae disc.

3. SCIATICA

Brief introduction

Sciatica refers to a syndrome marked mainly by radiating pain along the running course of the sciatic nerve (from the lumbar region, buttock, posterior side of the thigh, posterior lateral side of the leg to the lateral side of the foot).

Aetiology and pathogenesis

Lumbar sprain, contusion, muscular or traumatic injury may injure the tendons and meridians, leading to Qi and Blood stagnation, resulting in obstruction which causes pain; living in a Damp environment, walking in the rain, lack of warm clothing, exposure to Wind after sweating may all give rise to invasion of the body by Wind, Cold and Damp, which may block the circulation in the lower back and lower limbs; or retention of Damp Heat in the interior for a long time affects the Bladder Meridian of Foot-Taiyang, or Gallbladder Meridian of Foot-Shaoyang, resulting in lower back and leg pain. Sciatica includes syndromes of the Bladder and Gallbladder Meridians, as well as the muscle regions.

Syndrome differentiation

Sciatica is manifested by radiating pain, electric shock, burning pain in the lumbar region, buttock, posterior aspect of the thigh, posterior lateral aspect of the leg and lateral side of the foot. It is divided into two types: nerve root and nerve trunk affected syndromes. Clinically, sciatica with nerve root affected is more common.

1. **Sciatica with nerve root affected**: The nerve root inside the vertebral canal is affected, giving rise to secondary syndromes such as lumbar canal stenosis, protrusion of an intervertebral disc, spondylitis, spinal bifida (tuberculosis), etc. and is marked by a radiating pain from the lower back to one side of the buttock, posterior side of the thigh, posterior lateral aspect of the leg and lateral aspect of the foot, accompanied by fixed tenderness and pain during percussion in the lumbar sacral and spinal region; reduced sensory functions of the lateral side of the leg and dorsum of the foot; decreased functions or absence of knee and heel reflex; aggravation of pain when there is cough and sneezing, and when the abdominal pressure increases.

2. **Sciatica with nerve trunk affected**: The affected part is outside the vertebral canal where the sciatica nerve is distributed. It refers to hip joint arthritis, sacro-iliitis, injury of the buttock, pelvic inflammation, piriformis syndrome, etc. The pain is not obvious, but goes along the running course of the sciatic nerve, from the upper border of the sciatic foramen to the interspace between the sciatic tubercle and greater trochanter, middle of the popliteal fossa, below the small head of the fibula, and the posterior aspect of the lateral malleolus; reduced sensory functions of the lateral side of the leg and dorsum of the foot, decreased functions or absence of knee and heel reflex; but no changes when the abdominal pressure increases.

Treatment

Body acupuncture

1. **Principles of treatment**

    Unblock the meridians and collaterals, regulate Qi and relieve pain. Acupuncture is applied with reducing technique, combined with moxibustion.

2. **Prescription**

Points are mainly selected from the Bladder and Gallbladder Meridians. Bladder Meridian affected: Huantiao (GB30), Yanglingquan (GB34), Zhibian (BL54), Chengfu (BL36), Yinmen (BL37), Weizhong (BL40), Chengshan (BL57), Kunlun (BL60). Gallbladder Meridian affected: Huantiao (GB30), Yanglingquan (GB34), Fengshi (GB31), Xiyangguan (GB33), Yangfu (GB38), Xuanzhong (GB39), Zulinqi (GB41).

3. **Explanation**

Huantiao (GB30) is a meeting point of the two meridians. It is used to activate the circulation of the two meridians; Yanglingquan (GB34) is an Influential point of the tendons; it is used to relax the tendons and relieve pain.

4. **Modification**

- *To activate the meridian Qi in the lumbar region for lumbar and sacral pain*: + Shenshu (BL23), Dachangshu (BL25), Yaoyangguan (GV3), Ashi points.

- *To warm the meridians and alleviate pain for pain due to climatic changes*: + Dazhui (GV14), and Ashi points.

- *To remove Blood stasis for pain due to Blood stagnation*: + Geshu (BL17), Hegu (LI4), Taichong (LR3).

5. **Manipulation**

All points are punctured with routine needling techniques with the reducing method by lifting, thrusting and rotating the needles to produce a radiating needling sensation from the lower back downward to the foot along the Bladder or Gallbladder Meridians.

Other therapies

1. **Bleeding and cupping**

A plum blossom needle is used to tap on the lumbar sacral region or a three-edged needle used to prick the Ashi points to cause bleeding and followed by cupping.

2. **Electroacupuncture**

Jiaji points of L4–5, Yanglingquan (GB34), or Weizhong (BL40) for nerve root type, Zhibian (BL54) or Huantiao (GB30), Yanglingquan (GB34) or Weizhong (BL40) for nerve trunk type are punctured and stimulated by an electric apparatus of either dense wave or disperse and dense wave with its intensity gradually increasing from the moderate to strong.

3. **Point injection**

Prepare a mixture of 10–20ml Glucose 10% and vitamin B_1 100mg, vitamin B_{12} 100µg. Puncture the Jiaji points of L2–4 and Zhibian (BL54) with an injection needle. When there is a strong radiating needling sensation downward, lift the needle a bit, and inject the drug quickly into the point, 5–10ml for each point. For severe pain, 5–10ml of Procaine 1% can be injected into Ashi point or Huantiao (GB30).

Notes

1. Acupuncture is quite effective in treating sciatica. But if there is tumour or tuberculosis, the primary disease should be treated.

    Acupuncture can be combined with massage (Tuina) therapy in the treatment of sciatica caused by protrusion of the lumbar vertebral disc.

2. During an acute attack, the patient should stay in bed for rest; a hard wooden bed for sleep and a belt for holding the lower back are recommended for the patient suffering from protrusion of the lumbar vertebral disc.

3. When working, the patient should adopt an appropriate posture, and keep the body warm.

4. WEI SYNDROMES

Brief introduction

Wei syndromes are characterized by flaccidity, muscular atrophy or numbness of the limbs with motor impairment. They include multiple neuritis, sequellae of poliomyelitis, acute myelitis, or paralysis caused by injury of the motor neuron and peripheral nerve.

Aetiology and pathogenesis

Wei syndromes are mainly caused by deficiency of anti-pathogenic Qi with further attack of exogenous pathogenic Damp Heat, or high fever which may consume the Body Fluid. Consumption of Body Fluid fails to nourish the Zang Fu organs, tendons, muscles and meridians. Hence, the muscles and tendons become flaccid. Long-standing Damp due to living in a Damp environment, walking in the rain, or exposure to Cold may give rise to the accumulation of Damp which may turn into Heat; or retention of Damp Heat due to dysfunctions of the Spleen and Stomach caused by improper diet can affect the tendons and muscles, leading to flaccidity of the limbs; or a weakened constitution following a prolonged illness; consumption of Essence due to indulgent sexual activity may result in Liver and Kidney deficiency; Essence and Blood deficiency which fail to nourish the tendons and muscles, leading to muscular atrophy, weakness, and flaccidity. As a result a Wei syndrome occurs.

Syndrome differentiation

Wei syndromes are mainly marked by weakness of the limbs, flaccid tendons, paralysis or muscular atrophy.

1. **Consumption of Body Fluid by Lung Heat**: Fever with profuse sweating, sudden onset of weakness of the limbs when fever is reduced, accompanied by cough, restlessness, thirst, scanty deep yellow urine, dry stools; red tongue with yellow coating, thready and rapid pulse.

2. **Damp Heat**: Gradual onset of weakness and flaccidity of the limbs, especially the lower limbs, with numbness or Heat sensation of the lower limbs, accompanied by deep yellow urine, burning painful urination; yellow sticky tongue coating, soft and rapid pulse.

3. **Spleen and Stomach deficiency**: Weakness of the limbs over a long period, accompanied by poor appetite, shortness of breath, abdominal distension, loose stools, pale complexion, general lassitude; thin white tongue coating, and thready weak pulse.

4. **Liver and Kidney deficiency**: Slow onset, weakness and flaccidity of the lower limbs, accompanied by weakness and soreness of the lower back and knees, dizziness and tinnitus, seminal emission, prospermia, or irregular menstruation; red tongue with little coating, thready and rapid pulse.

Treatment
Body acupuncture

1. **Principles of treatment**

   Clear Heat, activate Qi and Blood by the reducing method of acupuncture without moxibustion for the syndrome of consumption of Body Fluid by Lung Heat; tonify Qi and benefit Blood, and nourish the tendons and muscles for the syndromes of Spleen and Stomach deficiency as well as Liver and Kidney deficiency syndromes by both acupuncture and moxibustion with the reinforcing method.

2. **Prescription**

   Points of the Large Intestine Meridian of Hand-Yangming and Stomach Meridian of Foot-Yangming and Jiaji points are selected.

   - *Upper limbs*: Jianyu (LI15), Quchi (LI11), Shousanli (LI10), Hegu (LI4), Waiguan (TE5), cervical and thoracic Jiaji points.

   - *Lower limbs*: Biguan (ST31), Futu (ST32), Zusanli (ST36), Fenglong (ST40), Fengshi (GB31), Yanglingquan (GB34), Sanyinjiao (SP6), and lumbar Jiaji points.

3. **Explanation**

   Points of the Yangming meridians of hand and foot are selected to unblock the circulation in the meridians and collaterals, regulate Qi and Blood, following the principle 'Only points along the Yangming meridians are selected in treating Wei syndromes'; Jiaji points can regulate Yin and Yang of the Zang Fu organs, activate Qi and Blood; Waiguan (TE5), and Fengshi (GB31) are selected to assist the Yangming meridians to promote Qi and Blood circulation; Yanglingquan (GB34), is an Influential point of the tendon which regulates the functions of the tendons; Sanyinjiao (SP6) can build up the Spleen, tonify the Liver, and nourish the Kidneys to strengthen the tendons, bones and treat flaccidity.

4. **Modification**

   - *To clear Heat and moisten the Dryness for Heat in the Lungs*: + Yuji (LU10), Chize (LU5) Feishu (BL13).

   - *To eliminate Damp Heat*: + Yinlingquan (SP9), Zhongji (CV3).

   - *To strengthen and tonify the Spleen and Stomach*: + Pishu (BL20), Weishu (BL21), Zhangmen (LR13), Zhongwan (CV12).

   - *To tonify and nourish the Liver and Kidneys*: + Ganshu (BL18), Shenshu (BL23), Taichong (LR3), Taixi (KI3).

5. **Manipulation**

   Yuji (LU10), Chize (LU5) are punctured with the reducing method, or by a three-edged needle to cause bleeding; points from the Large Intestine Meridian of Hand-Yangming are punctured to treat muscular atrophy of the upper limbs; points from the Stomach Meridian of Foot-Yangming are punctured to treat muscular atrophy of the lower limbs; the other points are punctured with routine needling techniques.

Other therapies

1. **Electroacupuncture**

   Puncture the points on the flaccid muscle, connect the needles with a pulse electroacupuncture stimulator with intermittent wave, moderate intensity, to cause regular contraction of the affected limb. The needles are retained for 20–30 minutes for each treatment.

2. **Cutaneous needle**

   A plum blossom needle is used to tap repeatedly on the Back-Shu points, such as Feishu (BL13), Pishu (BL20), Weishu (BL21) and points along the running course of both the hand and foot Yangming meridians. The treatment is given once every other day.

Notes

1. Acupuncture is effective to treat this disease, but for a prolonged case with deformity, other therapies should be combined.

2. Those patients who stay in bed should keep their four-limb functional posture normal so as to avoid foot drop or strephenopodia, or a nursing supporter or splints should be used. The body should be exercised appropriately to avoid bed sores.

3. During treatment, both active and passive functional exercises of the limbs are recommended for an earlier recovery.

5. WIND STROKE

Brief introduction

Wind Stroke is an emergency situation manifested by the patient falling down in a fit with loss of consciousness, deviation of mouth, slurred speech and hemiplegia; or deviation of mouth and hemiplegia without loss of consciousness. It is characterized by abrupt onset with pathological changes varying quickly like Wind (Wind in nature blows in gusts and is characterized by rapid changes), from which the term 'Wind Stroke' comes. In Western medicine, Wind Stroke refers to acute cerebrovascular diseases such as cerebral thrombosis, haemorrhage, embolism, subarachnoid haemorrhage, etc. In general, Wind Stroke can be divided into two categories: haemorrhage and ischaemia.

Aetiology and pathogenesis

Wind, Fire, Phlegm and stasis are the main aetiological factors; Wind Stroke is related to dysfunction of the Heart, Liver, Spleen, Kidney organs, etc. It is caused by either weak anti-pathogenic Qi leading to deficiency of defensive Qi; invasion of meridians due to exogenous pathogenic factors leading to Qi and Blood stagnation; or overstress and overstrain leading to Liver and Kidney Yin deficiency; upsurge of Liver Yang which makes Qi and Blood go upward; or irregular food intake, desire for fatty food leading to deficiency of Spleen; production of Phlegm and Heat; upward invasion of Wind and Phlegm disturbing the head (clear orifice); emotional changes affecting the Liver and inducing Heart Fire; or perversion of Qi and Blood caused by Wind and Fire. When Wind, Fire, and Phlegm attack the meridians, they cause Qi and Blood stagnation which impairs the meridian functions; adverse Qi circulation of Yin and Yang may give rise to a tense syndrome, while weakness of anti-pathogenic Qi leading to separation of Qi of Yin and Yang causes a flaccid syndrome.

Syndrome differentiation

The main symptoms are sudden disturbance of consciousness or loss of consciousness, and hemiplegia. Clinically, an attack on the Zang Fu organs and an attack on the meridians and collaterals are classified according to the symptom: being conscious or unconscious.

1. **Attack on the meridians and collaterals**: Numbness of the limbs, deviation of mouth, slurred speech, stiffness of tongue, hemiplegia, mostly no change of consciousness because of the shallow depth of the disease. If Wind enters the meridians and collaterals, there is thin tongue coating with white colour, and wiry and rolling or wiry and rapid pulse; if Liver and Kidney Yin deficiency causes upsurge of Wind Yang, there is dizziness, headache, tinnitus, blurred vision, red tongue with yellow coating, wiry, thready and rapid or wiry and rolling pulse.

2. **Attack on the Zang Fu organs**: Sudden falling down, loss of consciousness. The disease is severe because the pathogenic Qi enters deeply.

   - *Tense syndrome*: Clenched jaws, hemiplegia, trismus, tightly closed hands, flushed face, coarse breathing, rattling in the throat, retention of urine, constipation, wiry, rolling and rapid pulse.

   - *Flaccid syndrome*: Eyes closed and mouth agape, snoring but feeble breathing, hands opened and Cold sensation on four limbs, incontinence of urine and stools, thready and weak pulse; continuous and sticky sweating, mydriasis, or asymmetrical pupils on both sides; fading or large floating pulse indicating the danger that genuine Yang may separate from the body.

Treatment: Attack on the meridians and collaterals
Body acupuncture

1. **Principles of treatment**

   To promote meridians, regulate Qi and Blood; apply acupuncture mainly with even method.

2. **Prescription**

   Shuigou (GV26), Neiguan (PC6), Jiquan (HT1), Chize (LU5), Weizhong (BL40), Sanyinjiao (SP6), Zusanli (ST36).

3. **Explanation**

   The Heart dominates the Blood and vessels, Neiguan (PC6) adjusts Heart Qi and promotes Qi, Blood circulation; Sanyinjiao (SP6) is a meeting point of the three Yin meridians of the foot and can nourish Liver and Kidney Yin; Jiquan (HT1), Chize (LU5), Weizhong (BL40), Zusanli (ST36) can promote meridians on the limbs.

4. **Modification**

   - *Upsurge of Liver Yang*: + Taichong (LR3), Tiaxi (KI3) to reduce Liver Yang.
   - *Obstruction of meridians by Wind and Phlegm*: + Fenglong (ST40), Hegu (LI4) to eliminate Phlegm and dispel Wind.
   - *Fu organs affected by Phlegm and Heat*: + Quchi (LI11), Neiting (ST44), Fenglong (ST40) to clear Heat and remove Phlegm.
   - *Qi deficiency and Blood stagnation*: + Qihai (CV6), Xuehai (SP10) to benefit Qi and activate Blood.
   - *Yin deficiency stirring up Wind*: + Taixi (KI3), Fengchi (GB20) to nourish Yin and reduce Yang excess.
   - *Deviation of mouth*: + Jiache (ST6), Dicang (ST4).
   - *Hemiplegia of upper limbs*: + Quchi (LI11), Jianyu (LI15), Shousanli (LI10), Hegu (LI4).
   - *Hemiplegia of lower limbs*: + Huantiao (GB30), Yanglingquan (GB34), Yinlingquan (SP9), Fengshi (GB31).
   - *Dizziness*: + Fengchi (GB20), Wangu (GB12), Tianzhu (BL10).
   - *Strephenopodia*: + Juegu (GB39), Jiuneifan (Extra point), Qiuxu (GB40) penetrating to Zhaohai (KI6).
   - *Strephexopodia*: + Zhongfeng (LR4), Taixi (KI3), Jiuwaifan (Extra point).
   - *Foot drop*: + Jiexi (ST41), Jingshang (Extra point).

- *Constipation*: + Fenglong (ST40), Zhigou (TE6).

- *Incontinence of urine, retention of urine*: + Zhongji (CV3), Qugu (CV2), Guanyuan (CV4).

5. **Manipulation**

Reducing by rotating on Neiguan (PC6); reinforcing by lifting and thrusting on Sanyinjiao (SP6) and Zusanli (ST36); locating Jiquan (HT1) on 2 cun below original Jiquan (HT1) and running course of the Heart Meridian, avoiding armpit hair, inserting the needle with perpendicular direction, reducing by lifting and thrusting; puncturing Chize (LU5), Weizhong (BL40) with perpendicular direction, reducing by lifting and thrusting, making limbs feel a trembling sensation.

Treatment: Attack on the Zang Fu organs
Body acupuncture

1. **Principles of treatment**

To restore consciousness and open the orifices:

- *Tense syndrome*: To relieve the symptoms of tense type, acupuncture alone, no moxibustion with the reducing method.

- *Flaccid syndrome*: To recapture Yang from collapse, apply heavy moxibustion with the reinforcing method.

2. **Prescription**

Mainly points of the Governor Vessel. Shuigou (GV26), Suliao (GV25), Baihui (GV20), Neiguan (PC6).

3. **Explanation**

The brain is the palace of original spirit, and the Governor Vessel enters brain. Suliao (GV25), Shuigou (GV26) can restore consciousness and open the orifices; Baihui (GV20) is located on the vertex and has the function of restoring consciousness and opening the orifices; Neiguan (PC6) can regulate Heart Qi, and promote Qi and Blood circulation.

4. **Modification**

- *Tense syndrome*: + Shixuan (EX-UE11), Hegu (LI4), Taichong (LR3) to open the orifices and stop tenseness.

- *Flaccid syndrome*: + Guanyuan (CV4), Qihai (CV6), Shenque (CV8) to recapture Yang from collapse.

- *Respiratory failure:* + Qishe (ST11) to benefit pectoral Qi and promote respiration.

5. **Manipulation**

   Reducing by rotating on Neiguan (PC6); sparrow-pecking method on Suliao (GV25), Shuigou (GV26), stimulation depends upon change of the patient's facial expression; bleeding by three-edged needle pricking on Shixuan (EX-UE11); reducing with heavy stimulation on Taichong (LR3), Hegu (LI4); big moxa-cone on Guanyuan (CV4), Qihai (CV6); indirect salt moxa cone on Shenque (CV8).

Other therapies

1. **Auricular acupuncture**

   Points: Brain, Subcortex, Liver, Triple Burner by filiform needle puncturing, moderate stimulation and once a day; sequelae treated once every other day and retaining the needle for 30 minutes; also Vaccaria seeds to auricular points.

2. **Electroacupuncture**

   Choose 2 points separately from the upper and lower limbs. After the arrival of Qi by needling, connect to the electroacupuncture apparatus with disperse and dense wave and moderate-low stimulation until the muscle slightly trembles.

3. **Scalp acupuncture**

   Dingnie Qianxiexian (MS6), Dingpangxian I (MS8), Dingpangxian II (MS9), selecting No. 28–30 1.5–2.0 cun filiform needle, inserting the needle to form an angle of 30° with the skin surface. Rapidly insert needle to the scalp region, quickly rotating the needle for 2–3 minutes, retain the needle for 30 minutes, repeatedly rotating the needle 2–3 times during retaining. Tell the patient to move his limbs during the treatment; treatment performed once every other day.

Notes

1. Acupuncture and moxibustion are effective for the treatment of Wind Stroke, especially for the recovery of nerve functions such as limb movement, speech and swallowing, etc. Based on the principle 'The earlier the treatment, the better the result', patients should receive treatment early and combine treatment with physical exercise.

2. Comprehensive therapies should be taken for the acute stage of Wind Stroke manifested by high fever, loss of consciousness, Heart failure, high intracranial pressure, upper gastrointestinal bleeding, etc.

3. Patients with Wind Stroke should avoid bedsores and keep the respiratory tract flowing freely.

4. Wind Stroke focuses on prevention. When a person is over 40 years old, and often suffers from dizziness, headache, numbness of limbs, occasionally finds speech difficult, and has weakness of limbs, these symptoms indicate the aura of Wind Stroke. So prevention and treatment should be strengthened.

6. FACIAL PARALYSIS

Brief introduction

Facial paralysis is manifested by deviation of the mouth and eyes. This can occur in patients of any age, mostly in winter and summer. Facial paralysis is of sudden onset, mostly happens on one side of face. Both the Large Intestine Meridian of Hand-Yangming and the Stomach Meridian of Foot-Yangming pass through the head and face. When pathogenic factors obstruct the facial meridians, especially the muscle regions of the Small Intestine Meridian of Hand-Taiyang and the Stomach Meridian of Foot-Yangming, facial paralysis can occur. This condition is seen in peripheral facial paralysis or mostly Bell's palsy in Western medicine. Invasion of the face by Wind and Cold causes inflammation, ischaemia, oedema of facial canal and local tissues, or dysfunction of autonomic nervous system, local vasospasm, tissue oedema, and inflammatory change after facial neurothlipsis.

Aetiology and pathogenesis

TCM holds that overstrain, insufficient anti-pathogenic Qi, deficient defensive Qi, or invasion of facial meridians by Wind Cold or Wind Heat can cause Qi and Blood stagnation, dysfunction of muscle regions and failure to dominate tendons and muscles, as a result of which facial paralysis occurs. Peripheral facial paralysis has symptoms that are apparent in the tendons and muscles of the eye, mouth and cheek. The muscle regions of the Bladder Meridian of Foot-Taiyang and the Stomach Meridian of Foot-Yangming form a muscular net around the eye, so failure of eyelid to close is caused by dysfunction of the muscle regions of the Bladder Meridian of Foot-Taiyang and the Stomach Meridian of Foot-Yangming. The mouth and cheek are dominated by the muscle regions of the Small Intestine Meridian of Hand-Taiyang, the Large Intestine Meridian of Hand-Yangming and the Stomach Meridian of Foot-Yangming, and therefore facial paralysis is caused by dysfunction of the muscle regions mentioned above.

Syndrome differentiation

The main symptom is deviation of the mouth and eye. The patient usually suffers from a dull sensation of the muscles, wrinkles disappear, there is incomplete closure of the eye, tears, shallow nasal groove, drooping of the angle of the mouth deviating to healthy side, inability to frown, and failure to raise the eyebrow, close the eye, blow out the cheek, show the teeth or whistle on the affected side; in some cases, the patient initially feels pain in the mastoid region, the sense of taste decreases or disappears in the frontal one third of the tongue, and hearing becomes sensitive (hyperacusis), etc. Paralysis over a long time causes the patient to suffer from muscular contracture, the angle of the mouth deviated to affected side, and there can even be facial muscle spasm.

1. **Wind Cold syndrome**: In the early stages, history of Cold invasion on the face, pale tongue with thin and white coating, superficial and tense pulse.

2. **Wind Heat syndrome**: In the early stages, occuring after common cold and fever, combined with red tongue with thin and yellow coating, superficial and rapid pulse.

3. **Deficiency of Qi and Blood**: In the recovery period, in the case of a prolonged condition, combined with lassitude, pale complexion, dizziness, etc.

Treatment
Body acupuncture

1. **Principles of treatment**

   To promote Qi and Blood circulation, and regulate muscle regions, apply both acupuncture and moxibustion, even method.

2. **Prescription**

   Yangbai (GB14), Sibai (ST2), Quanliao (SI18), Dicang (ST4), Yifeng (TE17), Hegu (LI4).

3. **Explanation**

   Meridian points on the face can promote Qi and Blood circulation of the muscle regions, and activate Blood in local areas. Hegu (LI4) can treat all diseases of the face, and mouth and functions to dispel Wind and promote meridians when combined with nearby meridian points.

4. **Modification**

- *Wind Cold syndrome*: + Fengchi (GB20).
- *Wind Heat syndrome*: + Quchi (LI11).
- *Inability to frown*: + Zanzhu (BL2).
- *Shallow nasal groove*: + Yingxiang (LI20).
- *Deviation of philtrum*: + Shuigou (GV26).
- *Deviation of labial groove*: + Chengjiang (CV24).
- *Recovery period*: + Zusanli (ST36).

5. **Manipulation**

Apply the even method on facial points, adding moxibustion during the recovery period. In the acute period, mild stimulation on facial points and heavy reducing stimulation on limb points; in the recovery period, even method on Hegu (LI4) and the reinforcing method on Zusanli (ST36).

Other therapies

1. **Cutaneous needle**

Tap Yangbai (GB14), Quanliao (SI18), Dicang (ST4), Jiache (ST6) until local redness occurs. This is suitable for the recovery period.

2. **Blood-letting puncturing and cupping**

Prick Yangbai (GB14), Quanliao (SI18), Dicang (ST4) with a three-edged needle, then cup. Twice every week. It is suitable for recovery period.

3. **Electroacupuncture**

Select Taiyang (EX-HN5), Yangbai (GB14), Dicang (ST4), Jiache (ST6), connect to the electroacupuncture apparatus, apply intermittent wave and 10–20 minutes stimulation. The intensity is correct when the facial muscle is slightly trembling and this depends on the tolerance of patient. It is suitable for the recovery period.

4. **Point application**

Choose Taiyang (EX-HN5), Yangbai (GB14), Quanliao (SI18), Dicang (ST4), Jiache (ST6), grind Maqianzi (马钱子 *Semen Strychni*) into 0.3–0.6g powder and scatter the powder on the adhesive tape, and stick the tapes on the points, changing tapes once every 5 to 7 days; or pound castor bean and add a small amount of Shexiang (麝香 *Moschus*), take a piece about the size of a mung bean and stick this on the points, changing once every 3 to 5 days;

or grind Baifuzi (白附子 *Rhizoma Typhonii*) into powder, adding a small amount of borneol to make a cake, and stick cakes on the points once a day.

Notes

1. Acupuncture-moxibustion is effective in the treatment of facial paralysis, and it is safe, which makes it the first choice of treatment.

2. The patient should avoid invasion of the face by Wind and Cold. If necessary, the patient should wear a mask, and/or an eye patch; dust easily enters eye because of incomplete closure of the eye, so the patient should use eyedrops 2–3 times a day to prevent infection.

3. The prognosis of peripheral facial paralysis closely relates to the degree to which the facial nerve has been injured. In general, the prognosis is good if the facial paralysis is caused by aseptic inflammation; the prognosis is not good if the facial paralysis is caused by a virus (such as Hunt facial paralysis).

4. We should distinguish this condition from central facial paralysis.

7. TRIGEMINAL NEURALGIA

Brief introduction

Trigeminal neuralgia is a disease manifested by severe, burning and spasmodic pain, which is the most typical nerve pain seen in the clinic. It occurs most often in female patients over the age of 40, in both primary and secondary forms. It falls within the general area of 'Facial Pain' in TCM.

Aetiology and pathogenesis

According to TCM, trigeminal neuralgia is mostly associated with the invasion of exogenous Wind, emotional change, traumatic injury, etc. Exogenous Wind and Cold attack Yangming and Taiyang meridians on the face, which causes Qi and Blood stagnation because Cold is characterized by contraction; or Wind and toxic Heat invade the face and obstruct Qi and Blood circulation in the meridians. Traumatic injury, emotional change or prolonged illness can lead to Qi and Blood stagnation of the face and cause facial pain. Eye pain indicates a syndrome of the Bladder Meridian of Foot-Taiyang; pain of the upper jaw or lower jaw indicates a syndrome of the Large Intestine Meridian of Hand-Yangming, the Stomach Meridian of Foot-Yangming and the Small Intestine Meridian of Hand-Taiyang.

Syndrome differentiation

Onset is abrupt like an electric shock, and the pain is cutting, pricking and burning. It is combined with a flushed complexion, tears, salivation, nasal discharge, and muscular contracture of the face. Occurrence of trigeminal neuralgia is induced by speaking, swallowing, brushing the teeth, washing the face, Cold stimulation, or emotional change. It continues for from a few seconds to a few minutes; frequency is not fixed, and there are no symptoms during intermittent period.

1. **Wind Cold syndrome**: A history of Wind and Cold invasion, facial pain is worse after Cold attack, and better after warming, clear nasal discharge, white tongue coating, superficial and tense pulse.

2. **Wind Heat syndrome**: A burning sensation on the affected region, salivation, redness of the eyes, tears, thin and yellow tongue coating, superficial and rapid pulse.

3. **Qi and Blood stagnation**: Mostly associated with a history of traumatic injury, or a prolonged condition, many fixed painful points, purplish dark tongue or with ecchymosis, hesitant pulse.

Treatment
Body acupuncture

1. **Principles of treatment**

   To promote Qi and Blood in the meridians, dispel Wind and eliminate Cold, mainly apply acupuncture with the reducing method.

2. **Prescription**

   Points are selected mainly locally in the face and cheek, the Large Intestine Meridian of Hand-Yangming and the Stomach Meridian of Foot-Yangming meridians. Sibai (ST2), Xiaguan (ST7), Dicang (ST4), Zanzhu (BL2), Hegu (LI4), Neiting (ST44), Taichong (LR3).

3. **Explanation**

   Sibai (ST2), Xiaguan (ST7), Dicang (ST4), Zanzhu (BL2) can promote meridians of the face; Hegu (LI4) is a Yuan-Primary point, and all diseases of the face and mouth can be treated by Hegu (LI4); a combination of Hegu (LI4) with Taichong (LR3) can dispel Wind and promote the meridians, stop pain and relieve spasms; Neiting (ST44) can clear Heat and dispel Wind on Yangming meridians.

4. **Modification**

- *Eye branch*: + Sizhukong (TE23), Yangbai (GB14).
- *Upper jaw*: + Quanliao (SI18), Yingxiang (LI20).
- *Lower jaw*: + Chengjiang (CV24), Jiache (ST6), Yifeng (TE17).
- *Wind and Cold*: + Lieque (LU7) to dispel Wind and eliminate Cold.
- *Wind and Heat*: + Quchi (LI11), Waiguan (TE5) to dispel Wind and clear Heat.
- *Qi and Blood stagnation*: + Neiguan (PC6), Sanyinjiao (SP6) to activate Blood and eliminate stasis.

5. **Manipulation**

First puncture the distal points. Puncture deeply and penetrate with mild stimulation on all facial points. Moxibustion can be added for Wind Cold syndrome.

Other therapies

1. **Cutaneous needle**

Look for trigger points on the face, embed press needle and fix with adhesive tape. Change once every 2 to 3 days.

2. **Blood-letting puncturing and cupping**

Select Jiache (ST6), Dicang (ST4), Quanliao (SI18), prick with three-edged needle and apply flash cupping. Perform once every other day.

3. **Auricular acupuncture**

Points: Cheek, Forehead, Jaw, Ear-Shenmen. Puncture or embed.

Notes

1. Trigeminal neuralgia is stubborn and a condition that is difficult to treat. Acupuncture has a certain success in treating this disease. We should establish the origin of any secondary trigeminal neuralgia, and then apply a suitable method to treat the primary disease.

2. Mild manipulation and long retention are preferred on local regions, heavy manipulation is used on distal points, in particular, heavy and continuous stimulation is preferred on distal points during a period of attack.

8. HEADACHE

Brief introduction

Headache is a subjective symptom with pain in the head. It occurs in various diseases of Western medicine such as headache due to tension, vasoneurosis, meningitis, hypertension, cerebral arteriosclerosis, traumatic head injury, sequela of cerebral concussion, etc.

Aetiology and pathogenesis

The head is the 'Sea of Marrow', and is also the meeting place of all of the Yang meridians, the Palace of Clear Yang. The Qi and Blood of all of the five Zang and six Fu organs flow upward to the head. Invasion of the head by exogenous pathogenic factors and internal injuries can cause derangement and obstruction of Qi and Blood, then the loss of brain nourishment results in headache.

Syndrome differentiation

Headache mostly occurs on the forehead, vertex, the temporal region of one side, or repeatedly happens on left or right or whole head. The nature of pain includes boring pain, dull pain, distending pain, pricking pain or sharp pain.

1. **Yangming headache**: Frontal headache, including supraorbital bone pain, pain caused by eyes, nose and upper teeth disorders.

2. **Shaoyang headache**: Temporal headache, including pain caused by ear disorders.

3. **Taiyang headache**: Occipital headache, including pain caused by neck stiffness, cervical spondylosis.

4. **Jueyin headache**: Vertex headache, including pain caused by hypertension.

5. **Temporal and frontal headache**: Pain on the forehead and both sides of the head.

6. **Whole head pain**: Pain of the whole head, difficult to identify exact position of the pain.

Treatment
Body acupuncture

1. **Principles of treatment**

   To promote Qi and Blood circulation in the meridians, mainly apply acupuncture, use the reinforcing method for deficiency and reducing for excess.

2. **Prescription**

   Mainly local points, accompanied by distal points along related meridians.

   - *Yangming headache*: Yintang (EX-HN3), Shangxing (GV23), Yangbai (GB14), Zanzhu (BL2) penetrating to Sizhukong (TE23) through Yuyao (EX-HN4), Hegu (LI4), Neiting (ST44).

   - *Shaoyang headache*: Taiyang (EX-HN5), Sizhukong (TE23), Jiaosun (TE20), Shuaigu (GB8), Fengchi (GB20), Waiguan (TE5), Zulinqi (GB41).

   - *Taiyang headache*: Tianzhu (BL10), Fengchi (GB20), Houxi (SI3), Shenmai (BL62), Kunlun (BL60).

   - *Jueyin headache*: Baihui (GV20), Tongtian (BL7), Taichong (LR3), Xingjian (LR2), Taixi (KI3), Yongquan (KI1).

   - *Temporal and frontal headache*: Yintang (EX-HN3), Taiyang (EX-HN5), Taibai (SP3), Touwei (ST8), Yangbai (GB14), Hegu (LI4), Fengchi (GB20), Waiguan (TE5).

3. **Explanation**

   Mainly select local points accompanied by distal points to promote Qi and Blood circulation in the meridians.

4. **Modification**

   - *Invasion of exogenous Wind*: + Fengchi (GB20), Fengmen (BL12).

   - *Wind Cold*: Moxibustion towards Dazhui (GV14).

   - *Wind Heat*: Reducing on Quchi (LI11); Wind Dampness: reducing on Sanyinjiao (SP6) to dispel Wind, clear head and eyes.

   - *Invasion of head by Phlegm*: + Fenglong (ST40), Zusanli (ST36) to eliminate Phlegm, promote collaterals and stop pain.

   - *Qi and Blood stagnation*: + Hegu (LI4), Taichong (LR3), Geshu (BL17) to regulate Qi and activate Blood, eliminate stagnation and stop pain.

   - *Qi and Blood deficiency*: + Qihai (CV6), Xuehai (SP10), Zusanli (ST36) to benefit Qi and nourish Blood, reinforce deficiency and stop pain.

- *Upsurge of Liver Yang*: Same as treatment of Jueyin headache.

- *Headache with all parts affected*: + Ashi points.

5. **Manipulation**

Most head points are punctured horizontally, a few points perpendicularly, such as Taiyang (EX-HN5), Tianzhu (BL10), Fengchi (GB20), but strictly controlling the direction and depth of Fengchi (GB20) so as to prevent injury to the medulla; the reducing method for invasion of exogenous Wind, upward disturbance of Phlegm, Qi and Blood stagnation, upsurge of Liver Yang; prick to cause bleeding on Ashi points for Qi and Blood stagnation, upsurge of Liver Yang; reinforcing and moxibustion for Qi and Blood stagnation. Treat 1–2 times for acute headache, retaining the needles 30–60 minutes every time; treat once a day or every other day for chronic headache.

Other therapies

1. **Cutaneous needle**

Tap Yintang (EX-HN3), Taiyang (EX-HN5), Ashi points for 5–10 minutes until there is bleeding. This is used for invasion of Wind, Cold and Dampness or upsurge of Liver Yang.

2. **Three-edged needle**

Prick Yintang (EX-HN3), Taiyang (EX-HN5), Baihui (GV20), Dazhui (GV14), Zanzhu (BL2), etc. to cause bleeding with 3–5 drops for severe headache.

3. **Electroacupuncture**

Select Hegu (LI4), Fengchi (GB20), Taiyang (EX-HN5), Ashi points, etc., applying continuous wave and moderate stimulation. It is appropriate for Qi and Blood stagnation, and stubborn headache.

4. **Auricular acupuncture**

Points: Occiput, Temple, Forehead, Subcortex, Liver Yang, Ear-Shenmen. Apply 2 to 3 points each time, puncture by needle with strong stimulation, the duration of retaining the needles depending on when the headache is relieved; also Vaccaria seeds to auricular points; bleeding on the veins of the back auricle to treat stubborn headache.

5. **Point injection**

According to syndrome differentiation, respectively apply Chaihu (柴胡 *Radix Bupleuri*) injection, Danggui (当归 *Radix Angelicae Sinensis*) injection,

Danshen (丹参 *Radix Salviae Miltiorrhizae*) injection, Chuanxiong (川芎 *Rhizoma Ligustici Wallichii*) injection, vitamin B$_1$ or vitamin B$_{12}$ injection, routinely selecting 2 to 3 points with 0.5ml into each point.

Notes

1. Acupuncture and moxibustion are obviously effective in treating headache, and some functional headache can be cured. Acupuncture and moxibustion can relieve symptoms when headache is caused by organic diseases, but organic disease should also be treated to prevent further development of the disease.

2. Some patients have passive, pessimistic, worried and frightened feelings because they suffer from repeated headaches. So during acupuncture and moxibustion treatment, the doctor should comfort the patient.

9. DIZZINESS

Brief introduction

Dizziness is a largely subjective symptom with blurred vision, an illusion of bodily movement and rotatory sensation like sitting in a sailing boat or moving car, and is sometimes even accompanied by nausea, vomiting and sweating, which is mostly seen in Meniere's syndrome, cervical spondylosis, vascular diseases of the vertebro-basilar artery, anaemia, hypertension and cerebral vascular diseases in Western medicine.

Aetiology and pathogenesis

According to TCM, the brain is affected in dizziness, which relates to depression and anger, irregular food intake with a desire for greasy and fatty food, overstress and overstrain, Qi and Blood deficiency. Emotional change causes Liver Qi stagnation, Qi stagnation turns to Fire, hyperactivity of Liver Yang leads to upsurge and results in dizziness; desire for greasy and fatty food disturbs the function of the Spleen in the transportation and transformation of food and Water, then the obstruction of Phlegm and Dampness in Middle Burner causes dysfunction of clear Yang in ascending; overstress and overstrain causes Kidney Essence deficiency, so Kidney Essence can not fill up the brain; body weakness after illness, Qi and Blood deficiency, malnourishment of brain can also result in dizziness.

Syndrome differentiation

This disease is manifested in dizziness, blurred vision, and rotatory sensations. In mild cases, the patient feels as if they are sitting in a sailing boat, and this sensation can be relieved by closing the eyes; in severe cases, the patient feels blurred vision, unclear vision, continuous rotatory sensation, difficulty in standing, and easily falls down. The patient also suffers from nausea, vomiting, trembling sensation of the eyeball, tinnitus, deafness, sweating, pale complexion, etc.

1. **Upsurge of Liver Yang**: Dizziness, tinnitus, distension and pain of the head and eyes, easily irritated and angry, insomnia, dream disturbed sleep, flushed complexion, redness of eyes, bitter taste in the mouth, red tongue with yellow coating, wiry and rapid pulse.

2. **Obstruction of head by Phlegm**: A heavy and bandaged sensation of the head, rotatory sensation, fullness in the chest, nausea, vomiting, salivation, sticky sensation in the mouth, poor appetite, pale tongue with white and sticky coating, wiry and rolling pulse.

3. **Qi and Blood deficiency**: Dizziness, blurred vision, pale or sallow complexion, lassitude, palpitations, insomnia, abdominal distension, poor appetite, pale tongue with thin and white coating, weak pulse.

4. **Liver and Kidney Yin deficiency**: Prolonged dizziness, failing vision, insomnia, poor memory, irritability, dry mouth, tinnitus, lassitude, weakness and soreness of the lower back and knee joints, red tongue with thin coating, wiry and thready pulse.

Treatment

Body acupuncture

1. **Principles of treatment**

   - *Upsurge of Liver Yang*: To eliminate Liver Yang, clear head and eyes, apply acupuncture alone without moxibustion and using the reducing method.

   - *Obstruction of head by Phlegm*: To tonify Spleen and eliminate Dampness, eliminate Phlegm and promote meridians, apply both acupuncture and moxibustion, using the even method.

   - *Qi and Blood deficiency*: To tonify Qi and Blood, apply the reinforcing method.

   - *Liver and Kidney Yin deficiency*: To nourish Liver and Kidney, mainly apply acupuncture using even method.

2. **Prescription**

   Select mainly points from head and the Gallbladder Meridian of Foot-Shaoyang. Baihui (GV20), Fengchi (GB20), Touwei (ST8), Taiyang (EX-HN5), Xuanzhong (GB39).

3. **Explanation**

   Baihui (GV20) enters the brain through the collaterals, and can have the function of clearing the head and eyes, and stopping dizziness; Fengchi (GB20), Touwei (ST8), Taiyang (EX-HN5) are all located on the head and are near points to regulate Qi activities of head; Xuanzhong (GB39) fills up the Sea of Marrow and is a key point to stop dizziness.

4. **Modification**

   • *Upsurge of Liver Yang*: + Xingjian (LR2), Taichong (LR3), Taixi (KI3) to moisten Water for nourishment of Wood.

   • *Obstruction of head by Phlegm*: + Neiguan (PC6), Zhongwan (CV12), Fenglong (ST40) to tonify Spleen and harmonize Middle Burner, eliminate Dampness and remove Phlegm.

   • *Qi and Blood deficiency*: Qihai (CV6), + Xuehai (SP10), Zusanli (ST36) to tonify Qi and Blood, and regulate Spleen and Stomach.

   • *Liver and Kidney Yin deficiency*: + Ganshu (BL18), Shenshu (BL23), Taixi (KI3) to nourish Liver and Kidney Yin and strengthen the health.

5. **Manipulation**

   Pay attention to the direction, angle and depth when puncturing Fengchi (GB20). Routine puncturing methods are used for other points. Obstruction of the head by Phlegm can be treated by moxibustion towards Baihui (GV20).

Other therapies

1. **Three-edged needle**

   Severe dizziness: Prick to cause bleeding with 1 to 2 drops on Yintang (EX-HN3), Taiyang (EX-HN5), Baihui (GV20), etc.

2. **Scalp acupuncture**

   Select Dingzhongxian (MS5), Zhenxia Pangxian (MS14) with moderate stimulation, retain the needles for 20 minutes and treat once a day.

3. **Auricular acupuncture**

   Points: Adrenal, Subcortex, Occiput, Brain, Ear-Shenmen, Forehead, Inner Ear; add Liver and Gallbladder for upsurge of Liver Yang; add Spleen and Central Rim for obstruction of head by Phlegm; add Spleen and Stomach for Qi and Blood deficiency; add Liver and Kidney for Liver and Kidney Yin deficiency. Use 3 to 5 points on the one side every time, then puncture with moderate stimulation, retaining the needles for 20 to 30 minutes; or apply Vaccaria seeds to auricular points.

4. **Point injection**

   Choose 2 to 3 points from those used for acupuncture and moxibustion. Apply 0.5ml of either 5% Glucose liquid, vitamin B_1 injection, vitamin B_{12} injection, or Danggui (当归 *Radix Angelicae Sinensis*) injection to each point.

Notes

1. Acupuncture and moxibustion can be effective in treating dizziness, but we should distinguish a secondary from a primary condition, and whether it is chronic or acute. When dizziness is acute and severe, we will treat the secondary symptoms; when dizziness is mild or intermittent, we will treat the primary syndrome after differentiation.

2. To get a definite diagnosis, the patient should be examined through tests such as a blood pressure test, haemoglobin test, red blood cell count, ECG, electro-audiometer test, Brain Stem Evoked Potential, electronystagmograph, X-ray on cervical vertebra, and if necessary, CT or MRI during treatment.

3. When dizziness occurs, the patient should close his eyes and lie on the bed (or sit down), press Yintang (EX-HN3), Taiyang (EX-HN5), etc. by finger to promote Qi circulation in the meridians, then dizziness should be relieved.

4. If there is retention of Phlegm, the patient should take a light diet with less greasy and fatty food to prevent the occurrence of Dampness and Phlegm, Heat and Wind. The patient should also avoid hot and spicy food, stop smoking and drink no alcohol to prevent the upsurge of Liver Yang.

10. PRIMARY HYPERTENSION

Brief introduction

The main symptom of primary hypertension is continuously increased arterial blood pressure (BP: 140/90mmHg or 18.6/12kPa) while in a quiet state. Incidence of this condition is high and increasing, and seen in younger patients. So far the aetiology of this disease is unknown; currently it is thought that primary hypertension is caused by various factors based on genetic predisposition. Primary hypertension is related to inheritance, age, posture, career, emotion and food intake, etc.

Aetiology and pathogenesis

Plain Questions believes 'rotatory sensation, dizziness and blurred vision mostly are caused by dysfunctions of the Liver'. Primary hypertension relates to Kidney Yin deficiency. Liver Yang hyperactivity is mostly induced by mental factors, and irregular food intake.

Syndrome differentiation

In the early stage of hypertension, half of all patients do not have obvious symptoms; often hypertension is identified only on physical examination. When the fluctuation range of blood pressure is large, patients may experience more symptoms such as headache, dizziness, distension of the head, blurred vision, tinnitus, palpitations, insomnia and poor memory, etc. With the development of hypertension, blood pressure obviously continues to increase, and then patients suffer from organic injury and functional disturbances of brain, Heart, Kidneys and eyes, etc.

1. **Invasion of Liver Fire**: Dizziness, headache, palpitations, irritability, flushed complexion, redness of eyes, bitter taste in the mouth, yellow urination, constipation, red tongue with dry and yellow coating, wiry pulse.

2. **Hyperactivity of Yang due to Yin deficiency**: Dizziness, headache, heavy sensation of head and light on the feet, tinnitus, feverish sensation in the five centres, palpitations, insomnia, poor memory, red tongue with thin and white coating, wiry, thready and rapid pulse.

3. **Retention of Phlegm and Dampness**: Dizziness, headache, fullness in the chest, palpitations, poor appetite, vomiting and nausea, sputum and salivation, white and sticky tongue coating, rolling pulse.

4. **Qi deficiency and Blood stagnation**: Dizziness, headache, sallow complexion, palpitations, shortness of breath, lassitude, poor appetite, bluish and

purplish nails and lips, purplish dark tongue body with petechia, thready and hesitant pulse.

5. **Yin and Yang deficiency**: Dizziness, headache, sallow complexion, tinnitus, palpitations, shortness of breath and even cough and asthma after movement, weakness and soreness of the lower back and knee joints, insomnia or dream disturbed sleep, large amount of urine at night, sometimes swollen, pale or red tongue with white coating, thready pulse.

Treatment
Body acupuncture

1. **Principles of treatment**

   - *Liver Fire, hyperactivity of Yang due to Yin deficiency*: To nourish Yin and eliminate Fire, regulate the Liver to reduce Yang, apply acupuncture alone without moxibustion, use the reducing method.

   - *Retention of Phlegm and Dampness*: To tonify Spleen and eliminate Phlegm, clear head and eyes, apply both acupuncture and moxibustion, use even method.

   - *Qi deficiency and Blood stagnation*: To benefit Qi and nourish the Blood, eliminate stagnation and promote meridians, apply both acupuncture and moxibustion, use reinforcing and reducing method.

   - *Yin and Yang deficiency*: To nourish Yin and tonify Yang, and promote the Zang Fu organs, apply both acupuncture and moxibustion, use the reinforcing method.

2. **Prescription**

   Baihui (GV20), Quchi (LI11), Hegu (LI4), Taichong (LR3), Sanyinjiao (SP6).

3. **Explanation**

   Baihui (GV20) is located on the vertex, and is the meeting place of all the Yang meridians; it communicates with the Liver Meridian, so puncturing this point with the reducing method can eliminate Liver Fire; Quchi (LI11), Hegu (LI4) can clear and reduce Yangming; Taichong (LR3) is Yuan-Primary point of Liver Meridian and functions to regulate Liver Qi and reduce Liver Yang; Sanyinjiao (SP6) is the meeting point of all three Yin meridians of the foot, and functions to regulate and reinforce Liver, Spleen and Kidneys.

4. **Modification**
   - *Liver Fire*: + Fengchi (GB20), Xingjian (LR2) to reduce Liver Fire.
   - *Yang hyperactivity due to Yin deficiency*: + Taixi (KI3), Ganshu (BL18) to moisten Yin for reducing Yang.
   - *Retention of Phlegm and Dampness*: + Fenglong (ST40), Zusanli (ST36) to tonify the Spleen and remove Phlegm.
   - *Qi deficiency and Blood stagnation*: + Xuehai (SP10), Geshu (BL17) to benefit Qi and activate Blood.
   - *Both Yin and Yang deficiency*: + Guanyuan (CV4), Shenshu (BL23) to regulate Yin and Yang.
   - *Dizziness and heavy sensation of the head*: + Baihui (GV20), Taiyang (EX-HN5) to clear head and eyes.
   - *Palpitations*: + Neiguan (PC6), Shenmen (HT7) to calm down the Mind.

5. **Manipulation**

   Retention of Phlegm and Dampness, Qi deficiency and Blood stagnation, both Yin and Yang deficiency, add moxibustion towards Baihui (GV20); penetrating needle from Taichong (LR3) to Yongquan (KI1); apply ordinary manipulation on other points.

Other therapies

1. **Cutaneous needle**

   Tap the nape, lumbosacral region, and both sides of the trachea; the intensity of stimulation depends on the deficiency or excess of the disease and the body constitution of the patient. Treatment is performed once a day.

2. **Three-edged needle**

   Select Ear-Apex, Baihui (GV20), Dazhui (GV14), Yintang (EX-HN3), Taichong (LR3), Quchi (LI11), etc. Use 1 to 2 points every time, pricking to cause bleeding with 3 to 5 drops. Perform once every 2 to 3 days.

3. **Auricular acupuncture**

   Points: The groove for lowering blood pressure, Adrenal, Ear-Apex, Sympathetic Nerve, Heart, etc. Use 3 to 4 points every time with puncturing or embedding needles; or Vaccaria seeds to auricular points; pricking to cause bleeding on groove for lowering blood pressure and Ear-Apex if the blood pressure is very high.

Notes

1. Acupuncture and moxibustion are effective for the treatment of mild or moderate hypertension, and function to relieve symptoms of severe hypertension in combination with antihypertensives. Acupuncture and moxibustion should be carefully applied during the stage of hypertensive crisis.

2. If patient takes antihypertensives over a long period, he cannot suddenly stop taking the drugs during acupuncture and moxibustion treatment; he should gradually decrease the dosage of antihypertensives when the blood pressure is lowered to normal or near normal and subjective symptoms are obviously relieved or have disappeared after some period of treatment.

3. Hypertension can be a symptom of some diseases such as cardiocerebrovascular diseases, endocrine disease, urinary disease; this is known as 'symptomatic hypertension' or 'secondary hypertension', and should be distinguished from primary hypertension.

11. HYPOTENSION

Brief introduction

Hypotension is a condition where the blood pressure of an adult is continuously lower than 90/60mmHg (in the elderly, lower than 100/70mmHg). In Western medicine, hypotension is classified into physical hypotension, orthostatic hypotension, and secondary hypotension.

- Physical hypotension is commonly seen; generally, it is related to weak constitution and genetic inheritance. It mostly occurs in women of between 20 and 50 years old or in the elderly.

- Orthostatic hypotension means that blood pressure is suddenly lowered by over 20mmHg, accompanied by relevant symptoms due to dysfunction of blood pressure regulation when the patient stands for a long time or changes posture from lying to sitting or lying to standing.

- Secondary hypotension is mostly caused by diseases such as diarrhoea, haemorrhage, rheumatic cardiomyopathy, myocardial infarction, syringomyelia, Wind Stroke, or by drugs such as antihypertensives or antidepressants, etc.

Aetiology and pathogenesis

In TCM, hypotension is categorized with 'dizziness' or 'deficient syndrome'. It is based on Qi deficiency and relates to the Heart, Lungs, Spleen, Kidneys, etc. The Heart dominates the Blood and vessels, the Lungs link with hundred of vessels, so Heart and Lung Qi deficiency cannot push Blood to circulate in the vessels; Spleen Qi deficiency cannot produce Qi and Blood; Kidney Qi deficiency leads to weak circulation of Qi and Blood. Then Blood cannot fill up the vessels and hypotension occurs.

Syndrome differentiation

In mild cases, the patient has dizziness, headache, poor appetite, lassitude, a pale complexion, indigestion, is easily car sick or seasick, has little emotional self-control, dull responses, listlessness, etc. In severe cases, the patient has palpitations, dizziness on standing, shortness of breath, slurred speech, coordinative disturbance of motor activities, a cold sensation in the four limbs and even coma.

1. **Heart Yang deficiency**: Dizziness, poor memory, listlessness, lassitude, hypersomnia, pale complexion, weakness in the four limbs, cold sensation in the hands and feet, pale and flabby tongue body, deep and thready or slow and weak pulse.

2. **Qi deficiency in Middle Burner**: Dizziness, shortness of breath, spontaneous sweating, weakness and soreness in the four limbs, poor appetite, pale tongue with white coating, slow and weak pulse.

3. **Heart and Kidney Yang deficiency**: Dizziness, tinnitus, palpitations, shortness of breath, weakness and soreness of the lower back and knee joints, sweating and cold sensation in the four limbs, frequent night urination, pale tongue with thin and white coating, deep and thready pulse.

4. **Yang Qi collapse**: Dizziness, pale complexion, nausea and vomiting, sweating and cold sensation in the limbs, unstable walking, inability to stand, listlessness, even coma, pale tongue body, deep, thready and weak pulse.

Treatment
Body acupuncture

1. **Principles of treatment**

   To tonify and benefit the Heart and Spleen, regulate Qi and Blood, nourish the Kidneys and fill up the marrow, warm up Yang to produce Qi, apply both acupuncture and moxibustion, use the reinforcing method.

2. **Prescription**

Mainly select from Back-Shu points of the Bladder Meridian of Foot-Taiyang. Baihui (GV20), Qihai (CV6), Xinshu (BL15), Pishu (BL20), Shenshu (BL23), Zusanli (ST36).

3. **Explanation**

Baihui (GV20) is located on the vertex and belongs to the Governor Vessel; it is the meeting place of all of the Yang meridians, internally connects with the brain, and functions to lift up Yang Qi; Qihai (CV6) pertains to the Conception Vessel, functions to tonify Qi and increase blood pressure; Zusanli (ST36) reinforces the Spleen, produces Qi and Blood; Xinshu (BL15), Pishu (BL20), Shenshu (BL23) can promote the Heart, Spleen and Kidneys, and benefit Qi and nourish Blood to increase blood pressure.

4. **Modification**

- *Heart Yang deficiency*: + Tanzhong (CV17), Jueyinshu (BL14) to tonify Heart Yang.
- *Qi deficiency in Middle Burner*: + Zhongwan (CV12), Weishu (BL21) to tonify Qi in Middle Burner.
- *Heart and Kidney Yang deficiency*: + Neiguan (PC6), Taixi (KI3) to warm up Heart and Kidney Yang.
- *Yang Qi collapse*: + Shenque (CV8), Guanyuan (CV4) by moxibustion to recapture Yang from collapse.
- *Dizziness, headache*: + Yintang (EX-HN3), Taiyang (EX-HN5) to strengthen the brain and stop dizziness.
- *Insomnia, poor memory*: + Sishencong (EX-HN1) to calm down the Mind and benefit the intelligence.
- *Cold sensation in the four limbs*: + Dazhui (GV14), Mingmen (GV4) by moxibustion to warm up the meridians and promote Yang.
- *Acute stage*: + Neiguan (PC6), Suliao (GV25) to recapture Yang and increase blood pressure.

5. **Manipulation**

Apply ordinary manipulation of acupuncture and moxibustion with the reinforcing method; be careful with the direction, angle and depth of puncturing Back-Shu points; use heavy moxibustion towards Baihui (GV20). Moxibustion towards Zusanli (ST36) is applied all the year round.

Other therapies

1. **Auricular acupuncture**

   - *To increase blood pressure:* Select Heart and Adrenal points.
   - *Dizziness:* + Kidney, Occiput.
   - *Lassitude:* + Spleen.
   - *Poor memory:* + Subcortex, Central Rim.
   - *Palpitations, fullness in the chest:* + Chest, Ear-Shenmen.

   Use 3 to 5 points with Vaccaria seeds, moderate or slight stimulation. Treat once every 2 days on alternate ears.

2. **Cutaneous needle**

   Tap points according to acupuncture prescription 2 to 3 minutes on every point and every time.

Notes

1. Acupuncture and moxibustion are effective in increasing blood pressure. Because hypotension mostly accompanies or results from other diseases, it is important to make a precise diagnosis and actively treat the related diseases. Emergent treatment should be given when blood pressure is too low.

2. The elderly with hypotension should not move quickly or suddenly, but should change posture slowly from lying to sitting or standing.

3. Patients should actively take physical exercise to improve their constitution, increase nutrition, drink water and soup often, and eat less salt than the normal person.

12. ANAEMIA

Brief introduction

In anaemia the red blood cell count, haemoglobin and/or haematokrit per unit volume of Blood is lower than normal. The standard diagnosis of anaemia is that haemoglobin is less than 95% of the lower limit of normal reference values (normally, adult male haemoglobin is < 120g/L, adult female haemoglobin is < 110g/L, pregnant female haemoglobin is < 100g/L). According to the different levels, anaemia can be divided into mild anaemia (haemoglobin is between 90g/L of the lower limit of normal reference values), moderate anaemia (haemoglobin is between 60g/L to 90g/L), severe anaemia (haemoglobin is between 30g/L to 60g/L), extremely severe anaemia (haemoglobin is < 30g/L). Anaemia is a kind of syndrome or a symptom of various diseases due to insufficient Blood formation or Blood consumption; it often includes malnutrition anaemia, iron deficiency anaemia, haemolytic anaemia and aplastic anaemia, etc.

Aetiology and pathogenesis

According to TCM, anaemia is caused by dysfunction of the Spleen and Stomach, 'food in Stomach turns into fluid through Qi activity in the Middle Burner, then transforms into the red substance that is Blood'. Malnutrition or dysfunction of Spleen and Stomach in transportation and transformation can cause insufficient Qi and Blood formation; on the other hand, Essence and Blood are based on the same foundation, Kidneys produce marrow and store Essence, Kidney Qi deficiency disturbs the Kidneys in producing marrow and storing Essence, and Essence insufficiency can lead to Blood deficiency. Blood consumption mostly occurs due to bleeding, pregnancy, child growth, various parasitical worm diseases, and toxicity leading to weakness of the Zang Fu organs. Anaemia belongs to the 'Blood deficiency', 'deficiency' or 'yellow and swollen disease' category in TCM.

Syndrome differentiation

Symptoms are dizziness and blurred vision, palpitations and shortness of breath, lassitude, poor appetite, pale skin and mucosa, or is accompanied by glossitis, dry skin, dry hair and hair loss, dry nails or koilonychia, fever, mild oedema, low sex drive. Haemolytic anaemia can be related to jaundice, splenomegaly and protein in the urine, etc.

1. **Both Heart and Spleen deficiency**: Pale complexion, lassitude, dizziness, palpitations, pale and flabby tongue body with thin coating, soft and thready pulse.

2. **Both Spleen and Stomach deficiency**: Sallow or pale complexion, lassitude, listlessness, poor appetite, loose stools, pale tongue with thin and sticky coating, thready and weak pulse.

3. **Spleen and Kidney Yang deficiency**: Pale complexion, lassitude, listlessness, low voice, lazy speech, aversion to cold, cold sensation in the four limbs, spontaneous sweating, weakness and soreness of the lower back and knee joints, seminal emission, impotence, irregular menstruation, pale and flabby tongue with thin and white coating, deep and thready pulse.

4. **Kidney Yin deficiency**: Pale complexion, lassitude, listlessness, flushed cheeks, dizziness, blurred vision, weakness and soreness of the lower back and knee joints, sore throat, low fever, night sweating, feverish sensation in the five centres, insomnia, seminal emission, copious menstruation or functional uterus bleeding, red tongue with scanty coating, wiry and thready pulse.

Treatment

Body acupuncture

1. **Principles of treatment**

   To tonify the Heart, Spleen and Kidneys, regulate and nourish Qi and Blood, use both acupuncture and moxibustion, preferably with the reinforcing method (acupuncture alone with the even method and no moxibustion for Kidney Yin deficiency).

2. **Prescription**

   Mainly select from the Back-Shu point of the Bladder Meridian of Foot-Taiyang. Qihai (CV6), Xuehai (SP10), Geshu (BL17), Xinshu (BL15), Pishu (BL20), Shenshu (BL23), Xuanzhong (GB39), Zusanli (ST36).

3. **Explanation**

   Anaemia is mainly caused by deficiency, so reinforcing deficiency becomes the key point to treat anaemia. Qihai (CV6), Xuehai (SP10) can tonify both Qi and Blood; Geshu (BL17) is an Influential point for Blood and Xuanzhong (GB39) is an Influential point for marrow – they can reinforce Blood and nourish marrow; Xinshu (BL15), Pishu (BL20) and Shenshu (BL23) can nourish the Heart, Spleen and Kidneys; Zusanli (ST36) can regulate the Spleen and Stomach to produce Qi and Blood.

4. **Modification**

   - *Dizziness*: + Baihui (GV20) to benefit brain and stop dizziness.
   - *Palpitations*: + Neiguan (PC6) to calm down Mind and stop palpitations.
   - *Low fever and night sweating, feverish sensation in the five centres*: + Laogong (PC8) to clear Heat.
   - *Flushed cheeks*: + Taixi (KI3) to nourish Kidney Yin.
   - *Seminal emission and impotence*: + Guanyuan (CV4) to strengthen Kidney.

- *Irregular menstruation and large amount of menstruation:* Moxibustion towards Guanyuan (CV4), Sanyinjiao (SP6), Yinbai (SP1) to promote Spleen and regulate menstruation.

5. **Manipulation**

Routine treatment, i.e. acupuncture therapy.

Other therapies

1. **Auricular acupuncture**

   Points: Subcortex, Liver, Kidney, Diaphragm, Endocrine, Adrenal. Choose 3 to 4 points every time with moderate stimulation given by needle, or apply Vaccaria seeds to auricular points.

2. **Point injection**

   Select Xuehai (SP10), Geshu (BL17), Pishu (BL20), Zusanli (ST36). Use Danggui (当归 *Radix Angelicae Sinensis*) injection or Huangqi (黄芪 *Radix Astragali seu Hedysari*) injection, injecting 0.5ml in every point, or use vitamin B$_{12}$ injection, injecting 100 in every point, treating every day.

3. **Catgut implantation**

   Choose Xuehai (SP10), Shenshu (BL23), Pishu (BL20). Embed catgut into points. Use twice every month.

4. **Cutting therapy**

   Choose Geshu (BL17), Gongsun (SP4), Rangu (KI2). Use 1 to 2 points every time, cut 1cm skin, withdrawing a little fat, and then cover with sterile gauze.

Notes

1. Acupuncture and moxibustion are effective in relieving anaemia, but we should be sure to know the aetiology at the beginning of treatment. During acupuncture treatment, specific therapy according to the aetiology should be done, such as iron supplement for ischaemic anaemia, nutritional supplements for malnutrition anaemia, and stopping the bleeding for bleeding anaemia.

2. We should apply comprehensive therapies for the treatment of moderate and severe anaemia, blood transfusion if necessary.

13. LEUKOPENIA

Brief introduction

Leukopenia is a condition in which the white blood cell count in Blood is continuously less than $4.0 \times 10^9/L$, and is divided into primary and secondary types. Through body transformation reactions and direct toxicity to haematopoietic cells, physicochemical factors, infections and relevant diseases can inhibit haematopoiesis of the marrow, or disturb the white blood cells in the Blood, then leukopenia results. In TCM, it belongs to the 'deficient syndrome' category.

Aetiology and pathogenesis

Leukopenia is mainly caused by Spleen and Stomach Qi deficiency. When the Spleen and Stomach functions are weak, they cannot produce Qi and Blood, Blood cannot transform into Essence, deficient Essence cannot benefit the Kidneys to manufacture marrow, so insufficient Essence and Blood fail to nourish the body.

Syndrome differentiation

Leukopenia for most patients is of short duration and self-limited, with no obvious clinical symptoms. Patients with prolonged leukopenia suffer from dizziness, blurred vision, lassitude, low voice, lazy speech, weakness and soreness of the lower back and knee joints, hypersomnia, poor memory, tinnitus, spontaneous sweating and poor appetite, etc.

1. **Spleen Qi deficiency**: Sallow or pale complexion, dizziness and shortness of breath, hypersomnia, poor appetite and loose stools, pale tongue with thin coating, thready pulse.

2. **Spleen and Kidney Yang deficiency**: Apart from symptoms of Spleen Qi deficiency, also low voice, lazy speech, aversion to cold, cold sensation in the four limbs, spontaneous sweating, weakness and soreness of the lower back and knee joints, seminal emission and impotence, irregular menstruation, pale and flabby tongue with thin and white coating, deep and thready pulse.

Treatment

Body acupuncture

1. **Principles of treatment**

   To tonify Spleen Qi, warm up the Kidneys, apply both acupuncture and moxibustion, prefer the reinforcing method.

2. **Prescription**

   Qihai (CV6), Dazhui (GV14), Pishu (BL20), Shenshu (BL23), Gaohuangshu (BL43), Zusanli (ST36).

3. **Explanation**

   Qihai (CV6), Dazhui (GV14) can tonify Qi and communicate with Yang; Pishu (BL20), Shenshu (BL23) have the functions of tonifying Spleen and warming up the Kidneys; Gaohuangshu (BL43), Zusanli (ST36) can strengthen Qi and reinforce deficiency.

4. **Modification**

   - *Spleen Qi deficiency*: + Zhongwan (CV12), Weishu (BL21) to reinforce Stomach and tonify Spleen.

   - *Spleen and Kidney Yang deficiency*: Moxibustion towards Guanyuan (CV4), Mingmen (GV4) to warm up the Kidneys.

5. **Manipulation**

   Routine treatment; mainly moxibustion towards Gaohuangshu (BL43), Dazhui (GV14), 30 minutes for every treatment.

Other therapies

1. **Auricular acupuncture**

   Points: Spleen, Stomach, Kidney, Endocrine and Subcortex. Apply slight needling stimulation, rotating needles 2 to 3 times during retention, or use pills to auricular points once every 3 to 5 days and on alternate ears.

2. **Point injection**

   Select Zusanli (ST36), Xuehai (SP10). Applying Shenmai injection, Huangqi (黄芪 *Radix Astragali seu Hedysari*) injection, etc. Use ordinary dosage into every point, once every 2 to 3 days.

Notes

1. Acupuncture and moxibustion are effective in the treatment of leukopenia. But we should treat primary diseases at the same time.

2. Focus on prevention, avoiding drugs abuse, controlling dosages of radiotherapy and chaemotherapy, mostly minimizing stimulation given by physicochemical factors.

14. PALPITATIONS

Brief introduction

Palpitations refer to an unduly rapid action of the Heart which is felt by the patient and accompanied by nervousness and restlessness. In Western medicine, palpitations are commonly seen in arrhythmia due to various reasons including tachycardia, bradycardia, premature beat, atrial fibrillation or flutter, atrioventricular block, sick sinus syndrome, pre-excitation syndrome and cardiac functional insufficiency, neurosis, hyperthyroidism, iron-deficiency anaemia, etc.

Aetiology and pathogenesis

According to TCM, palpitations are caused by Heart dysfunctions, including Heart Qi deficiency, Heart Blood deficiency, Heart Yang deficiency, or invasion of the Heart by diseases of other Zang Fu organs, in which either the Heart cannot be well nourished or the Heart vessel is obstructed, as a result of which palpitations occur.

Syndrome differentiation

Subjectively abnormal heart beat such as a fast, slow, or heavy beat, or intermittent beat, both of sudden onset or continuous, listlessness, irritability, accompanied by dizziness, fullness in the chest, insomnia due to irritability, lassitude, etc. Middle aged or older patients also feel cardiac pain, asthma, sweating and cold sensation of the limbs, coma; rapid, abrupt, knotted, intermittent, slow pulses. Palpitations are often induced by emotional stimulation, fright and fear, overstrain and drinking alcohol, etc.

1. **Heart Yang deficiency**: Palpitations, made worse by moving, dizziness, pale complexion, fullness in the chest and shortness of breathing, aversion to cold and cold sensation in the limbs, pale and flabby tongue with white coating, deep, thready and slow pulse or intermittent, knotted pulse.

2. **Heart and Gallbladder Qi deficiency**: Palpitations induced by fright and fear, shortness of breathing and spontaneous sweating, listlessness and lassitude, insomnia and dream-disturbed sleep, pale tongue with thin and white coating, thready and wiry pulse.

3. **Heart and Spleen deficiency**: Palpitations, insomnia, poor memory, pale complexion, dizziness and lassitude, fullness in the chest and shortness of breath, spontaneous sweating, poor appetite, pale tongue with thin and white coating, weak pulse.

4. **Fire due to Yin deficiency**: Palpitations, worse after over-thinking, feverish sensation in the five centres, insomnia and dream-disturbed sleep, dizziness, blurred vision, tinnitus, dry mouth, feverish sensation on the face, red tongue with thin and yellow coating, thready and rapid pulse.

5. **Heart Blood stagnation**: Palpitations, fullness in the chest, sudden onset of cardiac pain, or purplish dark face and lips, darkish tongue body with petechia, thready and hesitant or intermittent, knotted pulse.

6. **Invasion of Heart by fluid retention**: Continuous palpitations, fullness in the chest and asthma, inability to lie with the face up, cough with a large amount of frothy sputum, swollen face and feet, scanty urine, white and sticky or white and watery tongue coating, wiry, rolling and rapid pulse.

Treatment

Body acupuncture

1. **Principles of treatment**

   To nourish Heart and calm down the Mind, stop palpitations, apply both acupuncture and moxibustion, prefer the reinforcing method (for Fire due to Yin deficiency use only acupuncture with even method).

2. **Prescription**

   Mainly points from the Heart Meridian of Hand-Shaoyin and the Pericardium Meridian of Hand-Jueyin, relative Back-Shu points and Front-Mu points. Use Shenmen (HT7), Neiguan (PC6), Tongli (HT5), Xinshu (BL15), Jueyinshu (BL14), Juque (CV14), Tanzhong (CV17).

3. **Explanation**

   Shenmen (HT7) is the Yuan-Primary point of the Heart Meridian of Hand-Shaoyin, has the function of calming down the Mind; Neiguan (PC6) is Luo-Connecting point of the Pericardium Meridian of Hand-Jueyin, Tongli (HT5) is Luo-Connecting point of the Heart Meridian of Hand-Shaoyin, they can calm the Mind, promote the meridians and stop palpitations; Xinshu (BL15), Jueyinshu (BL14), Juque (CV14), Tanzhong (CV17) are respectively Back-Shu points and Front-Mu points of the Heart Meridian of Hand-Shaoyin and the Pericardium Meridian of Hand-Jueyin; they can regulate and tonify Heart Qi for stopping palpitations.

4. **Modification**

- *Heart Yang deficiency*: + Guanyuan (CV4), Zusanli (ST36) to tonify Heart Yang.

- *Heart and Gallbladder deficiency*: + Baihui (GV20), Danshu (BL19) to tonify Heart and strengthen Gallbladder.

- *Heart and Spleen deficiency*: + Pishu (BL20), Zusanli (ST36) to tonify Heart and Spleen.

- *Fire due to Yin deficiency*: + Laogong (PC8), Taixi (KI3) to nourish Yin and remove Fire.

- *Heart Blood stagnation*: + Quze (PC3), Geshu (BL17) to activate Blood circulation and eliminate stagnation.

- *Invasion of Heart by fluid retention*: + Shuifen (CV9), Yinlingquan (SP9) to promote fluid circulation, and calm the Mind to stop palpitations.

5. **Manipulation**

Routine treatment is given with the reducing method for acute stage, 30–60 minutes retention of the needles until symptoms disappear or are relieved.

Other therapies

1. **Auricular acupuncture**

   Points: Heart, Sympathetic Nerve, Ear-Shenmen, Subcortex, Small Intestine. Apply puncturing with slight stimulation, 2 to 3 times manipulation while retaining the needles, once a day.

2. **Cutaneous needle**

   Choose both sides of trachea, lower mandibular region, nape, sacral region and Neiguan (PC6), Tanzhong (CV17), Sanyinjiao (SP6), Renying (ST9), apply moderate stimulation until there is flushed colour or little bleeding spots on the local region, twice a day for sudden onset.

3. **Point injection**

   Ordinary point selection. Using vitamin B_1 injection, vitamin B_{12} injection with 0.5ml on every point and once a day.

Notes

1. Palpitations can be caused by various diseases. We should actively find the primary diseases and treat them according to aetiology during acupuncture treatment.

2. Acupuncture and moxibustion treatment can not only relieve symptoms but also treat the disease itself. But for prevention of disease, comprehensive therapies should be adopted if there is heart failure caused by organic diseases.

3. During treatment, patient should maintain a good mood and avoid over-thinking, anger, fright and fear, etc.

15. INSOMNIA

Brief introduction

Insomnia or 'poor sleeping', is categorized under neurosis, neurasthenia and anaemia, etc. in Western medicine.

Aetiology and pathogenesis

According to TCM, insomnia is caused by a dysfunction of the Heart. Worry, over-thinking or overstrain can injure the Heart and Spleen, leading to Qi and Blood deficiency which fails to nourish the Heart and house the Mind, so insomnia occurs; indulgent sexual activity injures the Kidneys, Kidney Yin becomes insufficient, Fire comes due to Yin deficiency, resulting in disharmony between Heart and Kidneys that leads to insomnia; dysfunction of the Spleen and Stomach cause retention of Dampness and Phlegm which may turn into Heat, the Phlegm Heat may disturb the Heart in housing the Mind, so insomnia occurs; anger leads to Liver Qi stagnation, then upsurge of Liver Fire causes dysfunction of the Heart in housing the Mind, so insomnia occurs.

Syndrome differentiation

In mild cases, such as difficulty in falling asleep or being easily awakened then finding it difficult to go back to sleep; in severe cases, inability to sleep all night. These symptoms are accompanied by headache, dizziness, palpitations, poor memory, dream-disturbed sleep.

1. **Heart and Spleen deficiency**: Palpitations, easy fright and fear, dream-disturbed sleep and being easily awakened, pale tongue with thin coating, wiry and thready pulse.

2. **Heart and Gallbladder Qi deficiency**: Irritability, difficulty in falling asleep, easily awakened, feverish sensation in the five centres, dizziness, tinnitus, palpitations, poor memory, flushed cheeks region, dry mouth with scanty fluid, red tongue with scanty coating, thready and rapid pulse.

3. **Fire caused by Liver Qi stagnation**: Irritability, difficulty in falling asleep, listlessness and anger, fullness in the chest, hypochondriac pain, headache, dizziness, flushed complexion, red eyes, bitter taste in the mouth, constipation, yellow urine, red tongue with yellow coating, wiry and rapid pulse.

4. **Invasion of Phlegm and Heat**: Insomnia, irritability, suffocating feeling and distending pain in the epigastric region, bitter taste in the mouth, large amount of sputum, dizziness, blurred vision, red tongue with yellow and sticky coating, rolling and rapid pulse.

Treatment

Body acupuncture

1. **Principles of treatment**

   To regulate the Heart and calm down the Mind, clear Heart Heat and stop irritability.

2. **Prescription**

   Shenmen (HT7), Neiguan (PC6), Baihui (GV20), Anmian (Extra point).

3. **Explanation**

   Insomnia is mainly caused by dysfunction of the Heart in housing the Mind, so first we choose the Yuan-Primary point of the Heart Meridian of Hand-Shaoyin and Luo-Connecting point of the Pericardium Meridian of Hand-Jueyin to regulate the Heart and calm down the Mind. Baihui (GV20) can clear the head and eyes, and calm the Mind. Anmian (Extra point) is an often used and effective point to treat insomnia.

4. **Modification**

   * *Heart and Spleen deficiency*: + Xinshu (BL15), Pishu (BL20), Sanyinjiao (SP6) to tonify Heart and Spleen.

- *Heart and Gallbladder Qi deficiency*: + Xinshu (BL15), Danshu (BL19), Qiuxu (GB40) to reinforce the Heart and strengthen the Gallbladder, calm the Mind.

- *Fire due to Yin deficiency*: + Taixi (KI3), Taichong (LR3), Yongquan (KI1) to nourish Yin and remove Fire, calm the Mind.

- *Fire caused by Liver Qi stagnation*: + Xingjian (LR2), Taichong (LR3), Fengchi (GB20) to regulate the Liver and reduce Fire, eliminate stagnation and calm the Mind.

- *Phlegm and Heat*: + Zhongwan (CV12), Fenglong (ST40), Neiting (ST44) to clear Heat, remove Phlegm, harmonize the Stomach and calm the Mind.

5. **Manipulation**

Routine treatment. Perform treatment 2 hours before sleeping when patient is calm.

Other therapies

1. **Auricular acupuncture**

Points: Heart, Spleen, Ear-Shenmen, Subcortex, Sympathetic Nerve points. Use 2 to 3 points every time with slight stimulation and retain the needles for 30 minutes. Treat once a day.

2. **Cutaneous needle**

Tap Yintang (EX-HN3), Baihui (GV20), Back-Shu points located on the nape and lumbosacral region, stimulate 5 to 10 minutes on every point until the local skin turns red. Treat once a day.

Notes

1. Acupuncture and moxibustion are effective in treating insomnia, but we should find the definite aetiology through different examinations before treatment, and we should treat the primary diseases at the same time if insomnia is caused by fever, cough and asthma, pain, etc.

2. If insomnia is caused by temporary emotional tension, environmental noise or maladjustment of the bed, it is not a pathological disease, when the inducing factors return to normal, insomnia should stop. Older people are easily awakened because their normal sleeping time is shorter, if they do not have obvious symptoms, it is normal.

16. DEMENTIA

Brief introduction

Dementia is the condition in which, while the patient is clearly conscious, there is persistently general disturbance including of memory, the ability to solve problems of daily life, already learned skills, social skills and the ability to control the emotions and the reactions of the higher nerve functions caused by various physical diseases, and disturbance develops to an acquired syndrome with apsychosis at the end. Dementia often occurs in older people or children; it may be involved in senile dementia (genuine senile dementia), presenile dementia, cerebrovascular dementia and paediatric brain dysgenesis, etc., as diagnosed in Western medicine.

Aetiology and pathogenesis

According to TCM, the primary reasons leading to dementia include Liver and Kidney deficiency, Qi and Blood deficiency, malnourished meridians, insufficiency of the Sea of Marrow. There are also secondary causes such as obstruction of the meridians by retention of Phlegm, and Blood stagnation. The organs affected are mostly the Kidneys, Heart and Spleen, the Kidneys in particular.

Syndrome differentiation

Slow onset, mainly mental disturbance and symptoms of nervous system. In the early stages, there is only slightly decreased and slow memory, response and creativity, decreased adaptability to environment, difficulty in carrying out sustained work on some kinds of job, the patient is easily tired, worried and has low energy, etc. This develops to dysmnesia, cognitive disorder, personality change, affective disorder, dysphonia and psychosis, various disturbances of nervous functions such as limb apraxia, paralysis agitans, ataxia, epilepsy, pyramidal sign, etc. Finally, the patient is completely unable to take care of themselves, and there is no autonomic movement, no speech, and they are in a state of being brain-dead.

1. **Liver and Kidney deficiency**: Poor memory, explosive laughing and crying, easily angered, easily manic, accompanied by dizziness, blurred vision, numbness of the hands and feet, tremor, insomnia, epilepsy in the severe condition, red tongue with thin and yellow coating, wiry and rapid pulse.

2. **Qi and Blood deficiency**: Abnormal behaviour and expression, no speech during the whole day, or suddenly laughing or crying, easily changing moods, decreased memory or even loss of memory, unstable walking, pale complexion, shortness of breath, lassitude, pale tongue with white coating, thready and weak pulse.

3. **Obstruction of facial orifices due to retention of Phlegm**: Slow expression, slow behaviour, little speech, lying in bed all day, loss of memory, incontinence of urine and stools, flabby and pale tongue with teeth marks on the edge, white, sticky and thick coating, rolling pulse.

4. **Obstruction of meridians by Blood stagnation**: Indifferent expression, slow response, often no speech, or overactive imagination, poor memory and easily frightened, purplish dark tongue body with petechia, thready and hesitant pulse.

Treatment
Body acupuncture

1. **Principles of treatment**

   To tonify the Kidneys and fill up Essence, promote brain and benefit intelligence, apply both acupuncture and moxibustion with the reinforcing method for Liver and Kidney deficiency; Qi and Blood deficiency, mainly use acupuncture with even method for obstruction of the Middle Burner by retention of Phlegm, and obstruction of meridians by Blood stagnation.

2. **Prescription**

   Baihui (GV20), Sishencong (EX-HN1), Taixi (KI3), Dazhong (KI4), Xuanzhong (GB39), Zusanli (ST36).

3. **Explanation**

   Dementia is located in the brain, Baihui (GV20), Sishencong (EX-HN1) are located on the vertex, and have the function of restoring the brain and calming down the Mind; Taixi (KI3), Dazhong (KI4) can tonify the Kidneys and fill up Essence; Xuanzhong (GB39) is an Influential point for marrow, so puncturing this point with the reinforcing method can nourish the brain marrow, promote the brain and benefit the intelligence; Zusanli (ST36) can produce Qi and Blood.

4. **Modification**

   - *Liver and Kidney deficiency*: + Ganshu (BL18), Sanyinjiao (SP6) to nourish Liver and Kidney.

   - *Qi and Blood deficiency*: + Qihai (CV6), Geshu (BL17) to regulate Qi and tonify Blood.

   - *Obstruction of Middle Burner by retention of Phlegm*: + Fenglong (ST40), Zhongwan (CV12) to eliminate Phlegm and promote the meridians.

- *Obstruction of the meridians by Blood stagnation*: + Geshu (BL17), Weizhong (BL40) to activate Blood and eliminate stagnation.

5. **Manipulation**

   Routine treatment. The direction of puncturing Sishencong (EX-HN1) is to Baihui (GV20); adding moxibustion (heavy stimulation for 20 minutes) towards Baihui (GV20) after needling until a warming sensation penetrates to inside the skull and the deep layer of the point. Treat every day or once every other day.

Other therapies

1. **Scalp acupuncture**

   Select Dingzhongxian (MS5), Ezhongxian (MS1), Nieqianxian (MS10) and Niehouxian (MS11). Use 2 to 3 points every time with strong stimulation given by puncturing or disperse and dense wave, moderate stimulation given by electroacupuncture.

2. **Auricular acupuncture**

   Points: Heart, Liver, Kidney, Occiput, Brain, Ear-Shenmen, Adrenal. Use 3 to 5 points with shallow and gentle puncturing, retain needles for 30 minutes; or apply Vaccaria seeds to auricular points.

Notes

1. Western medicine believes that dementia is related to the neurotransmitters, receptors and neuropeptides. Experiment shows that acupuncture and moxibustion can adjust neurotransmitters and neuropeptides, and control and slow the progress of the disease, so it has certain treatment effects.

2. Acupuncture and moxibustion can be effective in the early stages, but not in the later stages. A primary disease should be treated if the diagnosis is made during acupuncture treatment.

3. Patient should avoid alcohol and use fewer sleeping and sedative drugs.

17. DEPRESSIVE DISORDER

Brief introduction

Depressive disorder is manifested by depression, mental dejection, reticence or incoherent speech, quiet and reduced movement. In TCM, it belongs to the category 'depressive syndrome'. The condition described here includes depression, obsessive-compulsive disorder and schizophrenia in Western medicine. It is mostly induced by emotional stimulation; the desire to fail, etc. and it has family history.

Aetiology and pathogenesis

According to TCM, depressive disorder is caused by hyperactivity of Yin Qi. In general, emotional changes such as worry, over-thinking, desire to fail lead to Liver Qi stagnation, disturbance of the Heart and Spleen, dysfunction of the Spleen in transportation and transformation in food and Water, retention of Phlegm, as a result of which there is upward disturbance of Phlegm to obstruct the Heart Mind. The dysfunction of the Heart in housing the Mind results in this disease.

Syndrome differentiation

Depression, doubt and worry, easily being frightened, idioglossia, few movements, crying easily, dementia, sighing, etc.

1. **Retention of Phlegm and stagnation of Qi**: Depression, even dull response, fullness in the chest, sighing, often doubting and worrying, idioglossia or muteness, poor appetite, thin and sticky tongue coating with white colour, wiry and thready or wiry and rolling pulse.

2. **Qi deficiency and Phlegm**: Depression, mental dejection, reticence, even appearing stunned and speechless, vain attempts at achievement, sallow complexion, loose stools, clear and profuse urine, flabby and pale tongue, rolling pulse.

3. **Heart and Spleen deficiency**: Confused Mind and speech, palpitations, easily becoming frightened, insomnia, poor appetite and lassitude, pale tongue with white coating, thready and weak pulse.

4. **Fire due to Yin deficiency**: Confused Mind, more speech than usual, easily becoming frightened, irritability, insomnia, dry mouth, red tongue with scanty coating, thready and rapid pulse.

Treatment

Body acupuncture

1. **Principles of treatment**

   To eliminate Phlegm and open the orifices, nourish the Heart and calm down the Mind. Apply both acupuncture and moxibustion with the reinforcing method for Heart and Spleen deficiency; acupuncture with reducing or even method for retention of Phlegm and stagnation of Qi, Qi deficiency and Phlegm, and Fire due to Yin deficiency.

2. **Prescription**

   Pishu (BL20), Fenglong (ST40), Xinshu (BL15), Shenmen (HT7).

3. **Explanation**

   The Spleen is the source of Phlegm production, Pishu (BL20) and Fenglong (ST40) function to tonify the Spleen and Stomach, eliminate Phlegm and Dampness; Xinshu (BL15) and Shenmen (HT7) can restore consciousness and open the orifices.

4. **Modification**

   - *Retention of Phlegm and stagnation of Qi:* + Zhongwan (CV12), Taichong (LR3) to regulate Qi and eliminate stagnation.

   - *Qi deficiency and Phlegm:* + Zusanli (ST36), Zhongwan (CV12) to tonify Spleen Qi.

   - *Heart and Spleen deficiency:* + Zusanli (ST36), Sanyinjiao (SP6) to tonify Spleen and nourish Heart, benefit Qi and calm the Mind.

   - *Fire due to Yin deficiency:* + Shenshu (BL23), Taixi (KI3), Daling (PC7), Sanyinjiao (SP6) to nourish Yin and reduce Fire.

5. **Manipulation**

   Routine treatment. Pay attention to direction, angle and depth of needling Back-Shu points to prevent injury of Zang Fu organs.

Other therapies

1. **Auricular acupuncture**

   Points: Heart, Subcortex, Kidney, Occiput, Ear-Shemen. Use 3 to 5 points each time, shallowly puncturing with slight stimulation, retaining needles for 30 minutes; or also apply Vaccaria seeds to auricular points.

2. **Electroacupuncture**

Selecting Baihui (GV20), Shuigou (GV26), Tongli (HT5), Fenglong (ST40), apply electroacupuncture on the points of the four limbs and using intermittent wave with long time stimulation.

3. **Point injection**

Select Xinshu (BL15), Geshu (BL17), Jianshi (PC5), Zusanli (ST36), Sanyinjiao (SP6). Using 1 to 2 points every time, apply 25–50mg chlorpromazine for injection, treating once a day.

Notes

1. Acupuncture and moxibustion are definitely effective in the treatment of this disease, but we should make a definite diagnosis before treatment, and distinguish the condition from depressive mental disorder or hysteria.

2. During treatment, a family member should actively nurse the patient; combine with psychological therapy for increased curative effect.

18. MANIC DISORDER

Brief introduction

Manic disorder is manifested in the patient being easily excited, shouting, restlessness and violent behaviours, which often occur in teenagers. The condition described here includes schizophrenia, manic syndrome, etc. in Western medicine. It is mostly induced by emotional stimulation, the desire to fail, cerebral trauma, etc., or a family history of the condition.

Aetiology and pathogenesis

According to TCM, manic disorder is caused by hyperactivity of Yang Qi, injury of the Liver and Gallbladder by anger and grief, Liver Qi stagnation leading to Fire, Phlegm and Fire caused by Fire consuming fluid, upsurge of Phlegm and Fire closing the Heart orifice, then mental confusion and restlessness resulting in manic mental disorder.

Syndrome differentiation

Confused Mind, uncontrolled crying and laughing, shouting, restlessness and violent behaviors.

1. **Disturbance of Mind by Phlegm and Fire**: No sleeping throughout the whole night, headache, flushed complexion, redness of eyes, violent behaviours, shouting, red or deep red tongue body with yellow and sticky coating, wiry, rolling and rapid pulse.

2. **Injury of Yin by excessive Fire**: Prolonged manic disorder, slow onset, sometimes restless, sometimes very talkative and easily frightened, irritability and insomnia, dry mouth, red tongue without coating, thready and rapid pulse.

3. **Qi and Blood stagnation**: Restlessness, anger and talkativeness, shouting, darkish complexion, fullness in the chest and hypochondriac region, headache, palpitations, purplish dark tongue body, wiry and rapid pulse.

Treatment

Body acupuncture

1. **Principles of treatment**

   To clear Heart Fire and calm down the Mind, apply acupuncture alone without moxibustion.

2. **Prescription**

   Points mainly from the Governor Vessel, the Pericardium Meridian of Hand-Jueyin. Shuigou (GV26), Dazhui (GV14), Fengchi (GB20), Laogong (PC8), Daling (PC7), Fenglong (ST40).

3. **Explanation**

   Shuigou (GV26), Dazhui (GV14) belong to the Governor Vessel, communicate with the brain, and have the function of restoring consciousness and opening the orifices, and calming down the Mind; Fengchi (GB20) is close to the brain and good for calming down the Mind; Laogong (PC8) can clear the Pericardium and reduce Heart Fire, and calm down the Mind; Fenglong (ST40) can remove Phlegm and promote the meridians, restore consciousness and open the orifices.

4. **Modification**

   - *Disturbance of Mind by Phlegm and Fire*: + Zhongwan (CV12), Shenmen (HT7) to clear the Heart and eliminate Phlegm.

   - *Injury of Yin by excessive Fire*: + Shenmen (HT7), Dazhong (KI4), Sanyinjiao (SP6) to nourish Yin and eliminate Fire, calm down the Mind.

- *Qi and Blood stagnation*: + Hegu (LI4), Taichong (LR3), Xuehai (SP10), Geshu (BL17) to activate Blood and eliminate stagnation, open the orifices and restore consciousness.

5. **Manipulation**

   Routine treatment. In the acute stage, retaining the needles for 30 minutes to 2 hours until the symptoms disappear and are relieved, combining with bleeding therapy.

Other therapies

1. **Three-edged needle**

   Bleeding on Dazhui (CV14), Shuigou (GV26), Baihui (GV20), Zhongchong (PC9).

2. **Electroacupuncture**

   Selecting Baihui (GV20), Shuigou (GV26), Tongli (HT5), Fenglong (ST40), apply electroacupuncture on the points of the four limbs and use continuous wave with long time stimulation.

3. **Auricular acupuncture**

   Points: Heart, Subcortex, Kidney, Occiput, Ear-Shenmen. Choose 3 to 4 points every time with heavy stimulation and retain the needles for 30 minutes.

4. **Point injection**

   Select Xinshu (BL15), Geshu (BL17), Jianshi (PC5), Zusanli (ST36), Sanyinjiao (SP6). Use 1 to 2 points every time, applying 25–50mg Chlorpromazine, injecting 0.5–1ml into every point, treating once a day.

Notes

1. Acupuncture and moxibustion are effective in treating this disease. During treatment, we should look after the patient to prevent suicide or their wounding others or the destruction of objects.

2. If this disease happens repeatedly, the patient should continue the treatment to strengthen effectiveness during the interval period during which symptoms are relieved.

19. EPILEPSY

Brief introduction

Epilepsy occurs in the form of seizures, manifested by falling down in a fit, loss of consciousness, foam on the lips, or screaming with the eyes staring upwards, and convulsions. After some minutes, consciousness returns, and the patient's condition becomes normal. Epilepsy is related to genetic inheritance. Epilepsy as described here refers to seizures, including both primary and secondary types recognised in Western medicine.

Aetiology and pathogenesis

According to TCM, epilepsy results from derangement of Qi and Blood obstructing the clear orifice caused by Phlegm, Fire, Blood stagnation and congenital factors.

Syndrome differentiation

Sudden onset, induced by fear and fright, overstress, emotional change, etc. Often preceded by an aura of dizziness, fullness in the chest, etc. During severe occurrences, loss of consciousness with sudden onset, stiffness in the neck and back, convulsions of the four limbs, foam on the lips, becoming normal after consciousness is restored, easily happening repeatedly; during mild occurrences, the eyes stare directly forward, there is no response to communication, the head is easily bent, there is weakness of four limbs; besides the typical seizures, there may be variations, such as convulsions of the mouth, eye and hand, etc., or heteroptics, or vomiting, copious sweating, dysphonia, or unconscious movement.

1. **Excessive type**: Mostly in the early stage of epilepsy, suddenly falling down, loss of consciousness, trismus, foam on the lips, or roaring. Soreness and pain of the four limbs after the occurrence, becoming normal after taking a rest.

   - *Disturbance of Mind by Phlegm and Fire*: Suddenly falling down, loss of consciousness, severe convulsions of the four limbs, roaring, foam on the lips, irritability, coarse voice, rattling voice in the throat, foul smell in the mouth, constipation, red or dark red tongue body with yellow and sticky coating, wiry and rolling pulse.

   - *Obstruction of orifice by Wind and Phlegm*: Suddenly falling down, eyes staring upwards, foam on the lips, convulsions of the hands and feet, rattling voice in the throat, white and sticky tongue coating, and rolling pulse.

- *Obstruction of collaterals by Blood stasis*: History of traumatic injury (or delivery injury), suddenly falling down during the onset, convulsions, or convulsions only at the corners of the mouth, the canthus and the limbs, purplish dark in the face and lips, purplish dark tongue body with petechia, wiry or hesitant pulse.

2. **Deficient type**: Mostly in the late stages of epilepsy, there is frequent occurrence, the convulsions are weakened, and there is lassitude after consciousness is restored, dull responses, hypophrenia.

   - *Blood deficiency stirring up Wind*: Suddenly falling down, feverish sensation of the face, or eyes staring, or limited convulsions (weakness and convulsions of the four limbs), incontinence of urine and stools, pale tongue with scanty coating, thready and weak pulse.

   - *Heart and Spleen deficiency*: Prolonged, suddenly falling down, or the head alone is easily bent, weakness in the four limbs. Accompanied by pale face, foam on the lips, convulsions and weakness of the four limbs, trismus, eyes closed, enuresis, and incontinence of stools. Pale tongue with white coating, weak pulse.

   - *Liver and Kidney Yin deficiency*: Suddenly falling down, or convulsions of the hands and feet, cold sensation in the four limbs, stiffness of the tongue, poor memory, insomnia, weakness and soreness of the lower back and knee joints, deep red tongue with scanty or no coating, wiry, thready and rapid pulse.

Treatment
Body acupuncture

1. **Principles of treatment**

   To eliminate Phlegm and open the orifices, dispel Wind and stop convulsions, acupuncture alone with the reducing method for excessive type; mainly acupuncture with even method for deficient type.

2. **Prescription**

   Mainly points from the Governor Vessel. Shuigou (GV26), Changqiang (GV1), Jinsuo (GV8), Jiuwei (CV15), Fenglong (ST40), Yanglingquan (GB34).

3. **Explanation**

Shuigou (GV26) can restore consciousness and calm down the Mind; Changqiang (GV1), Jiuwei (CV15), which are key points to treat epilepsy, can communicate between the Governor Vessel and the Conception Vessel, and balance Yin-Yang; Yanglingquan (GB34) is an Influential point of the tendons, and can relax tendons and muscles, relieve convulsions and stop pain in combination with Jinsuo (GV8); Fenglong (ST40) can harmonize the Stomach and descend turbid, clear Heat and eliminate Phlegm.

4. **Modification**

- *Disturbance of Mind by Phlegm and Fire*: + Xingjian (LR2), Neiguan (PC6), Hegu (LI4) to remove Phlegm, open the orifices, clear Liver Fire.

- *Obstruction of the orifices by Wind and Phlegm*: + Benshen (GB13), Fengchi (GB20), Taichong (LR3) to eliminate Liver Wind, remove Phlegm and open the orifices.

- *Obstruction of collaterals by Blood stasis*: + Baihui (GV20), Taiyang (EX-HN5), Geshu (BL17) to activate Blood and promote the collaterals, restore and keep consciousness.

- *Blood deficiency stirring up Wind*: + Xuehai (SP10), Sanyinjiao (SP6) to nourish Blood and soften the tendons, dispel Wind and stop convulsions.

- *Heart and Spleen deficiency*: + Xinshu (BL15), Pishu (BL20) to tonify Heart and Spleen, benefit Qi and nourish Blood.

- *Liver and Kidney Yin deficiency*: + Ganshu (BL18), Shenshu (BL23), Taixi (KI3) to promote Liver and Kidneys, reduce Yang and calm the Mind; attack at night: Zhaohai (KI6); attack at day: Shenmai (BL62) to regulate Yin-Yang.

- *Dizziness*: + Hegu (LI4), Baihui (GV20) to dispel Wind and open the orifices.

5. **Manipulation**

Deeply and strongly puncture Shuigou (GV26) to the nasal septum; bleed on Changqiang (GV1); take care of the direction, angle and depth of puncturing Jiuwei (CV15) to prevent injury to the Liver and Spleen, etc. Routine treatment on the other points.

Other therapies

1. **Auricular acupuncture**

   Points: Stomach, Subcortex, Ear-Shenmen, Heart, Occiput, Brain. Puncture 2 to 3 points every time with heavy stimulation, retain the needles for 30 minutes and manipulate the needles at intervals.

2. **Point injection**

   Select Zusanli (ST36), Neiguan (PC6), Dazhui (GV14), Fengchi (GB20). Choose 2 to 3 points every time with vitamin B_1 injection and 0.5ml into each point.

Notes

1. Acupuncture and moxibustion are quite effective in treating epilepsy, but the patient should have EEG to make an exact diagnosis. If it is possible, the patient should have CT and MRI scans to distinguish the condition from Wind Stroke, hysteria, etc. Primary diseases should be diagnosed and treated when secondary epilepsy occurs.

2. We should also make the differentiation to treat the primary disease even though the epilepsy is in the interval period.

3. Comprehensive therapies should be given when epilepsy occurs continuously and is accompanied by severe symptoms such as high fever and loss of consciousness.

4. The patient should avoid mental stimulation and overstress, and pay attention to food intake and daily life in order to prevent relapse.

20. HYSTERIA

Brief introduction

Hysteria is mainly manifested by depression, worry, restlessness, or quickness to anger and crying. Hysteria as described here refers to neurosis (formerly hysteria) in Western medicine; it is a type of psychogenic emotional disease.

Aetiology and pathogenesis

According to TCM, hysteria is mainly caused by emotional changes, injury of the Liver by depression and worry, or disturbance of the Spleen by worry. Liver Qi stagnation can transform into Fire, Spleen Qi stagnation can produce Dampness, disturbance of Qi activities can cause stagnation; prolonged stagnation can result in more depression, poor appetite, and Qi and Blood deficiency that cause pathological changes, including Spleen Qi deficiency or Kidney Yin deficiency. Spleen Qi deficiency means the Spleen Qi cannot promote the Stomach to circulate fluid; Kidney Yang deficiency cannot warm up Heart Fire, and this leads to Fire with deficient type that disturbs the Heart Mind, and dysfunction of the Qi activities of the five Zang organs eventually causes hysteria.

Syndrome differentiation

The patient often has a history of various emotional disturbances. Frequently worry, fullness in the chest, hypochondriac distension, sighs, poor appetite, insomnia, dream-disturbed sleep, easily becomes angry and cries, etc. Some patients may suffer from sudden blindness, hearing loss, aphasia, paralysis and consciousness disturbance, etc.

1. **Liver Qi stagnation**: Depression, fullness in the chest and hypochondriac distension, epigastric distension, frequent belching, sighs; or the sensation of a foreign body being in the throat; irregular menstruation; thin and white tongue coating, wiry pulse.

2. **Qi stagnation turning into Fire**: Easy irritability and anger, uncontrolled crying and laughing, fullness in the chest and hypochondriac distension, headache, redness of eyes, bitter taste in the mouth, acid regurgitation, constipation, yellow urine, red tongue with yellow coating, wiry and rapid pulse.

3. **Heart and Spleen deficiency**: Over-thinking and worry, fullness of the chest and palpitations, insomnia and poor memory, sallow complexion, dizziness and blurred vision, lassitude, easily sweating, poor appetite, pale tongue with thin and white coating, wiry and thready pulse.

4. **Fire caused by Yin deficiency**: Prolonged, poor sleeping, irritability and easily angered, uncontrolled crying and laughing, dizziness and palpitations, redness of the cheeks, feverish sensation in the five centres, dry mouth and sore throat, or night sweating, red tongue with thin coating, wiry and thready or thready and rapid pulse.

Treatment

Body acupuncture

1. **Principles of treatment**

   To regulate Qi and eliminate stagnation, nourish the Heart and calm down the Mind, acupuncture alone with the reducing method for Liver Qi stagnation and Qi stagnation turning into Fire; acupuncture alone with even method for Fire due to Yin deficiency; both acupuncture and moxibustion with the reinforcing method for Heart and Spleen deficiency.

2. **Prescription**

   Mainly points from the Pericardium Meridian of Hand-Jueyin and the Liver Meridian of Foot-Jueyin. Shenmen (HT7), Daling (PC7), Neiguan (PC6), Qimen (LR14), Xinshu (BL15), Hegu (LI4), Taichong (LR3).

3. **Explanation**

   Shenmen (HT7), Daling (PC7) can calm down the Mind; Neiguan (PC6) can open the chest and eliminate stagnation; Xinshu (BL15) can tonify Heart Qi and calm down the Mind; Qimen (LR14), Taichong (LR3) can regulate Liver Qi and eliminate stagnation; Hegu (LI4) and Taichong (LR3) are 'the Four Gates' points to restore consciousness and open the orifices.

4. **Modification**

   - *Liver Qi stagnation*: + Xingjian (LR2), Ganshu (BL18) to regulate Liver Qi and eliminate stagnation.

   - *Qi stagnation turning into Fire*: + Xingjian (LR2), Neiting (ST44), Zhigou (TE6) to remove Liver Fire, eliminate stagnation and harmonize Stomach.

   - *Heart and Spleen deficiency*: + Pishu (BL20), Sanyinjiao (SP6), Zusanli (ST36), Zhongwan (CV12) to tonify Spleen Qi, nourish the Heart and calm down the Mind.

   - *Fire due to Yin deficiency*: + Sanyinjiao (SP6), Taixi (KI3), Shenshu (BL23) to nourish Yin and reduce Fire, nourish Heart and calm down the Mind.

   - *Foreign body sensation in the throat*: + Tiantu (CV22), Lieque (LU7), Zhaohai (KI6) to benefit throat.

   - *Blindness*: + Taiyang (EX-HN5), Sibai (ST2), Guangming (GB37) to open the orifices and restore vision.

   - *Hearing loss*: + Ermen (TE21), Tinggong (SI19) to open orifice and promote hearing.

- *Aphasia*: + Lianquan (CV23), Fengchi (GB20) to benefit the tongue orifice.

- *Paralysis of the limbs*: + Quchi (LI11), Zusanli (ST36), Yanglingquan (GB34) to promote meridians.

- *Consciousness disturbance*: + Shuigou (GV26), Baihui (GV20) to restore consciousness and open the orifices.

5. **Manipulation**

Oblique or horizontal insertion of needle on Qimen (LR14) without perpendicular and deep puncturing to avoid pneumothorax or injury to a live organ; be careful of direction, depth and angle in puncturing Back-Shu points to prevent injury of the internal Zang Fu organs; routine treatment on the other points.

Other therapies

1. **Auricular acupuncture**

Points: Heart, Occiput, Brain, Liver, Endocrine, Ear-Shenmen. Choose 3 to 5 points every time with shallow puncturing or application of electric stimulator with strong stimulation, retain the needles for 20 minutes. Imbed needles or Vaccaria seeds to auricular points during recovery period.

2. **Electroacupuncture**

Select Zusanli (ST36), Neiguan (PC6), Taichong (LR3), Sanyinjiao (SP6). Choose 2 to 3 points every time with 10 to 20 minutes connection to electric stimulator.

3. **Point injection**

Select Fengchi (GB20), Xinshu (BL15), Pishu (BL20), Zusanli (ST36). Apply injection of either Water, Danshen (丹参 *Radix Salviae Miltiorrhizae*) injection, or Shenmai (参脉) injection, injecting 0.3–0.5ml on every point. Injection before sleeping is recommended to treat insomnia.

4. **Catgut Implantation**

Select Ganshu (BL18), Xinshu (BL15), Pishu (BL20), Zusanli (ST36). Apply catgut implantation and fix with sterile gauze.

Notes

1. Hysteria is a psychogenic emotional disease. We cannot ignore the function of verbal suggestion during treatment. We should relax patients and help them gain the confidence to overcome the disease.

2. Body system examinations and lab tests need to be taken to exclude organic disorders. Distinguish these from mental symptoms caused by depressive mental disorder, manic mental disorder, cerebral arteriosclerosis and brain trauma, etc.

21. PARKINSON'S DISEASE

Brief introduction

Parkinson's disease belongs to 'Tremor syndrome' in TCM. Parkinson's disease is commonly seen as an extrapyramidal disease of central nervous system degeneration; it is mainly manifested by static tremor, myotonia, bradykinesia.

Aetiology and pathogenesis

Parkinson's disease is mostly caused by Liver and Kidney deficiency, Qi and Blood insufficiency, obstruction of the meridians by Dampness and Phlegm, malnutrition of tendons, stirring up of Wind by deficiency. It locates in the brain, and the affected organs are mainly the Liver, Kidneys and Spleen. The syndrome is a complicated one with deficiency as the root cause, and excess displaying in the symptoms.

Syndrome differentiation

Parkinson's disease is of slow onset; most patients have a diagnosis after 2 years. It is mainly manifested by static tremor, myotonia and bradykinesia. Tremor mostly begins from one side in the hand and arm, and presents as 'pill-rolling'. Tremor is worse after emotional change, better after the movement of limbs and disappear during sleep. Myotonia is manifested in increased tension of the whole body muscle, and presents as 'lead-pipe rigidity'. Tremor and myotonia together present as 'cogwheel rigidity'; facial rigidity reduces expression and the ability to wink, and presents as 'mask face'; rigidity of lingualis and throat muscle is manifested in slow and unclear speech, and difficulty swallowing in severe cases. Bradykinesia presents as difficult volitional movement, slow and reduced movement; the initial stage is manifested in 'festinating gait'; the hands do not both swing back and forth during walking because the patient loses the facility for combined activities; there is difficulty in standing when sitting, difficulty in turning the body when lying; 'micrographia' during writing. Some patients have other autonomic nervous symptoms such as aversion to Heat, copious sweating, seborrhoea, difficulty in urinating, intractable constipation, orthostatic hypotension, etc. Some patients have mental symptoms including insomnia, depression, dull response, hypophrenia and dementia, etc.

1. **Liver and Kidney deficiency**: Contracture, muscular rigidity, wooden motions, tremor of the head and four limbs (obvious when quiet, severe during emotional change, relieved or disappearing during volitional movement), dizziness and blurred vision, tinnitus, insomnia and dream-disturbed sleep, soreness of the lumbar region and weakness of the four limbs, numbness of the limbs, thin tongue body with purplish dark colour, thready and wiry pulse.

2. **Qi and Blood deficiency**: Contracture, muscular rigidity, reduced movement, tremor of the limbs, weakness of the four limbs, lassitude, dizziness and blurred vision, lustreless complexion, pale tongue with white coating, thready and weak pulse.

3. **Phlegm stirring up the Wind**: Contracture, muscular rigidity, difficult movement (tremor comes and goes, is often under self-control), fullness in the chest, epigastric distension, dizziness and blurred vision, flabby tongue with pale colour and teeth mark, sticky coating, wiry and rolling pulse.

Treatment
Body acupuncture

1. **Principles of treatment**

   To benefit the Liver and Kidneys, regulate Qi and nourish Blood, eliminate Phlegm and promote collaterals, dispel Wind and stop contracture, apply both acupuncture and moxibustion. Use the reinforcing method for Liver and Kidney deficiency, Qi and Blood deficiency; even method for Phlegm stirring up the Wind.

2. **Prescription**

   Baihui (GV20), Sishencong (EX-HN1), Fengchi (GB20), Hegu (LI4), Taichong (LR3), Yanglingquan (GB34).

3. **Explanation**

   Baihui (GV20) and Sishencong (EX-HN1) function to restore consciousness, calm down the Mind and stop contracture; Fengchi (GB20) can dispel Wind, calm down the Mind and stop contracture; Taichong (LR3) can regulate the Liver and dispel Wind, and combined with Hegu (LI4) they 'open the Four Gates' that can promote Qi and Blood circulation and balance Yin and Yang; Yanglingquan (GB34) is the Influential point for tendons, and has the functions of nourishing Blood and softening the tendons, relaxing the tendons and promoting the collaterals.

4. **Modification**

   - *Liver and Kidney deficiency*: + Ganshu (BL18), Shenshu (BL23), Sanyijiao (SP6) to benefit Liver and tonify Kidney.

   - *Qi and Blood deficiency*: + Qihai (CV6), Xuehai (SP10), Zusanli (ST36) to promote Qi and nourish Blood.

   - *Phlegm stirring up the Wind*: + Fenglong (ST40), Zhongwan (CV12), Yinlingquan (SP9) to eliminate Phlegm and promote collaterals.

   - *Severe tremor*: + Dazhui (GV14) to stop tremor.

   - *Rigidity*: + Dabao (SP21), Qimen (LR14) to stop rigidity.

5. **Manipulation**

   Routine treatment on every point; puncture Sishencong (EX-HN1) with needle tip direction to Baihui (GV20); deeply insert needle on Dazhui (GV14) for tremor to get an electric shock sensation radiating to the four limbs, then withdraw needle when feeling this sensation without lifting and thrusting, rotate and retain the needle, or bleed on Dazhui (GV14) to cause a small amount of Blood by three-edged needle and cupping, perform treatment once a week; apply moxibustion on Dabao (SP21), Qimen (LR14) for rigidity with 10 minutes on each point; use strong moxibusion for 20 minutes on Baihui (GV20), Dazhui (GV14) so that the patient can feel a warming sensation to the encephalic region and deep layer of the point.

Other therapies

1. **Auricular acupuncture**

   Points: Subcortex, Central rim, Ear-Shenmen, Occiput, Neck, Elbow, Wrist, Finger, Knee. Use 2 to 4 points every time with moderate stimulation given by needle; or apply electroacupuncture, Vaccaria seeds to auricular points.

2. **Electroacupuncture**

   After puncturing, select 2 to 3 pairs of points on the head connected by electroacupuncture with a disperse and dense wave and 20 minutes heavy stimulation.

3. **Scalp acupuncture**

   Select Dingzhongxian (Middle Line of Vertex), Dingnie Qianxiexian (Anterior Oblique Line of Vertex-Temporal), Dingpangxian I (Lateral Line 1 of Vertex), Dingpangxian II (Lateral Line 2 of Vertex). Manipulate and retain the needles for 30 minutes.

4. **Point injection**

   Choose Tianzhu (BL10), Dazhui (GV14), Quchi (LI11), Shousanli (LI10), Yanglingquan (GB34), Zusanli (ST36), Sanyinjiao (SP6) and Fengchi (GB20), etc. Apply Shaoyao (芍药 *Paeonia Lactiflora*) Gancao (甘草 *Radix Glycyrrhizae*) injection or Danggui (当归 *Radix Angelicae Sinensis*) injection, Danshen (丹参 *Radix Salviae Miltiorrhizae*) injection, Huangqi (黄芪 *Radix Astragali seu Hedysari*) injection, etc. or 10% Glucose injection or 0.25% Procaine injection (taking skin test before using) into 2 to 3 points with 0.5ml to 2ml on each point every time.

Notes

1. This disease is difficult to treat. There is no very effective treatment method up to now. Western medicine cannot stop its development, and the patient should take Western medicine for the rest of their life, but the side effects of Western medicine are very obvious. Acupuncture and moxibustion can produce a marked effect, they are better used for short duration; improvement of rigidity as a result of treatment is more obvious than of tremor.

2. Apart from the routine treatment, the patient should take proper physical exercise and combine with exercise therapy and physical therapy. Patients in the late stages should strengthen their health care and life care, enhance their nutrition, and generally try to prevent complications and delay the occurrence of systemic failure.

3. Since the aetiology of degeneration of cerebral tissue caused by primary Parkinson's disease is not clear, prevention becomes difficult. Generally speaking, we should ask the patient to calm the Mind, keep a pleasant mood, avoid emotional changes such as worry, melancholy and anger, etc., have a regular daily life, keep to a light diet, with appropriate work and rest, and participate in physical exercises. Besides, we should pay attention to environmental protection, and avoid disturbance from carbon monoxide, manganese, mercury, cyanide and usage of drugs such as antidepressants and reserpine, etc.

22. COMMON COLD

Brief introduction

The common cold is commonly seen as a respiratory disease; it can be classified into cold, severe cold and influenza. Common cold can occur in all four seasons, especially in winter and autumn.

Aetiology and pathogenesis

According to TCM, the common cold often results from the invasion of exogenous pathogenic factors and lowered superficial resistance. It is mostly caused by an irregular daily lifestyle, abnormal cold and warmth, becoming wet or being caught by the rain, overstress and overstrain, invasion of Wind after drinking alcohol, etc. leading to a weak constitution, and it easily occurs in patients with chronic diseases. Wind accompanied with Cold, Heat, Dampness and summer Heat can enter the body through the skin, hair, mouth and nose to attack the Lungs and Wei defence, causing a series of Lung and Wei-defence symptoms.

Syndrome differentiation

The symptoms include nasal obstruction, nasal discharge, cough, headache, aversion to cold and fever, soreness of the body, etc.

1. **Wind Cold syndrome**: Nasal obstruction, clear nasal discharge, cough, clear and dilute sputum, slight itching in the throat, sneezing, more aversion to cold than fever, no sweating, headache, soreness and heaviness of the limbs, no thirst or thirst with preference for drinking warming water, thin and white tongue coating, superficial or tense pulse.

2. **Wind Heat syndrome**: Nasal obstruction and dry nose, scanty or sticky nasal discharge, heavy cough, yellow and sticky sputum, sore throat, more fever than aversion to cold, sweating, headache or head distension, redness of face and eyes, dry mouth with preference for drinking cold water, thin and yellow tongue coating, superficial and rapid pulse.

3. **Summer Heat and Dampness syndrome**: Heavy cough, white and sticky sputum, fever, difficult sweating, soreness and heaviness of the limbs, heaviness and distension of the head, fullness in the chest, poor appetite, abdominal distension, loose stools, scanty urine with yellow colour, white and sticky or slightly yellow and sticky tongue coating, soft pulse.

Treatment

Body acupuncture

1. **Principles of treatment**

   - *Wind Cold syndrome:* To dispel Wind and eliminate Cold, clear the Lungs and remove exogenous pathogenic factors, apply both acupuncture and moxibustion with the reducing method.

   - *Wind Heat syndrome:* To dispel Wind and clear Heat, benefit Lung Qi.

   - *Summer Heat and Dampness syndrome:* To clear summer Heat and remove Dampness, both types can be treated by acupuncture alone with the reducing method without moxibustion.

2. **Prescription**

   Fengchi (GB20), Dazhui (GV14), Lieque (LU7), Hegu (LI4), Waiguan (TE5).

3. **Explanation**

   Dazhui (GV14), Fengchi (GB20), Waiguan (TE5) can dispel Wind and eliminate exogenous pathogenic factors; Hegu (LI4) can dispel Wind and clear summer Heat, eliminate exogenous pathogenic factors and clear Heat; Lieque (LU7) can promote the Lungs to stop the cough. Hegu (LI4) and Lieque (LU7) are a combination of Yuan-Primary and Luo-Connecting points, and they strengthen the function of promoting the Lungs and eliminating exogenous pathogenic factors.

4. **Modification**

   - *Wind Cold syndrome:* + Fengmen (BL12), Feishu (BL13) to dispel Wind and eliminate Cold.

   - *Wind Heat syndrome:* + Quchi (LI11), Chize (LU5) to dispel Wind and clear Heat.

   - *Summer Heat and Dampness syndrome:* + Zhongwan (CV12), Zusanli (ST36) to harmonize the Middle Burner and eliminate Dampness.

   - *Excessive pathogenic factors and weak body constitution:* + Feishu (BL13), Zusanli (ST36) to tonify anti-pathogenic Qi and eliminate pathogenic factors.

   - *Nasal obstruction and discharge:* + Yingxiang (LI20) to promote Lung Qi in descending and dispersing, and opening the orifices.

   - *Headache:* + Yintang (EX-HN3), Taiyang (EX-HN5) to dispel Wind and stop pain.

   - *Sore throat:* + Shaoshang (LU11) to clear Heat and benefit the throat.

5. **Manipulation**

  • *Wind Cold syndrome:* Both acupuncture and moxibustion on Dazhui (GV14), Fengmen (BL12), Feishu (BL13) and Zusanli (ST36).

  • *Wind Heat syndrome:* Bleeding on Dazhui (GV14), Shaoshang (LU11) by three-edged needle, and routine treatment on other points. Treat once a day for cold, 1 or 2 times a day for severe cold and influenza.

Other therapies

1. **Three-edged needle**

  Points: Ear-apex, Weizhong (BL40), Chize (LU5), Taiyang (EX-HN5), Shaoshang (LU11). Bleed 1 to 2 points every time. This method is suitable for Wind Heat syndrome.

2. **Cupping**

  Select Feishu (BL13), Fengmen (BL12), Dazhui (GV14), Shenzhu (GV12). Choose 2 to 3 points every time retaining the cups for 10 minutes. Or move cup on the Bladder Meridian of the back. This method is suitable for Wind Cold syndrome.

3. **Auricular acupuncture**

  Points: Lung, Internal Nose, Trachea, Throat, Forehead, and Adrenal points. Choose 2 to 3 points with shallow puncturing and retaining the needles for 30 minutes, also apply Vaccaria seeds to auricular points.

Notes

1. We should distinguish this disease from infectious diseases such as idemic encephalitis, epidemic encephalitis B and mumps, etc.

2. Acupuncture and moxibusion are effective in treating this disease, but we should apply comprehensive therapies when there is continuous high fever, severe cough, haemoptysis and haematemesis, etc.

3. During the epidemic period of the common cold, we should stay indoors with good ventilation and avoid public places. We can apply moxibustion towards Dazhui (GV14) and Zusanli (ST36) for prevention.

23. COUGH

Brief introduction

Cough in Chinese is called Ke Sou. Ke refers to upper perversion of Lung Qi; there is rattling in the throat but no sputum. Sou means sticky sputum but no rattling in the throat. Clinically, sputum and rattling are mostly present together, so we call cough Ke Sou. Cough may result from either the attack of the body by exogenous pathogenic factors or internal injuries. Cough due to attack by exogenous pathogenic factors is mostly an acute disease that can be transformed into a chronic one if treatment is not given in time; cough caused by internal injuries is mainly a chronic disease but with acute attacks if there is the invasion of the body by exogenous pathogenic factors. If the cough is prolonged, and occurs in old or weak persons, Lung Qi can be consumed, and then cough and asthma may happen together. Cough is commonly seen in upper respiratory tract infection, acute or chronic bronchitis, bronchiectasis in Western medicine.

Aetiology and pathogenesis

Cough due to exogenous pathogenic factors is mostly caused by Wind and Cold, Wind and Heat, Dryness and Heat, etc. Exogenous pathogenic factors first attack the Lung organ, then there is dysfunction of Lung Qi in descending and dispersing, Body Fluid cannot be distributed, accumulation of fluid turns into Phlegm which obstructs the passage of Qi, and finally cough and sputum occur. Cough due to internal injuries is prolonged and caused by dysfunctions of the Lungs, Spleen and Kidneys. Lung deficiency can cause dysfunction of Lung Qi in descending and dispersing; Spleen deficiency can result in retention of Water leading to Dampness and Phlegm; Kidney deficiency can cause dysfunction of the Kidneys in receiving the Qi, so there is shortness of breath. When Liver Fire attacks the Lungs, Lung Heat can consume fluid, then the cough is frequent and may even occur with bloody sputum. Cough due to exogenous pathogenic factors is mostly an excess syndrome, while cough due to internal injuries is mainly a deficient syndrome or a complicated syndrome of both deficiency and excess.

Syndrome differentiation

1. **Cough due to exogenous pathogenic factors**: Sudden onset, dry cough in the early stages, itching or pain in the throat, small amount of sticky or dilute sputum after a few days, accompanied by exterior syndromes such as fever, aversion to cold, nasal discharge, soreness and pain in the head and body, etc.

- *Invasion of the Lungs by Wind and Cold*: Cough with white sputum, nasal obstruction and discharge, aversion to cold and fever, headache, soreness and weakness in the whole body, pale tongue with thin and white coating, superficial and rapid pulse.

- *Invasion of the Lungs by Wind and Heat*: Cough with yellow sputum, difficult expectoration because of sticky, dry mouth and sore throat, headache and fever, red colour on the tongue tip with thin and yellow coating, superficial and rapid pulse.

- *Invasion of the Lungs by Dryness and Heat*: Dry cough without sputum, even bloody sputum, difficult expectoration, dry nose and throat, headache and fever, dry stools and yellow urine, red tongue with scanty fluid, thin and white coating, thready and rapid pulse.

2. **Cough due to internal injuries**: Prolonged, repeated cough and expectoration, or asthma. Generally, worse in autumn and winter, alleviated in spring and summer.

   - *Obstruction of Lung by Phlegm and Dampness*: Heavy cough, large amount of frothy and easily spat out sputum of white colour, pale tongue with white and sticky coating, soft and rolling pulse.

   - *Lung and Kidney Yin deficiency*: Dry cough without sputum, bloody sputum, feverish sensation in the five centres, afternoon fever and night sweating, red tongue with scanty coating, thready and rapid pulse.

   - *Lung and Kidney Yang deficiency*: Cough and asthma, dilute sputum, pale face, chills, pale tongue with thin and white coating, deep and thready pulse.

   - *Liver Fire burning Lung*: Frequent cough, scanty and sticky sputum, difficult expectoration, hypochondriac distension and pain, redness of eyes, bitter taste in the mouth, constipation, yellow urine, red tongue tip with thin and yellow coating, wiry and rapid pulse.

Treatment
Body acupuncture

1. **Principles of treatment**

   Cough due to exogenous pathogenic factors: to promote Lung Qi, eliminate exogenous pathogenic factors and stop the cough, mainly apply acupuncture (add moxibustion for Wind and Cold syndrome) with the reducing method. Cough due to internal injuries: to regulate the Zang Fu organs, tonify the Lungs, strengthen the Spleen, benefit the Kidneys, clear the Liver, eliminate Phlegm and stop the cough, apply both acupuncture and moxibustion with the reducing method for obstruction of the Lungs by Phlegm and Dampness, use both acupuncture and moxibustion with the reinforcing method for Spleen and Kidney Yang deficiency; apply acupuncture alone with even method without moxibustion for Lung and Kidney Yin deficiency, use acupuncture alone with the reducing method without moxibustion for Liver Fire burning the Lungs.

2. **Prescription**

Mainly points from the Lung Meridian of Hand-Taiyin, Back-Shu and Front-Mu points of Lung. Feishu (BL13), Zhongfu (LU1), Lieque (LU7), Taiyuan (LU9).

3. **Explanation**

Cough is due to dysfunctions of the Lungs, therefore use a combination of Back-Shu and Front-Mu points, selecting Feishu (BL13), Zhongfu (LU1) to regulate Qi activities of Lung organ, promote functions of Lung Qi in descending and dispersing, and eliminate Phlegm. Lieque (LU7) is Luo-Connecting point of the Lung Meridian of Hand-Taiyin, and in combination with Feishu (BL13) can promote Lung Qi; Taiyuan (LU9) is Yuan-Primary point of the Lung Meridian of Hand-Taiyin, and in combination with Feishu (BL13) can promote the Lungs and remove Phlegm.

4. **Modification**
   - *Invasion of the Lungs by Wind and Cold*: + Fengmen (BL12), Hegu (LI4) to disperse Wind and promote the Lungs.
   - *Invasion of the Lungs by Wind and Heat*: + Dazhui (GV14), Quchi (LI11), Chize (LU5) to disperse Wind and clear Heat.
   - *Invasion of the Lungs by Dryness and Heat*: + Taixi (KI3), Zhaohai (KI6) to moisten Dryness and stop the cough.
   - *Obstruction of the Lungs by Phlegm and Dampness*: + Zusanli (ST36), Fenglong (ST40) to eliminate Phlegm and stop the cough.
   - *Liver Fire burning the Lungs*: + Xingjian (LR2), Yuji (LU10) to reduce Liver and clear the Lungs.
   - *Lung and Kidney Yin deficiency*: + Shenshu (BL23), Gaohuangshu (BL43), Taixi (KI3) to nourish Yin and reduce Fire.
   - *Spleen and Kidney Yang deficiency*: + Pishu (BL20), Shenshu (BL23), Guanyuan (CV4), Zusanli (ST36) to tonify Spleen and Kidney.
   - *Pain in the chest*: + Tanzhong (CV17) to open the chest and regulate Qi.

- *Hypochondriac pain*: + Yanglingquan (GB34) to regulate Shaoyang.

- *Dry and itching sensation in the throat*: + Zhaohai (KI6) to nourish Yin and benefit the throat.

- *Bloody sputum*: + Kongzui (LU6) to clear the Lungs and stop bleeding.

- *Night sweating*: + Yinxi (HT6) to nourish Yin and stop sweating.

- *Oedema, difficult urination*: + Yinlingquan (SP9), Sanyijiao (SP6) to tonify Spleen and eliminate Dampness.

5. **Manipulation**

Avoid the radial artery when puncturing Taiyuan (LU9); do not use perpendicular and deep insertion on Zhongfu (LU1), Fengmen (BL12), Feishu (BL13), Pishu (BL20), Shenshu (BL23) so as to prevent injury of the internal organs. Routine treatment on the other points. Treat 1 to 2 times a day for cough due to exogenous pathogenic factors, apply once a day or every other day for cough due to internal injuries.

Other therapies

1. **Cutaneous needle**

Select points on the nape, the Bladder Meridian of Foot-Taiyang from level of first thoracic vertebra to second lumbar vertebra, the Stomach Meridian of Foot-Yangming on both sides of Adam's apple. Tap to the point of slight bleeding 1 to 2 times a day for cough due to exogenous pathogenic factors; tap to skin redness once a day or every other day for cough due to internal injuries.

2. **Cupping**

Points: Feishu (BL13), Fengmen (BL12), Gaohuangshu (BL43), etc., retaining cups 10 to 15 minutes. This method is suitable for cough caused by exogenous Wind and Cold.

3. **Point application**

Points: Feishu (BL13), Gaohuangshu (BL43), Dazhui (GV14), Dazhu (BL11), Shenzhu (GV12), Dingchuan (EX-B1), Tiantu (CV22), Zhongfu (LU1), Tanzhong (CV17). Apply Baijizi (白芥子 *Brassica Alba Boiss*), Gansui (甘遂 *Radix Kansui*), Xixin (细辛 *Asarum*), Yanhusuo (延胡索 *Rhizoma Corydalis Yanhusuo*), Rougui (肉桂 *Cortex Cinnamomi*), Tiannanxing (天南星 *Rhizoma Arisaematis*), etc. to make plaster, using 3 to 4 points every time and changing plasters once every 3 days. This method is suitable for cough due to internal injuries.

4. **Auricular acupuncture**

   Points: Lung, Spleen, Kidney, Trachea, Ear-Shenmen, Adrenal, Subcortex. Puncture 2 to 3 points every time, preferring strong stimulation for cough due to exogenous pathogenic factors and moderate stimulation for cough due to internal injuries; retain the needles 30 minutes, also apply Vaccaria seeds to auricular points.

5. **Electroacupuncture**

   Modify points according to acupuncture prescription. Using 2 to 3 points every time, apply dense wave and rapid frequency for cough due to exogenous pathogenic factors; use disperse and dense wave, stimulating 20 to 30 minutes for cough due to internal injuries. Treat 1 to 2 times a day for cough due to exogenous pathogenic factors, once a day or every other day for cough due to internal injuries.

6. **Point injection**

   Select Feishu (BL13), Tiantu (CV22), Dingchuan (EX-B1), Jiaji (EX-B2) from T1 to T7. Using 2 to 3 points every time.

   - *Cough due to exogenous pathogenic factors*: Antibiotics including Penicillin, Streptomycin, etc., treatment dosage every time is not more than 1/5 to 1/2 of intramuscular injection dosage and a skin test is necessary; or select Banlangen (板蓝根 *Radix Isatidis*), Yuxingcao (鱼腥草 *Herba Houttuyniae*) injection; treating once a day or every other day.

   - *Cough due to internal injuries*: Selecting Compound Danggui (当归 *Radix Angelicae Sinensis*) injection, Huangqi (黄芪 *Radix Astragali seu Hedysari*) injection, placenta injection, mixing with ratio of 4:2:1 and injecting 0.5ml to 1ml on each point; treating once every 3 days.

Notes

1. Cough due to internal injuries is prolonged and reoccurs easily, so patient should take long-term treatment. Both of primary and secondary should be treated during the acute stage; during remission stage, Lung, Spleen and Kidney should be promoted to treat the primary.

2. Comprehensive therapies should be given for severe symptoms such as high fever, sticky sputum, fullness of the chest, asthma, shortness of breath, etc.

3. Do not often go outdoors during the epidemic period of common cold to avoid inducing cough. Please take rest during the attack of cough to avoid further development.

4. Please take physical exercise to enhance constitution, strengthen the anti-pathogenic Qi and increase the body ability to adapt Cold.

24. ASTHMA

Brief introduction

Asthma is a kind of paroxysmal allergic disease. The clinical manifestations are paroxysmal wheezing, dyspnoea and orthopnoea. In Western medicine, this condition includes bronchial asthma, asthmatic bronchitis, and obstructive pulmonary emphysema. The disease may occur at any age. It is commonly seen during Cold season.

At the early stage, patients often get itching nose and throat, cough, sneezing and chest distress. This disease often occurs with sudden chest distress, dyspnoea, wheezing, prolonged exhalation, orthopnoea, dysphoria, sweating as well as cyanic lips and fingers. It can last for several minutes or even longer. At the resolving stage, abundant watery sputum may appear, then rapid respiration becomes alleviated.

Aetiology and pathogenesis

Its main pathogenic factor is long-retained Phlegm. Climatic changes, emotional changes, overstrain and diet will provoke the latent Phlegm. Then the Phlegm ascends with Qi that obstructs the trachea and causes asthma. Recurrent asthma will result in simultaneous deficiency of the Lungs, Spleen, Kidneys and Heart.

Syndrome differentiation

In the early stage, patients often get an itching nose and throat, cough, sneezing and chest distress. Asthma often presents with sudden chest distress, dyspnoea, wheezing, prolonged exhalation, orthopnoea, dysphoria, sweating, and cyanic lips and fingers. Attacks can last for several minutes or longer. At the resolving stage, abundant watery sputum may appear, and then respiration becomes alleviated.

1. **Cold Phlegm obstructing the Lungs**: This occurs after a Cold attack, dyspnoea, or sputum roaring in the throat, expectoration of thin and white sputum, accompanied by aversion to cold, fever, headache without sweating, pale tongue with slippery coating and floating pulse.

2. **Phlegm Heat obstructing the Lungs**: Dyspnoea and chest oppression, sputum roaring in the throat, yellow and sticky sputum, unsmooth expectoration, accompanied by fever, thirst, red tongue, yellow and greasy coating, slippery and rapid pulse.

3. **Lung-Spleen Qi deficiency**: Cough, asthma and shortness of breath, aggravation on exertion, low voice in cough, thin sputum, aversion to Wind and spontaneous sweating, pale tongue with thin and white coating, soft and thin pulse.

4. **Lung-Kidney Yin deficiency**: Shortness of breath and dyspnoea, cough with scanty sputum, dizziness and tinnitus, aching and weakness of loins and knees, tidal fever and night sweating, red tongue with scanty coating, thin and rapid pulse.

5. **Heart-Kidney Yang deficiency**: Shortness of breath and asthma, more exhalation and less inhalation, aversion to cold and cold limbs, profuse cold sweating, purple tongue with spots, thin and white coating, deep and thin pulse.

Treatment
Body acupuncture

1. **Principles of treatment**

   For Cold Phlegm obstructing the Lungs, both needling and moxibustion can be used with the reducing method. For Phlegm Heat obstructing the Lungs, needling is used with the reducing method. For Lung-Kidney Yin deficiency, more needling and less moxibustion can be used with reinforcing or even method. For Lung-Spleen Qi deficiency, both needling and moxibustion can be used.

2. **Prescription**

   Points of the Lung Meridian of Hand-Taiyin together with Front-Mu and Back-Shu points of the Lung meridian are selected as the principal points. Feishu (BL13), Zhongfu (LU1), Tiantu (CV22), Tanzhong (CV17), Kongzui (LU6), Dingchuan (EX-B1) and Fenglong (ST40).

3. **Explanation**

   Feishu (BL13) and Zhongfu (LU1) are selected to regulate the function of the Lungs. The function of Tiantu (CV22) is to descend Qi. Tanzhong (CV17) is the Qi point of the Eight Influential Points. Kongzui (LU6), the Xi-Cleft point of the Lung Meridian, is effective for acute diseases.

4. **Modification**

   - *Cold Phlegm obstructing the Lung*: + Fengmen (BL12) and Taiyuan (LU9) are added to disperse Wind and diffuse the Lungs.

- *Phlegm Heat obstructing the Lung*: + Dazhui (GV14), Quchi (LU11) and Taibai (SP3) are added to clear Heat and resolve Phlegm.

- *Lung-Spleen Qi deficiency*: + Pishu (BL20) and Zusanli (ST36) are added to strengthen the Lungs (Metal) by reinforcing the Spleen (Earth).

- *Lung-Kidney Yin deficiency*: + Shenshu (BL23), Guanyuan (CV4) and Taixi (KI3) are added to nourish the Lungs and Kidneys.

- *Heart-Kidney Yang deficiency*: + Xinshu (BL15), Shenshu (BL23), Qihai (CV6), Guanyuan (CV4) and Neiguan (PC6) are added to tonify Heart Qi.

- *Hectic fever and night sweating*: + Yinxi (HT6) and Fuliu (KI7) are added to enrich Yin and check sweating.

5. **Manipulation**

Fengmen (BL12), Feishu (BL13), Pishu (BL20), Shenshu (BL23) and Xinshu (BL15) should not be punctured perpendicularly nor deeply to avoid hurting the organs. For Heart-Kidney Yang deficiency, moxibustion is applied on Qihai (CV6) and Guanyuan (CV4). The routine method is used on the rest of the points. For obstinate asthma, scarring moxibustion is added. In the attack stage, the treatment is given twice or several times a day. In the remission stage, the treatment is given once every 1 to 2 days.

Other therapies

1. **Cutaneous needle**

Tap along *m. sternocleidomastoideus*, the first lateral line of the Bladder Meridian (T7-L2) on the back and the Lung Meridian from Chize (LU5) to Yuji (LU10) on both sides until the skin becomes red or bleeds slightly. This is applicable in the attack stage.

2. **Point application**

Baijiezi (*Semen Sinapis Albae*), Gansui (*Radix Euphordiae Kansui*), Xixin (*Herba Asari*), Rougui (*Cortex Cinnamomi*) and Tiannanxing (*Rhizoma Arisaematis*) are prepared into paste which is applied to Feishu (BL13), Gaohuang (BL43), Tanzhong (CV17), Pishu (BL20) and Shenshu (BL23) in the hot summer days. It is applicable in the remission stage.

3. **Auricular acupuncture**

Points: Antitragic Apex (AT1,2,4i), Adrenal Gland (TG2p), Trachea (CO16), Lung (CO14), Subcortex (AT4) and Sympathetic (AH6a). Each time 3 points are selected. The filiform needles are used with strong stimulation.

The needles are retained for 30 minutes. In the attack stage, the needling is done once or twice a day. In the remission stage, the needling is done with mild stimulation twice a week.

4. **Electroacupuncture**

   Each time 2–3 points are selected and disperse and dense wave is chosen with strong stimulation for 30 to 40 minutes.

5. **Point injection**

   In the stage of attack, Tiantu (CV22), Dingchuan (EX-B1) are selected. Each point is injected 0.2ml of 0.1% Adrenalin. The treatment is given once a day. In the remission stage, Jiaji (EX-B2) (T1~T7), Feishu (BL13), Gaohuang (BL43), Pishu (BL20), Shenshu (BL23) are selected. Each time 2–3 points are chosen. Each point is injected 0.5–1ml liquid with a mixture of the injection of placenta and the injection of Huangqi (黄芪 *Radix Astragali seu Hedysari*) (the ratio of the injection of placenta to the injection of Huangqi (黄芪 *Radix Astragali seu Hedysari*) is 1 to 2). The treatment is given 2 to 3 times a week.

Notes

1. The effect of acupuncture and moxibustion on this disease is certain. At the period of the attack, the therapy is selected to control the symptoms. At the remission stage, the treatment is selected to reinforce the resistance of the body.

2. In severe cases, the combined treatment will be needed.

3. In the remission stage, Fengmen (BL12), Feishu (BL13), Gaohuang (BL43), Pishu (BL20), Shenshu (BL23), Guanyuan (CV4), Qihai (CV6) and Zusanli (ST36) are selected and moxibusted once a day. Each time 3–5 points are used and moxibusted until the skin becomes red. The moxibustion should continue for 3 to 6 months. It is effective in preventing asthma.

4. Exercise the body to strengthen the constitution. Proper diet, including the avoidance of smoking, alcohol, fat and seafood are effective in treating the disease.

25. MALARIA

Brief introduction

Malaria is a type of infectious disease which is caused by the invasion of plasmodia. It is characterized by paroxysms of shivering chills and high fever occurring at regular intervals. It occurs mostly in summer and autumn.

Aetiology and pathogenesis

The disease is caused mainly by the malarial pestilential factor together with pathogenic Wind Cold, summer Heat or Dampness that invades the body, residing in the area between the exterior and interior, moving outward and inward between Ying-nutrient and Wei defence. When they move inward to struggle with Yin, there are chills, while when they move outward to fight with Yang, there is fever. If the pathogenic factors avoid fighting with the Ying-nutrient and Wei defence, there appears to be an interval between the paroxysms. The chronic cases with a mass formed in the hypochondriac region is due to deficiency of Qi and Blood and stagnation of excessive Phlegm in the meridians and collaterals.

Syndrome differentiation

Paroxysms of shivering chills and high fever with a generally hot sensation, preceded by yawning and lassitude. An intolerable headache develops, flushed face, red lips, and dire thirst. Eventually, the patient will break out in profuse perspiration and the fever subsides with the body feeling cool.

1. **Warm malaria**: Higher fever and slight chills, uneven sweating, thirst with desire to drink, dry stools and brown urine, red tongue with sticky and yellow coating, wiry and slippery pulse.

2. **Cold malaria**: Severe chills and low fever, chest and hypochondriac stuffiness, nausea and vomiting, lassitude, pale complexion, light-coloured tongue with thin and white coating, wiry and slow pulse.

3. **Prolonged malaria**: Occurrence after overstrain or improper diet, spontaneous sweating, sallow complexion, fatigue, poor appetite, dry or loose stools, light-coloured tongue with thin coating, thin and weak pulse.

4. **Hypochondriac mass**: A mass in the left hypochondriac region is usually found with dull pain, or paroxysms of shivering chills and high fever, emaciation, fatigue, pale lips and nails, light-coloured tongue, wiry and thin pulse. In chronic cases delirium and convulsions may occur.

Treatment

Body acupuncture

1. **Principles of treatment**

   A Shaoyang disorder is an intermediate syndrome in which pathogenic factors remain between the exterior and interior. They should be treated by harmonizing Shaoyang through mediation, to expel malarial pathogen and prevent the attack. For warm malaria, needling can be used with the reducing method. For cold malaria, prolonged malaria and hypochondriac mass, both needling and moxibustion are applied with reinforcing or even method.

2. **Prescription**

   Dazhui (GV14), Taodao (GV13), Zhongzhu (TE3), Jianshi (PC5) and Houxi (SI3).

3. **Explanation**

   Dazhui (GV14), the meeting point of the three Yang meridians and the Governor Vessel, in combination with Taodao (GV13), is selected for activating the Yang Qi. They are considered the key points for arresting malaria attack. Regular attack of chills and fever is the chief symptom of Shaoyang disease. So Zhongzhu (TE3) of the Triple Burner Meridian of Hand-Shaoyang and Jianshi (PC5) of Pericardium Meridian are used for harmonizing and releasing the Shaoyang. Houxi (SI3) is used for dispersing Qi of Taiyang Meridian to lead pathogenic Qi outwards. The joint use of above points may harmonize the Shaoyang and eliminate pathogenic factors to arrest the attack of malaria.

4. **Modification**

   - *Warm malaria*: + Quchi (LU11) and Waiguan (TE5) are added to clear Heat.
   - *Cold malaria*: + Zhiyang (GV9) and Qimen (LR14) are added to reinforce Yang and eliminate the pathogenic factors.
   - *Prolonged malaria*: + Pishu (BL20), Zusanli (ST36) and Sanyinjiao (SP6) are added to tonify the Spleen.
   - *Hypochondriac mass*: + Pigen (EX-B4), Zhangmen (LR13) and Taichong (LR3) are added to soften hardness and dissipate binding.
   - *Vomiting*: + Neiguan (PC6) and Gongsun (SP4) are added to harmonize the Stomach and check vomiting.

- *High fever*: + Shixuan (EX-UE11) and Weizhong (BL40) are added to eliminate Heat.

- *Abdominal pain and diarrhoea*: + Tianshu (ST25), Qihai (CV6) and Zusanli (ST36) are added to move Qi and check diarrhoea.

- *Coma and delirium*: + Shuigou (GV26), Zhongchong (PC9), Laogong (PC8) and Yongquan (KI1) are added to open the orifices.

- *Feverish sensation and night sweating*: + Taixi (KI3) and Fuliu (KI7) are added to nourish Yin and clear Heat.

- *Fatigue and spontaneous sweating*: + Guanyuan (CV4) and Qihai (CV6) are added to tonify Qi and promote Yang.

- *Pale lips and nails*: + Geshu (BL17), Pishu (BL20) and Sanyinjiao (SP6) are added to fortify the Spleen and nourish Blood.

5. **Manipulation**

Zhangmen (LR13), Qimen (LR14), Pishu (BL20) and Geshu (BL17) should not be needled perpendicularly and deeply to avoid pricking the organs. For fatigue and spontaneous sweating, moxibustion is added on Guanyuan (CV4) and Qihai (CV6). The routine method is used on the rest of the points. For warm and cold malaria, acupuncture is applied 1–2 hours before the disease attacks. The treatment is given once a day. For prolonged malaria and hypochondriac mass, the treatment is given once every 2–3 days.

Other therapies

1. **Cutaneous needle**

One hour before the attack stage, tap on Dazhui (GV14), Taodao (GV13), Shenzhu (GV12), Fengfu (GV16), Jianshi (PC5), Hegu (LI4), Taichong (LR3), Dazhu (BL11) and Jiaji (EX-B2) (T5-L5) until the skin becomes red.

2. **Three-edged needle**

Before the attack of chills, prick Dazhui (GV14), Shixuan (EX-UE11), Weizhong (BL40) and Quze (PC3) for bleeding.

3. **Auricular acupuncture**

Points: Adrenal Gland (TG2p), Subcortex (AT4), Endocrine (CO18), Spleen (CO13) and Liver (CO12). The needles are used with strong stimulation 1–2 hours before the attack. The needles are retained for one hour and manipulated once every 10 minutes.

4. **Point injection**

   Dazhui (GV14), Taodao (GV13), Jianshi (PC5), Hegu (LI4), Taichong (LR3) and Quchi (LI11) are selected. Each point is injected with 1ml of water for injection 2–3 hours before attack.

Notes

1. The effect of acupuncture and moxibustion on this disease is certain in China. It is considered that the acupuncture and moxibustion applied 1–2 hours before an attack can achieve better results. During the attack stage, acupuncture and moxibustion is also effective.

2. In the attack stage, patients should stay in bed and get sufficient rest.

3. In the stage of malaria with splenomegaly, the mass region should not be needled perpendicularly and deeply to avoid pricking the Spleen.

4. Pernicious malaria should be treated by acupuncture in combination with medicine.

5. In summer and autumn, Guanyuan (CV4), Qihai (CV6) and Zusanli (ST36) are selected and moxibusted with moxa roll for 10 minutes. Or 3–5 moxa cones are applied on each point. This is effective in preventing malaria.

26. STOMACH ACHE

Brief introduction

Stomach ache refers to a painful sensation located between the lower margin of the sternum and the infracostal margins. The relevant diseases are acute and chronic gastritis, gastric ulcer, gastrospasm, volvulus of Stomach, gastroptosis, prolapse of gastric mucosa and gastric neurosis.

Aetiology and pathogenesis

It is mainly caused by pathogenic Cold attacking the Stomach, retention of food, disharmony between the Liver and Stomach and deficiency in the Spleen and Stomach that leads to a disorder of Stomach Qi, stasis in the Stomach collateral and malnourishment of the Stomach. It may become aggravated because of improper diet, emotional upsets, overstrain and pathogenic Cold.

Syndrome differentiation

The main clinical manifestation includes pain in the epigastrium, usually accompanied with distension, nausea, vomiting, anorexia, acid regurgitation and gastric discomfort.

1. **Yang deficiency in the Spleen and Stomach**: Dull stomach ache, preference for warmth and pressure, relieved by intake of food, pale tongue with white coating, thin and weak pulse.

2. **Yin deficiency in the Stomach**: Burning pain in the gastric area, hunger without appetite, dry mouth, dry stools, red tongue with scanty coating, wiry and thin or thin and rapid pulse.

3. **Pathogenic Cold attacking the Stomach**: Sudden onset of stomach ache, aversion to cold and preference for warmth, thin white tongue coating, taut and tense pulse.

4. **Retention of food**: Distension, fullness and pain in the epigastrium, acid regurgitation, alleviation of pain after vomiting, thick and greasy tongue coating, and slippery pulse.

5. **Disharmony between the Liver and Stomach**: Epigastralgia involving the rib-sides, frequent belching and sighing, wiry pulse.

6. **Blood stasis blocking the collaterals**: Stabbing epigastralgia with fixed and impressible pain, purplish tongue or with ecchymosed and unsmooth pulse.

Treatment
Body acupuncture

1. **Principles of treatment**
   - For Yang deficiency in the Spleen and Stomach and pathogenic Cold attacking the Stomach, both needling and moxibustion are applied to disperse Cold, warm the meridian and relieve pain. For deficiency type, the reinforcing method is applied, while for excess type, the reducing method is applied.

   - For Yin deficiency in the Stomach, needling is applied with reinforcing or even method to nourish Yin, clear away Heat, strengthen the Stomach and relieve pain. For disharmony between the Liver and Stomach, needling with the reducing method is applied to soothe the Liver, normalize the function of the Stomach and relieve pain. For retention of food, needling is applied with the reducing method to promote digestion.

For Blood stasis blocking the collaterals, needling is applied with the reducing method to invigorate Blood circulation, remove Blood stasis and relieve pain.

2. **Prescription**

Zhongwan (CV12), Neiguan (PC6), Gongsun (SP4) and Zusanli (ST36).

3. **Explanation**

The Stomach governs descent. Zhongwan (CV12) is the Front-Mu point of the Stomach and the Influential point of the Fu organs. Zusanli (ST36) is the He-Sea point of the Stomach. They are the key points selected to treat the disorders of the Stomach. Neiguan (PC6) is the Luo-Connecting point of the Pericardium Meridian and one of the confluent points of eight extra meridians. It is connected with the Yin Link Vessel as well as the Stomach, Heart and thorax. Gongsun (SP4) is one of the confluent points of the eight extra meridians, and in combination with Neiguan (PC6) is effective to treat the disorders of the Stomach, Heart and thorax.

4. **Modification**

- *Yang deficiency in the Spleen and Stomach*: + Shenque (CV8), Qihai (CV6), Pishu (BL20) and Weishu (BL21) are added to disperse Cold and warm the Middle Burner.

- *Pathogenic Cold attacking the Stomach*: + Shenque (CV8) and Liangqiu (ST34) are added to disperse Cold and relieve pain.

- *Retention of food*: + Liangmen (ST21) and Jianli (CV11) are added to promote digestion.

- *Disharmony between the Liver and Stomach*: + Qimen (LR14) and Taichong (LR3) are added to soothe the Liver.

- *Blood stasis blocking the collaterals*: + Geshu (BL17) and Ashi points are added to remove Blood stasis and relieve pain.

5. **Manipulation**

For Yang deficiency in the Spleen and Stomach and pathogenic Cold attacking the Stomach, Zhongwan (CV12), Qihai (CV6), Shenque (CV8), Zusanli (ST36), Pishu (BL20), Weishu (BL21) and Ashi points are selected and moxibusted with moxa roll or ginger-isolated moxa. cupping is also applied on these points. Qimen (LR14) and Geshu (BL17) should not be needled perpendicularly nor deeply to avoid hurting the organs. Routine method is used for the rest of the points. For acute epigastric pain, the treatment is given 1–2 times a day. For chronic epigastric pain, the treatment is given once a day or every other day.

Other therapies

1. **Finger pressure**

   The points selected are Zhongwan (CV12), Zhiyang (GV9) and Zusanli (ST36). Press these points with thumbs or middle fingers for 3–5 minutes with the intensity that patients can bear. At the same time, let patients do abdominal breathing.

2. **Auricular acupuncture**

   Points: Stomach (CO4), Duodenum (CO5), Spleen (CO13), Liver (CO12), Shenmen (TF4) and Sympathetic Nerve (AH6a) are selected. The points are punctured superficially. Each time 3–5 points are selected. The needles are retained for 30 minutes, or Vaccaria seeds are applied to auricular points.

3. **Point injection**

   Danggui (当归 *Radix Angelicae Sinensis*) injection, Shengmai (invigoration of the vessels) injection, Danshen (丹参 *Radix Salviae Miltiorrhizae*) injection, Shenfu (人参 *Radix Ginseng*; 附子 *Radix Aconiti Lateralis Preparata*) injection, the injection of vitamin B_1 and the injection of vitamin B_{12} are used. 2–3 points are selected each time. Each point is injected with 2–4ml of liquid.

4. **Herbal Bag**

   Biba (荜茇 *Fructus Piperis Lonngi*) 15g, Ganjiang (干姜 *Rhizoma Zingiberis*) 15g, Gansong (干松 *Radix et Rhizoma Nardostachyos*) 10g, Shannai (山奈 *Rhizoma Kaempferiae*) 10g, Xixin (细辛 *Herba Asari*) 10g, Yuanhu (元胡 *Rhizoma Corydalis*) 10g, Rougui (肉桂 *Cortex Cinnamomi*) 10g, Wuzhuyu (吴茱萸 *Fructus Evodiae*) 10g, Baizhi (白芷 *Radix Angelicae Dahuricae*) 10g, Huixiang (茴香 *Fructus Foeniculi*) 6g, and Aiye (艾叶 *Folium Artemisiae Argyi*) 30g. Grind them into powder. Make a 15cm × 15cm square cloth packet with a piece of soft cotton cloth, sew the packet tight so as to prevent heaping up or leakage of the powder. Put the packet on the gastric area. It is applicable to treat gastric pain with deficiency of Spleen and Stomach Yang.

Notes

1. The treatment of this disease by acupuncture and moxibustion is effective. Usually several treatments can achieve a curative effect.

2. Proper diet, good mood and avoidance of cold food are effective in treating this disease.

3. It is necessary to rule out Liver and Gallbladder disease, pancreatitis and cardiac infarction.

4. For ulcerative bleeding and gastric perforation, the combined treatment of the primary disease is needed.

27. GASTROPTOSIS

Brief introduction

Gastroptosis refers to the condition in which the location of the Stomach is lower than normal position due to looseness of the ligament supporting the Stomach and decline of the gastrotonia. This disease is usually seen among women with emaciation.

Aetiology and pathogenesis

This disease is usually caused by improper diet and overstrain that lead to hypofunction of the Spleen and Stomach as well as sinking of Spleen Qi.

Syndrome differentiation

The clinical manifestations are dragging distension in the upper abdomen and stomach ache, which are immediately alleviated when the patient lies flat. It is usually accompanied by distension, anorexia, nausea, belching, diarrhoea or constipation.

1. **Spleen insufficiency with sinking of Qi**: Emaciation, pale complexion, palpitations, dizziness, dull stomach ache, dragging distension in the epigastrium and abdomen, aggravation after meal, alleviation after lying flat, light-coloured tongue with thin coating, thin and weak pulse.

2. **Liver depression and Qi stagnation**: Belching and deep sighing.

3. **Spleen Qi failing to ascend**: Fullness and mass in the abdomen, as well as nausea.

Treatment

Body acupuncture

1. **Principles of treatment**

   Fortify the Spleen and replenish Qi, as well as elevate Yang to cure drooping. Both needling and moxibustion can be used with the reinforcing method.

2. **Prescription**

   Points of the Conception Vessel together with Back-Shu points of the Spleen and Stomach are selected as the principal points. Zhongwan (CV12), Qihai (CV6), Baihui (GV20), Weishu (BL21), Pishu (BL20) and Zusanli (ST36).

3. **Explanation**

   Weishu (BL21) is the Back-Shu point of the Stomach. Zhongwan (CV12) is the Front-Mu point of the Stomach. Zusanli (ST36) is the Lower He-Sea point of the Stomach. They are the key points selected to nourish the Stomach Qi. Pishu (BL20) and Qihai (CV6) are added to fortify the Spleen and replenish Qi, as well as harmonize the Middle Burner. Baihui (GV20) is added to lift up the prolapse.

4. **Modification**

   - *Stuffiness, fullness and nausea*: + Gongsun (SP4) and Neiguan (PC6) are added.

   - *Deep sighing*: + Taichong (LR3) and Qimen (LR14) are added.

5. **Manipulation**

   Routine method is used on all the acupoints. The reinforcing method is applied on the main points, while even method is applied on added points. Moxibustion or cupping can be added on upper abdomen and back.

Other therapies

1. **Auricular acupuncture**

   Points: Stomach (CO4), Spleen (CO13), Sympathetic Nerve (AH6a) and Subcortex (AT4) are selected. Needle with routine techniques or embed with needles, or Vaccaria seeds are applied to auricular points.

2. **Point injection**

The points selected are the same as in body acupuncture. Inject these points with an injection of Huangqi (黄芪 *Radix Astragali seu Hedysari*) and Shengmai (invigoration of the vessels) injection. 1–3 points are selected each time. Each point is injected with 1 ml of liquid.

3. **Catgut implantation**

Zhongwan (CV12), Pishu (BL20), Weishu (BL21), Qihai (CV6), and Zusanli (ST36) are selected.

Routine method is used on all the acupoints. The treatment is given once every 2 weeks.

Notes

1. The effect of acupuncture and moxibustion on this disease is certain.

2. Proper diet and good mood are effective in treating this disease.

28. VOMITING

Brief introduction

Vomiting is due to the reversed flow of Stomach Qi. Heaving (ou) is vomiting with ejection of emesis accompanied by sound, while disgorgement (tu) is the ejection of emesis without any sound, and retching (gan ou) is vomiting accompanied by sound without actual emesis. The relevant diseases are acute gastritis, pylorospasm (pylorochesis), prolapse of the gastric mucosa, duodenal stasis, gastric neurosis, cholecystitis and pancreatitis.

Aetiology and pathogenesis

Vomiting is divided into excess and deficiency syndromes. The deficiency syndrome is mainly caused by insufficiency of the Stomach. The excess syndrome is caused by exogenous pathogenic Qi, food retention, Phlegm-fluid retention, Qi stagnation and Blood stasis, resulting in reversed flow of the Stomach Qi. The organs involved are the Stomach, Spleen and Liver. The deficiency syndrome is mainly caused by dysfunction of the Spleen, while the excess syndrome is usually caused by dysfunction of the Liver. Its main pathogenic factors are improper diet, anxiety, motion sickness, drug reaction and pregnancy.

Syndrome differentiation

The main clinical manifestation includes vomiting and retching, usually accompanied by discomfort in the epigastrium, nausea, anorexia, acid regurgitation and gastric discomfort.

1. **Exterior pathogens attacking the Stomach**: Sudden vomiting, fever, aversion to cold, headache and general body ache, white tongue coating, soft and slow pulse.

2. **Food retention**: Acid fermented vomiting, epigastric and abdominal distension, relieved by vomiting, thick greasy tongue coating, rolling and forceful pulse.

3. **Stagnant Liver Qi overacting on the Stomach**: Frequent belching, acid regurgitation, distension in the chest and hypochondriac regions, wiry pulse.

4. **Phlegm-fluid retention**: Vomiting clear liquids, fullness of the epigastrium, poor appetite, dizziness, palpitations, white greasy tongue coating, and slippery pulse.

5. **Hypofunction of the Spleen and Stomach**: Repeated vomiting induced by improper diet, pale complexion, lack of strength, loose stools, pale tongue with thin coating, and weak pulse.

6. **Stomach Yin deficiency**: Repeated vomiting or dry heaves, hunger without desire to eat, dry mouth and throat, dry red tongue with scanty coating, rapid and thready pulse.

Treatment

Body acupuncture

1. **Principles of treatment**

   Descend the rebellious Qi and harmonize the Stomach. For food retention and stagnant Liver Qi overacting on the Stomach, needling is applied with the reducing method. For exterior pathogens attacking the Stomach, hypofunction of the Spleen and Stomach, as well as Phlegm-fluid retention, both needling and moxibustion are selected with the reinforcing method. For Stomach Yin deficiency, needling is applied with even method.

2. **Prescription**

   Zhongwan (CV12), Weishu (BL21), Neiguan (PC6) and Zusanli (ST36).

3. **Explanation**

The disease is due to the rebellion of the Stomach Qi. Weishu (BL21) is the Back-Shu point of the Stomach. Zhongwan (CV12) is the Front-Mu point of the Stomach. Neiguan (PC6) is the Luo-Connecting point of the Pericardium Meridian, and is able to relieve the fullness of the chest and Stomach. Zusanli (ST36) is the Lower He-Sea point of the Stomach. These are the key points selected to descend the rebellious Qi and harmonize the Stomach.

4. **Modification**

- *Exterior pathogens attacking the Stomach*: + Waiguan (TE5) and Dazhui (GV14) are added to release the exterior.

- *Food retention*: + Liangmen (ST21) and Tianshu (ST25) are added to reduce food retention.

- *Stagnant Liver Qi overacting on the Stomach*: + Taichong (LR3) and Qimen (LR14) are added to soothe Liver Qi.

- *Phlegm-fluid retention*: + Fenglong (ST40) and Gongsun (SP4) are added to resolve and transform congested fluids.

- *Hypofunction of the Spleen and Stomach*: + Pishu (BL20) and Gongsun (SP4) are added to fortify the Spleen and Stomach.

- *Stomach Yin deficiency*: + Pishu (BL20) and Sanyinjiao (SP6) are added to nourish and replenish Stomach Yin.

5. **Manipulation**

The routine method is used on all the acupoints. For hypofunction of the Spleen and Stomach, moxa stick, ginger-isolated moxa or warm needling can be added. cupping can be added on upper abdomen and Back-Shu points. The treatment is given once a day. For serious cases, the treatment can be given twice a day.

Other therapies

1. **Auricular acupuncture**

Points: Stomach (CO4), Cardia (CO3), Duodenum (CO5), Gallbladder (CO11), Spleen (CO13), Liver (CO12), Ear-Shenmen (TF4) and Sympathetic Nerve (AH6a). Each time 2–4 points are selected. The points are punctured superficially, or embedded with needles. Or Vaccaria seeds are applied to auricular points.

2. **Point injection**

The points selected are Zusanli (ST36), Zhiyang (GV9) and Lingtai (GV8). Each point is injected with 1–2ml of normal saline.

3. **Point application**

Shenque (CV8), Zhongwan (CV12), Neiguan (PC6), and Zusanli (ST36) are selected. Put a piece of ginger on each point, fix it with adhesive tape. This method is also applicable for vomiting due to motion sickness.

Notes

1. Acupuncture and moxibustion can produce satisfactory effects for this condition.

2. Vomiting due to obstruction of digestive tract and cancer will need to be combined with treatment of the primary disease.

3. Proper diet and avoidance of hot, cold and fat food are effective in treating the disease.

29. HICCUPS

Brief introduction

Hiccups are caused by Stomach Qi ascending to disturb the diaphragm. The condition is characterized by an involuntary short and frequent cough. The relevant diseases are phrenospasm, gastric neurosis, gastritis, gastrectasia, gastric carcinoma, end stage of cirrhosis, cerebrovascular disease, uraemia and hiccups caused by the Stomach or oesophagus operation.

Aetiology and pathogenesis

Its main aetiology and pathogenesis is reversed flow of Stomach Qi. When the Lung Qi is insufficient, the Lung fails to descend, leading to hiccups. If the Stomach Qi is stagnated, it will ascend and disturb the diaphragm. Liver Qi stagnation can cause ascending of Qi. If the Kidney is insufficient, it fails to receive Qi, causing hiccups. In clinical practice, Stomach Qi rebelling upwards to disturb the diaphragm is commonly seen. It is mainly caused by improper diet, emotional stress and Cold air.

Syndrome differentiation

Main symptoms are continual short hiccups in the glottis, which are uncontrollable. This is usually accompanied by a stifling sensation in the chest and hypochondriac regions, discomfort in the epigastrium and anxiety.

1. **Cold in the Stomach**: Deep, slow and rigorous hiccups relieved by warmth and aggravated by cold, white and thin tongue coating, slow and decelerating pulse.

2. **Stomach Fire blazing upwards**: Loud rigorous hiccups with bad breath and intense thirst, desire for cold drinks, dark scanty urine and constipation, dry yellow tongue coating, slippery and rapid pulse.

3. **Liver Qi stagnation**: Persistent hiccups aggravated by emotional stress, stifling sensation in the chest and hypochondriac regions, thin white tongue coating, wiry pulse.

4. **Spleen and Stomach Yang deficiency**: Low and weak hiccups, shortness of breath, discomfort in the epigastrium, cold limbs, fatigue, poor appetite, pale tongue with thin coating, thready and forceless pulse.

5. **Stomach Yin deficiency**: Abrupt intermittent hiccups, dry mouth and throat, hunger without desire to eat, dry red tongue with little coating, thready and rapid pulse.

Treatment

Body acupuncture

1. **Principles of treatment**

   - *Cold in the Stomach, Spleen and Stomach Yang deficiency*: Both needling and moxibustion are selected to warm the Middle Burner, expel Cold and calm hiccups. The reducing method in excess patterns; the reinforcing method in deficient patterns.

   - *Liver Qi stagnation and Stomach Fire blazing upwards*: Needling is applied with the reducing method to descend rebellious Qi.

   - *Stomach Yin deficiency*: Needling is selected with even method to nourish the Stomach and calm hiccups.

2. **Prescription**

   Geshu (BL17), Neiguan (PC6), Zhongwan (CV12), Tiantu (CV22), Tanzhong (CV17), Zusanli (ST36).

3. **Explanation**

Geshu (BL17) is selected to normalize the diaphragm and stop the hiccups. Neiguan (PC6) is the Luo-Connecting point of the Pericardium Meridian. It is connected with the Yin Link Vessel. It is used to relieve depression in the chest and diaphragm and subdue ascending Qi. Zhongwan (CV12) and Zusanli (ST36) are used to regulate the Stomach to descend the adverse Qi. Tiantu (CV22) lies on the throat, and is used to ease the throat. Tanzhong (CV17) lies near the diaphragm, is the Influential point of Qi. It is selected to descend the adverse Qi.

4. **Modification**

- *Cold in the Stomach, Stomach Fire blazing upwards, Stomach Yin deficiency*: + Weishu (BL21).
- *Spleen and Stomach Yang deficiency*: + Pishu (BL20), Weishu (BL21).
- *Liver Qi stagnation*: + Qimen (LR14), Taichong (LR3).

5. **Manipulation**

Routine method is used on all the acupoints. Geshu (BL17) and Qimen (LR14) should not be needled deeply to avoid pricking the organs. For Cold in the Stomach, Spleen and Stomach Yang deficiency, moxa stick or ginger-isolated moxa can be added. cupping or warm needling can be added on Zhongwan (CV12), Neiguan (PC6), Zusanli (ST36) and Weishu (BL21).

Other therapies

1. **Finger pressure**

The points selected are Yifeng (TE17), Cuanzu (BL2), Yuyao (EX-HN4) and Tiantu (CV22). Press any one point from the selected points with the thumb or middle finger for 1–3 minutes with the intensity that the patient can bear. At the same time, let the patient do deep breathing, then hold his breath.

2. **Auricular acupuncture**

Points: Middle Ear (HX1), Stomach (CO4), Ear-Shenmen (TF4), Lung (CO14), Spleen (CO13), Liver (CO12) and Kidney (CO10) are selected. The points are punctured with strong stimulation, or embedded with needles, or Vaccaria seeds are applied to auricular points.

3. **Point application**

Grind 0.5g of Shexiang (麝香 *Moschus*) into powder, put it into the umbilicus, fix it with adhesive tape. This treatment is applicable for excess patterns.

Grind 10g of Wuzhuyu (吴茱萸 *Fructus Evodiae*) into powder, mix it with vinegar to make paste, then put it on Yongquan (KI1) on both sides, fixing it with adhesive tape. It is applicable for all kinds of hiccups.

Notes

1. Acupuncture and moxibustion can produce immediate effects for this disease.

2. For hiccups caused by organic diseases, combined treatment of the primary disease will be needed.

3. Hiccups due to prolonged disease may be life-threatening if Stomach Qi is depleted.

30. ABDOMINAL PAIN

Brief introduction

Abdominal pain refers to any painful sensation in the area from beneath the epigastrium to the suprapubic margin. The abdomen includes many organs and meridians. Any disorder of these organs and meridians can cause this condition.

Aetiology and pathogenesis

It is a very common condition, which may be seen in internal medical, surgical and gynaecological disorders. The relevant diseases are acute and chronic enteritis, gastrospasm, enterospasm and irritable bowel syndrome.

Syndrome differentiation

It is due to long-term emotional disturbance, improper diet and over exertion.

1. **Food retention**: Abdominal distension and pain, aggravated by pressure, belching, acid regurgitation, anorexia, relieved by diarrhoea and vomiting, greasy tongue coating and slippery pulse.

2. **Liver Qi stagnation**: Pain and distension in the lateral abdomen relieved by belching or passing gas and aggravated by emotional stress, deep sighing, thin white tongue coating and wiry pulse.

3. **Cold invasion**: Sudden and urgent onset of severe abdominal pain, alleviated by warmth, aggravated by Cold, white tongue coating, deep and tight pulse.

4. **Spleen Yang deficiency**: Intermittent dull pain in the abdomen, preference for pressure and warmth, aggravated by hunger and exertion, pale tongue with thin coating, deep and thready pulse.

Treatment

Body acupuncture

1. **Principles of treatment**

   - *Food retention and Liver Qi stagnation*: Needling is applied with the reducing method to regulate the flow of Qi.

   - *Cold invasion*: Both needling and moxibustion are used with the reducing method to warm the Middle Burner and disperse Cold.

   - *Spleen Yang deficiency*: Both needling and moxibustion are added with the reinforcing method to tonify the Spleen Yang.

2. **Prescription**

   Zhongwan (CV12), Tianshu (ST25), Guanyuan (CV4), Zusanli (ST36).

3. **Explanation**

   Zhongwan (CV12) is the Front-Mu point of the Stomach and the confluent point of the Fu organs. Tianshu (ST25) is the Front-Mu point of the Large Intestine. Guanyuan (CV4) is the Front-Mu point of the Small Intestine. Zusanli (ST36) is the Lower He-Sea point of the Stomach. They are the key points selected to treat the disorders of the abdominal pain.

4. **Modification**

   - *Food retention*: + Neiting (ST44) to relieve food stagnation.

   - *Liver Qi stagnation*: + Taichong (LR3) to soothe the Liver.

   - *Cold invasion*: + Qihai (CV6) to warm the Middle Burner and disperse Cold.

   - *Spleen Yang deficiency*: + Pishu (BL20) to tonify the Spleen Yang.

5. **Manipulation**

   The routine method is used on all the acupoints. For Cold invasion and Spleen Yang deficiency, moxa or warming needle can be added. Moxibustion on salt can be added on Shenque (CV8).

Other therapies

1. **Auricular acupuncture**

   Points: Abdomen (AH8), Large Intestine (CO7), Small Intestine (CO6), Ear-Shenmen (TF4), Spleen (CO13), Liver (CO12) and Sympathetic Nerve (AH6a). Each time 3–5 points are selected. The points are punctured with strong stimulation, or embedded with needles, or Vaccaria seeds are applied to auricular points.

2. **Point injection**

   Tianshu (ST25) and Zusanli (ST36) are selected. Each point is injected with 0.5ml liquid mixed with 50mg Phenergan and 50mg Atropine.

3. **Topical application of drug**

   Stir-bake 50g Maifu (麦麸 wheat bran), 30g Congbai (葱白 *Bulbus Allii Fistulosi*), 30g Shengjiang (生姜 *Rhizoma Zingiberis Recens*), 15g salt, with 15ml vinegar and 30ml white spirit. Fill a bag with these. Press the area of pain with the bag and change it when it turns cool. This is applicable for the Cold invasion pattern.

Notes

1. Acupuncture and moxibustion can produce immediate effects for this condition. For abdominal pain caused by organic disease, combining treatment of the primary disease will be needed.

2. Abdominal pain with severe acute attack should be observed carefully and treated by combined therapies or surgery.

31. DIARRHOEA

Brief introduction

Diarrhoea is characterized by frequent passage of loose or watery stools. The relevant diseases are acute or chronic enteritis, intestinal tuberculosis, IBS and chronic nonspecific ulcerative colitis.

Aetiology and pathogenesis

This disease involves Spleen, Stomach, intestines, Kidneys and Liver. The dysfunction of the organs causes the failure of the Small Intestine to receive food and the failure of the Large Intestine in transportation. The pure and turbid substances mix together, and run down to the intestines. The pathogenesis is excessive Dampness and the dysfunction of the Spleen and Stomach. It is due to invasion of exogenous pathogenic factors, improper diet and emotional disturbance.

Syndrome differentiation

1. **Cold Dampness**: Acute onset, thin clear or loose watery stools with severe abdominal pain and borborygmus, abdominal pain relieved by defecation, aversion to cold, poor appetite, white greasy tongue coating, and soft pulse.

2. **Damp Heat**: Urgent defecation with severe abdominal pain, yellow-brown and sticky stools with an unpleasant smell, burning sensation of the anus, fever, abdominal pain relieved by defecation, yellow greasy tongue coating, soft rapid pulse.

3. **Food-retention**: Frequent loose stools with a rotten smell after improper diet, abdominal pain relieved by defecation, belching with a foul smell, acid regurgitation, poor appetite, thick turbid or greasy tongue coating, and slippery pulse.

4. **Liver Qi stagnation**: Recurrent painful diarrhoea induced by emotional strain, red tongue with thin white coating, and wiry pulse.

5. **Spleen Qi deficiency**: Loose stools containing undigested food, increased frequency of bowel movements with improper diet, fatigue, pale tongue with thin white coating, and thready pulse.

6. **Kidney Yang deficiency (daybreak diarrhoea)**: Diarrhoea before dawn that contains undigested food, Cold abdominal pain, cold limbs, pale tongue with white coating, deep and thready pulse.

Treatment
Body acupuncture

1. **Principles of treatment**
   - *Cold Dampness, Spleen Qi deficiency, and Kidney Yang deficiency*: Both needling and moxibustion are selected to strengthen the Spleen and Kidneys, drain Dampness. The reinforcing method is applied in the deficiency patterns; the reducing method is applied in the excess patterns.
   - *Liver Qi stagnation, food-retention, and Damp Heat*: Needling is selected with the reducing method to soothe the Liver.

2. **Prescription**

Front-Mu and Back-Shu and Lower He-Sea points of the Large Intestine are selected as the principal points. Shenque (CV8), Tianshu (ST25), Dachangshu (BL25), Shangjuxu (ST37), Sanyiiao (SP6).

3. **Explanation**

Dachangshu (BL25), the Back-Shu point and Tianshu (ST25), the Front-Mu point of the Large Intestine are used in the Shu-Mu combination of the prescription. Shangjuxu (ST37), the Lower He-Sea point of the Large Intestine, is selected to regulate the Stomach and intestine. Shenque (CV8) is moxibusted with moxa to warm Yang. Sanyinjiao (SP6) is used to invigorate the Spleen, and eliminate Dampness.

4. **Modification**

- *Cold Dampness*: + Pishu (BL20) and Yinlingquan (SP9) to strengthen the Spleen and drain Dampness.

- *Damp Heat*: + Hegu (LI4) and Xiajuxu (ST39) to clear Heat and eliminate Dampness.

- *Food-retention*: + Zhongwan (CV12) and Jianli (CV11) to reduce food retention and guide out stagnation.

- *Liver Qi stagnation*: + Qimen (LR14) and Taichong (LR3) to soothe the Qi.

- *Spleen Qi deficiency*: + Pishu (BL20) and Zusanli (ST36) to strengthen the Spleen.

- *Collapse of Spleen Qi*: + Baihui (GV20) to lift Spleen Yang.

- *Kidney Yang deficiency*: + Shenshu (BL23), Mingmen (GV4) and Guanyuan (CV4) to warm the Kidney.

5. **Manipulation**

The routine method is used on all the acupoints. Moxibustion on ginger and moxibustion on salt can be added on Shenque (CV8). For Cold Dampness and Spleen Qi deficiency, moxibustion on ginger, gentle moxibustion or warming needle can be added. For Kidney Yang deficiency, moxibustion on Fuzi (附子 *Radix Aconiti Lateralis Preparata*) cake. For acute cases, the treatment is given once or twice a day. For chronic cases the treatment is given once a day or once every other day.

Other therapies

1. **Auricular acupuncture**

   Points: Large Intestine (CO7), Small Intestine (CO6), Abdomen (AH8), Stomach (CO4), Spleen (CO13) and Ear-Shenmen (TF4). Each time 3–5 points are needled with mild stimulation, or Vaccaria seeds are applied to auricular points.

2. **Umbilicus therapy**

   Grind some Wubeizi (五倍子 *Galla Chinensis*) into powder, mix it with vinegar to make paste, put the paste into umbilicus, and fix it with adhesive tape. Change it every 1–2 days. It is applicable to long-term diarrhoea.

3. **Point injection**

   The points selected are Tianshu (ST25) and Shangjuxu (ST37). The injection of vitamin B_1, the injection of vitamin B_{12}, and Berberine injection are used. Each point is injected with 0.5–1ml liquid.

Notes

1. Acupuncture and moxibustion can produce an immediate effect for this condition. Transfusion is administered for cases with severe vomiting and heavy dehydration.

2. Proper diet and avoidance of cold and fatty food are effective in treating the condition.

32. DYSENTERY

Brief introduction

Dysentery is characterized by abdominal pain, tenesmus and frequent discharge of stools containing Blood and mucous. It is a common epidemic disease in summer and autumn. This condition includes bacillary and amoebic dysentery.

Aetiology and pathogenesis

The disease is often due to the invasion of epidemic Damp Heat and internal injury by intake of raw, cold and unclean food, which hinders and damages the Stomach and intestines.

Syndrome differentiation

The main manifestations are abdominal pain, diarrhoea with discharge of Blood, pus or mucous and tenesmus.

1. **Cold Damp**: Diarrhoea with discharge of Blood, pus and mucous, more pus and mucous than Blood in the stools, abdominal distension, general heaviness, white greasy tongue coating, soft and decelerating pulse.

2. **Damp Heat**: Diarrhoea with discharge of Blood and pus, burning pain at the perianal region and dark scanty urine; yellow greasy tongue coating, slippery and rapid pulse.

3. **Food-resistant**: Diarrhoea with discharge of Blood and pus, nausea, vomiting, complete loss of appetite, greasy tongue coating and slippery pulse.

4. **Intermittent dysentery**: Recurrent, intermittent dysentery, discharge of Blood and mucous.

Treatment
Body acupuncture

1. **Principles of treatment**

   - *Cold Damp*: Both needling and moxibustion are selected with the reducing method to warm and transform Cold Dampness.

   - *Damp Heat*: Needling is applied with the reducing method to clear Heat.

   - *Epidemic dysentery*: Needling is applied with the reducing method to clear Heat and relieve toxicity.

   - *Food-resistant*: Needling is applied with even method to arrest vomiting.

   - *Intermittent dysentery*: Both needling and moxibustion are applied with both reinforcing and the reducing method to tonify the Spleen.

2. **Prescription**

   Front-Mu and Lower He-Sea points of the Large Intestine are selected as the principal points. Hegu (LI4), Tianshu (ST25), Shangjuxu (ST37), Yinlingquan (SP9).

3. **Explanation**

   Hegu (LI4) is the Yuan-Primary point of the Large Intestine Meridian. Tianshu (ST25) is the Front-Mu point of the Large Intestine Meridian. Shangjuxu (ST37) is the Lower He-Sea point of the Large Intestine Meridian. All these points are selected to regulate the Stomach and intestine. Yinlingquan (SP9) is used to invigorate the Spleen, and eliminate Dampness.

4. **Modification**

- *Cold Damp*: + Guanyuan (CV4) and Sanyinjiao (SP6) to warm and transform Cold Dampness.

- *Damp Heat*: + Quchi (LI11) and Neiting (ST44) to clear Heat.

- *Epidemic dysentery*: + Dazhui (GV14), Zhongchong (PC9) and Shuigou (GV26) to clear Heat and relieve toxicity.

- *Food-resistant*: + Neiguan (PC6) and Zhongwan (CV12) to arrest vomiting.

- *Intermittent dysentery*: + Pishu (BL20), Shenque (CV8) and Zusanli (ST36) to tonify Spleen and Kidney.

- *Prolapse of rectum*: + Qihai (CV6) and Baihui (GV20) to lift Spleen Yang.

5. **Manipulation**

Routine method is used. For Cold Damp and intermittent dysentery, gentle moxibustion, warming needle, moxibustion on ginger or moxibustion on Fuzi (附子 *Radix Aconiti Lateralis Preparata*) cake can be added.

Other therapies

1. **Auricular acupuncture**

Points: Large Intestine (CO7), Rectum (HX2), Small Intestine (CO6), Abdomen (AH8), Spleen (CO13) and Kidney (CO10). Each time 3–5 points are needled with mild stimulation, or Vaccaria seeds are applied to auricular points.

2. **Point injection**

The points selected are Tianshu (ST25) and Shangjuxu (ST37). The injection of vitamin B_1, Berberine injection or 5% Glucose injection is used. Each point is injected with 1ml liquid.

Notes

1. The effect of acupuncture and moxibustion on this disease is certain.

2. For toxic bacillary dysentery, combined treatment is necessary.

3. During the attack stage of acute dysentery, the isolation ward is indispensable.

33. CONSTIPATION

Brief introduction

Constipation refers to dry impacted faeces, infrequent and difficult defecation. The disorder can be seen in functional constipation, IBS, diseases of the rectum and anus, diseases of endocrinal and metabolic systems, and constipation due to the side effects of drugs in Western medicine.

Aetiology and pathogenesis

The pathogenesis of constipation is mainly due to the dysfunction of the Large Intestine in transmission and also related to the dysfunction of the Spleen, Stomach, Liver and Kidneys. The disorder is mainly caused by improper diet, excessive anxiety and deficiency of Qi and Blood.

Syndrome differentiation

Reduced bowel movements, prolonged circle of defecation, or hard stools and difficulty in emptying the bowels. Accompanied symptoms include abdominal distension, abdominal pain, dizziness and bloody stools.

1. **Heat accumulation**: Dry impacted faeces, fever, red face, bad breath, dark scanty urine, red tongue with dry yellow coating, rapid and slippery pulse.

2. **Qi stagnation**: Dry stools, focal distension in the chest and hypochondrium, relieved after passing gas, frequent belching, sighing, thin greasy tongue coating and wiry pulse.

3. **Cold invasion**: Dry stools, abdominal cold pain, cold limbs, moist white tongue coating, deep and slow pulse.

4. **Deficiency of Qi and Blood**: Desire to defecate, ineffective straining to force bowel movements, great effort required for defecation, shortness of breath, pale tongue, thready and weak pulse.

Treatment
Body acupuncture

1. **Principles of treatment**

   Unblock obstruction of the bowel movement.

   - *Heat accumulation, Qi stagnation*: Needling is applied with the reducing method.

- *Cold invasion*: Both needling and moxibustion are applied with the reducing method.

- *Deficiency of Qi and Blood*: Both needling and moxibustion are applied with the reinforcing method.

2. Prescription

Front-Mu and Back-Shu and Lower He-Sea points of the Large Intestine Meridian are selected as the principal points. Tianshu (ST25), Dachangshu (BL25), Shangjuxu (ST37), Zhigou (TE6), Zhaohai (KI6).

3. Explanation

Tianshu (ST25), the Front-Mu point; Dachangshu (BL25), the Back-Shu point of the Large Intestine and its Lower He-Sea point, Shangjuxu (ST37) are applied to descend Qi and promote defecation. Zhigou (TE6) is used to soothe the Qi of the Triple Burner. Zhaohai (KI6) is applied to moisten the intestine and promote defecation.

4. Modification

- *Heat accumulation*: + Hegu (LI4) and Quchi (LI11) to drain Heat and unblock the bowel obstruction.

- *Qi stagnation*: + Zhongwan (CV12) and Taichong (LR3) to promote the movement of Qi.

- *Cold invasion*: + Shenque (CV8) and Guanyuan (CV4) to warm the Yang.

- *Deficiency of Qi and Blood*: + Pishu (BL20) and Qihai (CV6) to strengthen the Spleen and benefit the Qi.

5. Manipulation

The routine method is used. For Cold invasion and deficiency of Qi and Blood, gentle moxibustion, warming needle, moxibustion on ginger or moxibustion on Fuzi (附子 *Radix Aconiti Lateralis Preparata*) cake can be added.

Other therapies

1. Auricular acupuncture

Points: Large Intestine (CO7), Rectum (HX2), Triple Burner (CO17), Abdomen (AH8), Liver (CO12), Spleen (CO13) and Kidney (CO10). Each time 3–5 points are applied with mild stimulation, or Vaccaria seeds are applied to auricular points.

2. **Umbilicus therapy**

Dahuang (大黄 *Radix et Rhizoma Rhei*) 10g, Mangxiao (芒硝 *Natrii Sulfas*) 10g, Houpo (厚朴 *Cortex Magnoliae Officinalis*) 6g, Zhishi (枳实 *Fructus Aurantii Immaturus*) 6g, Zhuyazao (猪牙皂 *Fructus Gleditsiae*) 6g and Bingpian (冰片 *Borneolum Syntheticum*) 3g. Grind them into powder, mix it with honey to make paste, put the paste into umbilicus, and fix it with adhesive tape. Change it every 1–2 days.

Notes

1. Acupuncture and moxibustion can produce an immediate effect for this disease.

2. Exercise the body to strengthen the constitution. Proper diet and good mood are effective in treating this disease.

34. HYPOCHONDRIA PAIN

Brief introduction

Hypochondria pain refers to bilateral or unilateral pain in the infracostal regions. The disorder can be seen in acute or chronic hepatitis, hepatocirrhosis, liver cancer, cholecystitis, cholelithiasis, biliary ascariasis and intercostal neuralgia.

Aetiology and pathogenesis

The organs involved are the Spleen, Stomach, Liver and Gallbladder. The causes of hypochondriac pain are Liver Qi stagnation, Blood stasis, Dampness and Liver Yin deficiency.

Syndrome differentiation

The main manifestations are bilateral or unilateral pain in the infracostal regions. The characteristics of the pain are distending, stabbing, dull and wandering pain.

1. **Liver Qi stagnation**: Distending and migrating hypochondriac pain, aggravated by emotional stress, chest stuffiness, frequent belching, thin white tongue coating and wiry pulse.

2. **Blood stasis in the Liver channels**: Stabbing hypochondriac pain with fixed location, aggravated at night, purple tongue, deep and choppy pulse.

3. **Damp Heat in the Liver and Gallbladder**: Stuffy sensation and pain in the hypochondria, bitter taste in the mouth, distension of the chest, poor appetite, nausea and vomiting, yellow sclera, skin and urine, yellow greasy tongue coating, wiry, slippery and rapid pulse.

4. **Liver Yin deficiency**: Persistent vague hypochondriac pain, aggravated by exertion, dry mouth and throat, dizziness, red tongue with scanty coating, thready, wiry and rapid pulse.

Treatment
Body acupuncture

1. **Principles of treatment**

   Unblock the obstruction to alleviate pain. Needling is added with the reducing method. (For Liver Yin deficiency, even method is applied.)

2. **Prescription**

   Qimen (LR14), Zhigou (TE6), Yanglingquan (SP9), Zusanli (ST36).

3. **Explanation**

   Qimen (LR14) and Yanglingquan(GB34) are selected to ease the Liver and relieve pain in the hypochondriac region. Zhigou (TE6) is used to soothe the Qi of the Triple Burner. Zusanli (ST36) strengthens the function of the Spleen and Stomach.

4. **Modification**

   - *Liver Qi stagnation*: + Xingjian (LR2) and Taichong (LR3) to soothe the Liver and regulate Qi.

   - *Blood stasis in the Liver channels*: + Geshu (BL17) and Ashi points to dispel stasis.

   - *Damp-Heat in the Liver and Gallbladder*: + Zhongwan (CV12) and Sanyinjiao (SP6) to clear Heat and drain Dampness.

   - *Liver Yin deficiency*: + Ganshu (BL18) and Shenshu (BL23) to tonify Liver and Kidney.

5. **Manipulation**

   The routine method is used on all the acupoints. Qimen (LR14), Pishu (BL20), Geshu (BL17) and Ganshu (BL18) should not be needled perpendicularly and deeply to avoid pricking the organs. For Blood stasis in the Liver channels, Bleeding and cupping can be added on Geshu (BL17), Qimen (LR14) and Ashi points.

Other therapies

1. **Cutaneous needle**

    Tap the skin over the affected hypochondriac area and Jiaji (EX-B2) (T7-T10), and then apply cupping. It is applicable for pain due to Blood stasis.

2. **Auricular acupuncture**

    Points: Liver (CO12), Gallbladder (CO11), Chest (AH10) and Ear-Shenmen (TF4) are needled with mild stimulation, or Vaccaria seeds are applied to auricular points.

3. **Point injection**

    Jiaji (EX-B2) points from the affected area are selected. Inject 10ml of 10% Glucose, or with 1ml of vitamin B_1 added in it. It is applicable for intercostal neuralgia.

Notes

1. The effect of acupuncture and moxibustion on this disease is certain. Combined treatment of the primary disease will be needed at the same time.

2. Proper diet and avoidance of fatty foods are effective in treating the disease.

35. JAUNDICE

Brief introduction

Jaundice is mainly manifested by yellow discolouration of the sclera, skin and urine. Yellow discolouration of the sclera is the main symptom for diagnosis of jaundice.

Aetiology and pathogenesis

Dampness in the Spleen and Heat in the Stomach lead to abnormal circulation of the bile which spreads to the skin surface. This is divided into Yang jaundice and Yin jaundice according to its nature.

Syndrome differentiation

It is characterized by a yellowish discolouration of the sclera, skin and urine. Yellowish discolouration of the sclera is the marker for diagnosis of jaundice.

1. **Yang jaundice**: Bright yellow sclera, skin and urine, fever, intense thirst, scanty urination, constipation, yellow greasy tongue coating, slippery and rapid pulse.

2. **Yin jaundice**: Dusky, smoky yellow discolouration of the sclera, skin and urine, fatigue, poor appetite, loose stools, pale tongue with greasy coating, soft and deep or soft and slow pulse.

Treatment

Body acupuncture

1. **Principles of treatment**

   - *Yang jaundice*: Needling is applied with the reducing method to clear Heat and drain Dampness.

   - *Yin jaundice*: Both needling and moxibustion with reducing or mild reinforcing and the reducing method to warm the Middle Burner and drain Dampness.

2. **Prescription**

   Danshu (BL19), Yanglingquan (GB34), Yinlingquan (SP9), Zhiyang (GV9).

3. **Explanation**

   The Zang Fu organs impaired are the Spleen, Stomach, Liver and Gallbladder. Danshu (BL19) is the Back-Shu point of the Gallbladder. Yanglingquan (GB34) is the Lower He-Sea point of the Gallbladder. They are used to regulate the flow of Qi in the Liver and Gallbladder. Yinlingquan (SP9) is selected to strengthen the Spleen and remove Dampness.

4. **Modification**

   - *Yang jaundice*: + Neiting (ST44) and Taichong (LR3) to clear Heat and drain Dampness.

   - *Yin jaundice*: + Pishu (BL20), Zhongwan (CV12) and Zusanli (ST36) to strengthen the Spleen and drain Dampness.

   - *Fever*: + Dazhui (GV14).

   - *Nausea and vomiting*: + Neiguan (PC6).

   - *Constipation or diarrhoea*: + Tianshu (ST25) to descend Qi and promote defecation.

   - *Severe jaundice*: + Wangu (SI4) to drain Dampness.

5. **Manipulation**

The routine method is used on all the acupoints. Danshu (BL19) should not be needled perpendicularly and deeply. Or Vaccaria seeds are applied to acupoints.

Other therapies

1. **Auricular acupuncture**

   Points: Liver (CO12), Gallbladder (CO11), Spleen (CO13) and Stomach (CO4) are needled. Or Vaccaria seeds are applied to auricular points.

2. **Point injection**

   The points selected are as same as the acupuncture prescription. Each time 1–3 points are chosen. The injection of Banlangen (板蓝根 *Radix Isatidis*) and the injection of Tianzhuhuang (天竺黄 *Concretio Silicea Bambusae*) or the injection of vitamin B$_1$ and the injection of vitamin B$_{12}$ are used. Each point is injected 0.5–1ml liquid.

Notes

1. Acupuncture can produce an immediate effect for this condition.

2. Combined treatment of the primary disease will be needed at the same time.

36. OEDEMA

Brief introduction

Oedema refers to the subcutaneous retention of fluid which leads to puffiness of the head, face, eyelids, limbs, abdomen and/or the whole body. The relevant diseases are acute and chronic nephritis, chronic congestive heart failure, hepatocirrhosis, anaemia, endocrine dyscrasia and dystrophy.

Aetiology and pathogenesis

The functional derangement of the Lungs, Spleen, Kidneys and three Burners may lead to oedema. Clinically, oedema is divided into two patterns. These are Yin oedema and Yang oedema.

Syndrome differentiation

1. **Yang oedema**: Acute onset, oedema starting from the eyelids and spreading to the limbs and the entire body, shiny thin skin tone, insignificant or no pitting on pressure, wheezing, scanty urine, aversion to cold, fever, sore throat, white and greasy tongue coating, floating and slippery or slippery and rapid pulse.

2. **Yin oedema**: Systemic pitting oedema especially in the lower part of the body, decreased or increased urine output, distension of the epigastrium, poor appetite, loose stools, soreness and heaviness sensation in the lower back and knees, pale tongue with white coating, deep and thready or slow pulse.

Treatment

Body acupuncture

1. **Principles of treatment**

   - *Yang oedema*: Needling is applied with the reducing method to dispel Wind and eliminate water retention.

   - *Yin oedema*: Both needling and moxibustion are added with the reinforcing method to warm Yang and resolve water retention.

2. **Prescription**

   Shuifen (CV9), Shuidao (ST28), Sanjiaoshu (BL22), Weiyang (BL39), Yinlingquan (SP9).

3. **Explanation**

   Shuifen (CV9) and Shuidao (ST28) are applied to promote the Water circulation. Weiyang (BL39) and Sanjiaoshu (BL22) are applied to regulate the Qi activity of the Triple Burner and water passages. Yinlingquan (SP9) is used to remove Dampness and promote diuresis.

4. **Modification**

   - *Yang oedema*: + Feishu (BL13), Lieque (LU7) and Hegu (LI4) to dispel Wind and disperse Lung Qi.

   - *Yin oedema*: Spleen Yang deficiency + Pishu (BL20), Zusanli (ST36) and Sanyinjiao (SP6) to strengthen the Spleen and resolve Dampness.

   - *Kidney Yang deficiency*: + Shenshu (BL23), Guanyuan (CV4) and Zusanli (ST36) to warm Yang and resolve water retention.

5. **Manipulation**

The routine method is used on all the acupoints. Feishu (BL13) and Pishu (BL20) should not be needled perpendicularly and deeply. For Kidney Yang deficiency, moxibustion is added.

Other therapies

1. **Cutaneous needle**

Tap along the first and second lateral line of the Bladder Meridian on the back until the skin becomes slightly red. The treatment is given once every other day.

2. **Three-edged needle**

Prick Yaoshu (GV2), Shenshu (BL23), Weizhong (BL40) and Yinlingquan (SP9) for bleeding. It is applicable to oedema caused by chronic nephritis.

3. **Auricular acupuncture**

Points: Lung (CO14), Spleen (CO13), Kidney (CO10) and Bladder (CO9) are selected. The points are punctured with medium stimulation, or embedded with needles, or Vaccaria seeds are applied to auricular points.

4. **Point application**

Crush Cheqianzi (车前子 *Semen Plantaginis*) 10g, Dasuan (大蒜 *Bulbus Allii*) 5 cloves and Tianluo (田螺 *Viviparus seu Cipangopaludina*) into a mash, then apply it on the umbilicus. Or crush Bimazi (蓖麻子 *Semen Ricini*) 50 cloves and Xiebai (薤白 *Bulbus Allii Macrostemonis*) 3–5 cloves into a mash, then apply on Yongquan (KI1). The treatment is given once a day.

Notes

1. Acupuncture and moxibustion can produce satisfying effects for this disease. Combined treatment of the primary disease will be needed at the same time.

2. The recommendation is to avoid salt intake during the initial stage of oedema. As oedema is gradually reduced, a low-sodium diet can be resumed.

3. Exercise the body to strengthen the constitution. Avoidance of overstrain and too much sexual activity are effective in treating the disease.

37. RETENTION OF URINE

Brief introduction

Retention of urine is a condition manifested by difficult urination. The mild case refers to difficulty in urination and dripping of urine, while the severe case refers to failure in urination. The relevant disease is urinary retention.

Aetiology and pathogenesis

The location of this disease is in the Bladder. It is usually caused by Damp Heat accumulation, Liver Qi stagnation, substantial obstruction and Kidney deficiency.

Syndrome differentiation

It is manifested by difficult urination and distending pain in the lower abdomen.

1. **Damp Heat accumulation in the Bladder**: Scanty urine, distension in the lower abdomen, bitter taste and sticky sensation in the mouth, thirst without desire to drink, a sense of incomplete defecation, red tongue with yellow coating, deep and rapid pulse.

2. **Liver Qi stagnation**: Enuresis or difficult urination, distension in the lower abdomen, pain in the hypochondriac region, bitter taste in the mouth, thin white tongue coating, and wiry pulse.

3. **Substantial obstruction in the urinary passage**: Dribbling or weak urine stream, interrupted urination, or total urinary retention, distension and pain in the lower abdomen, purple tongue with spots, and choppy pulse.

4. **Kidney Qi deficiency**: Anuria or dribbling and weak urine stream, soreness and weakness of the lower back and knees, pale tongue, deep, thready and weak pulse.

Treatment

Body acupuncture

1. **Principles of treatment**

    Facilitate the Qi flow and unblock obstruction.

    *   *Damp Heat accumulation in the Bladder, Liver Qi stagnation, and substantial obstruction in the urinary passage*: Needling is applied with the reducing method.

- *Kidney Qi deficiency*: Both needling and moxibustion are applied with the reinforcing method.

2. **Prescription**

   Guanyuan (CV4), Sanyinjiao (SP6), Yinlingquan (SP9), Pangguangshu (BL28).

3. **Explanation**

   Guanyuan (CV4) and Sanyinjiao (SP6) are used to tonify the Spleen, Liver and Kidneys, and assist Qi transformation. Yinlingquan (SP9) is used to tonify the Spleen and promote urination. Pangguangshu (BL28) is used to assist Qi transformation.

4. **Modification**

   - *Damp Heat accumulation in the Bladder*: + Zhongji (CV3) and Xingjian (LR2) to clear Heat and drain Dampness.

   - *Liver Qi stagnation*: + Taichong (LR3) and Zhigou (TE6) to spread constrained Liver Qi.

   - *Substantial obstruction in the urinary passage*: + Xuehai (SP10) and Geshu (BL17) to transform stasis.

   - *Kidney Qi deficiency*: + Guanyuan (CV4), Shenshu (BL23) and Taixi (KI3) to tonify the Kidney and promote urination.

5. **Manipulation**

   Zhongji (CV3) is needled with the pinpoint downward. This point should not be needled deeply to avoid pricking the Bladder. The routine method is used on the rest of the points.

Other therapies

1. **Umbilicus therapy**

   Stir-bake some salt until it turns crisp, put it into the umbilicus when it becomes cool, and then add two pieces of Congbai (*Bulbus Allii Fistulosi*) cake on the salt. Finally, moxa cone is applied on the cake. The treatment continues until the patient is able to urinate.

2. **Auricular acupuncture**

   Points: Bladder (CO9), Kidney (CO10), Triple Burner (CO17) and Urethra (HX3). Each time 1–3 points are selected and needled with medium stimulation. Or Vaccaria seeds are applied to auricular points.

3. **Electroacupuncture**

   Weidao (GB28) on both sides is needled with the pinpoint towards Qugu (CV2). It is needled horizontally 2–3 cun. The electricity is attached to the needles for 40–60 minutes.

Notes

1. Acupuncture and moxibustion can produce satisfying effects for this disease. Combined treatment of the primary disease will be needed at the same time.

2. The patient who suffers from this disease is usually suffering from mental stress at the same time. During treatment, let him (her) contract and relax abdominal muscles.

3. For retention of urine accompanied with asthma and coma, the combined treatment is necessary.

38. URINATION DISTURBANCE

Brief introduction

Urination disturbance refers to urgency, increased frequency, oliguria, painful urination, spasmodic pain in the lower abdomen. This condition includes acute urinary tract infection, urinary calculus, urinary tuberculosis, tumour, prostatitis, cystitis, and chyluria.

Aetiology and pathogenesis

The impaired parts are the Bladder and Kidneys, often involving the Spleen and Liver. The causes of this disease are retention of Damp Heat in the Lower Burner and obstruction of Qi activities in the Bladder, Kidney deficiency, or Yin deficiency with empty Fire.

Syndrome differentiation

The main manifestations are urgency, increased frequency, oliguria, painful urination, spasmodic pain in the lower abdomen.

1. **Dysuria caused by Heat**: Frequent urination with burning pricking pain, yellow and red urine, distending pain in the lower abdomen, aversion to cold, fever, bitter taste in the mouth, nausea, vomiting, yellow greasy tongue coating, slippery and rapid pulse.

2. **Dysuria caused by calculi**: Difficult urination with sand or stones in the urine, urgent spasmodic pain in the urethra while urinating midstream, spasmodic pain in the lower abdomen, urine mixed with Blood, red tongue with thin coating, wiry and rapid pulse.

3. **Painful urination with Blood**: Frequent urination with burning, pricking pain, red urine containing blood clots, fever, irritability, red tongue with yellow coating, wiry and choppy pulse.

4. **Dysuria caused by Qi dysfunction**: Difficulty in urinating and distension of the lower abdomen, thin white tongue coating, deep and wiry pulse.

5. **Dysuria with milky urine**: Turbid, milky and oily urine, possibly with clots, difficult urination accompanied by burning and pricking pain, red tongue with yellow greasy coating, slippery and rapid pulse.

6. **Dysuria caused by overstrain**: Difficult urination with continuous dribbling exacerbated by exertion, soreness and weakness of the lower back and knees, fatigue, lassitude, pale tongue and weak pulse.

Treatment
Body acupuncture

1. **Principles of treatment**

   Clear Heat and drain Dampness, unblock urinary obstruction, improve the movement of Qi, and strengthen the Spleen and benefit the Qi. For deficiency type, needling is applied with the reinforcing method, while for excess type, needling is applied with the reducing method.

2. **Prescription**

   Points of the Spleen Meridian of Foot-Taiyin together with Back-Shu and Front-Mu points of the Bladder are selected as the principal points. Zhongji (CV3), Pangguangshu (BL28), Sanyinjiao (SP6), Yinlingquan (SP9).

3. **Explanation**

   Pangguangshu (BL28), the Back-Shu point and Zhongji (CV3), the Front-Mu point of the Bladder are used in the Shu-Mu combination of the prescription to promote Qi activity of the Bladder. Yinlingquan (SP9), the He-Sea point of the Spleen Meridian of Hand-Taiyin and Sanyijiao (SP6), the Crossing point of the Spleen, Liver and Kidney Meridian, are used to promote urination.

4. **Modification**

- *Dysuria caused by Heat*: + Xingjian (LR2).
- *Dysuria caused by calculi*: + Zhibian (BL54), Shuidao (ST28) and Weiyang (BL39).
- *Dysuria caused by Qi dysfunction*: + Ganshu (BL18) and Taichong (LR3).
- *Painful urination with Blood*: + Xuehai (SP10) and Geshu (BL17).
- *Dysuria with milky urine*: + Qihai (CV6) and Zusanli (ST36).
- *Dysuria caused by overstrain*: + Pishu (BL20), Shenshu (BL23), Guanyuan (CV4) and Zusanli (ST36).

5. **Manipulation**

   Zhongji (CV3) is needled after urination. It should not be needled deeply to avoid pricking the Bladder. For acute cases, the treatment is given 1–2 times a day. For chronic cases, the treatment is given once a day or once every other day.

Other therapies

1. **Auricular acupuncture**

   Points: Bladder (CO9), Kidney (CO10), Sympathetic Nerve (AH6a) and Adrenal Gland (TG2p). Each time 2–4 points are selected and needled with strong stimulation.

2. **Electroacupuncture**

   Shenshu (BL23) and Sanyinjiao (SP6) are selected. After the needling sensation is felt, the high frequency pulse current is attached to the needles for 5–10 minutes.

3. **Cutaneous needle**

   Tap on Sanyinjiao (SP6), Ququan (LR8), Guanyuan (CV4), Qugu (CV2), Guilai (ST29), Shuidao (ST28), inguinal region and Jiaji (EX-B2) (L3-L4) until the skin becomes red or bleeds slightly.

Notes

1. In the acute stage, acupuncture and moxibustion can produce an immediate effect.

2. Patients suffering dysuria caused by calculi should drink more water and exercise the body to strengthen their constitution. If there is renal dysfunction, combined treatment will be needed.

3. For dysuria with milky urine and dysuria caused by overstrain, combined treatment with Chinese herbs will be necessary.

39. INCONTINENCE OF URINE

Brief introduction

Incontinence of urine refers to any involuntary leakage of urine. There are five major categories of incontinence of urine: overflow, urgent, functional, stress and reflex. Overflow incontinence occurs when the patient's Bladder is always full so that it frequently leaks urine. Weak Bladder muscles, resulting in incomplete emptying of the Bladder, or a blocked urethra can cause this type of incontinence. Functional incontinence occurs when a person recognizes the need to urinate, but cannot physically make it to the bathroom in time due to limited mobility. The urine discharge may be more than usual. Urgent incontinence is involuntary loss of urine occurring for no apparent reason while suddenly feeling the need or urge to urinate. The most common cause of urgent incontinence is involuntary and inappropriate detrusor muscle contractions. Stress urinary incontinence is due, essentially, to insufficient strength of the pelvic floor muscles. It is the discharge of small amounts of urine associated with coughing, laughing, sneezing, exercising or other movements that increase intra-abdominal pressure and thus increase pressure on the Bladder. Reflex incontinence is losing control of Bladder without warning. This kind of patient typically suffers from neurological impairment.

Aetiology and pathogenesis

It is mainly caused by deficiency of the Kidney Qi with the inability of the Bladder to restrain the urine discharge. The retention of Damp Heat and Blood stasis in the Bladder also can cause this disease.

Syndrome differentiation

This refers to any involuntary leakage of urine. It may be associated with coughing, laughing, sneezing, exercising or other movements.

1. **Kidney Qi deficiency**: Urinary incontinence, lassitude, cold intolerance, soreness and weakness of the lower back and knees, weakness of the feet, pale tongue with thin coating, deep, thready and weak pulse.

2. **Qi deficiency of Spleen and Lung**: Urinary incontinence may be exacerbated by cough, urinary urgency, distension and heaviness in the lower abdomen, pale complexion, short breath, pale tongue, soft and weak pulse.

3. **Damp-Heat accumulation in the Bladder**: Urinary incontinence, frequent urination with burning sensation, red tongue with yellow greasy coating, thin, slippery and rapid pulse.

4. **Substantial obstruction in the urinary passage**: Urinary incontinence, distension and pain in the lower abdomen, purple tongue with spots, thin coating and choppy pulse.

Treatment
Body acupuncture

1. **Principles of treatment**
   - *Kidney Qi deficiency and Qi deficiency of Spleen and Lung*: Both needling and moxibustion are applied with the reinforcing method to tonify Qi.

   - *Damp Heat accumulation in the Bladder and substantial obstruction in the urinary passage*: Needling is applied with the reducing method to clear Heat, drain Dampness and transform stasis.

2. **Prescription**

   The Back-Shu and Front-Mu points of the Kidney and Bladder Meridians are selected as the principal points. Zhongji (CV3), Pangguangshu (BL28), Shenshu (BL23), Sanyinjiao (SP6).

3. **Explanation**

   Pangguangshu (BL28), the Back-Shu point and Zhongji (CV3), the Front-Mu point of the Bladder Meridian are used in the Shu-Mu combination of the prescription to promote Qi activity of the Bladder. Shenshu (BL23) is applied to tonify the Kidneys. Sanyijiao (SP6), the Crossing point of the Spleen, Liver and Kidney Meridians, are used to regulate Qi of the Spleen, Liver and Kidneys.

4. **Modification**
   - *Kidney Qi deficiency*: + Guanyuan (CV4) and Mingmen (GV4) to tonify the Kidney.

   - *Qi deficiency of Spleen and Lung*: + Feishu (BL13), Pishu (BL20) and Zusanli (ST36) to tonify the Spleen and Lung.

- *Damp Heat accumulation in the Bladder:* + Yinlingquan (SP9) and Xingjian (LR2) to clear Heat and drain Dampness.

- *Substantial obstruction in the urinary passage:* + Ciliao (BL32) and Taichong (LR3) to transform stasis.

5. **Manipulation**

   Zhongji (CV3) and Guanyuan (CV4) are needled with the pinpoint downward. Feishu (BL13) and Pishu (BL20) should not be needled perpendicularly and deeply. Moxibustion is applied on Guanyuan (CV4) and Mingmen (GV4). The routine method is used on the rest of the points.

Other therapies

1. **Auricular acupuncture**

   Points: Bladder (CO9), Kidney (CO10) and Urethra (HX3) are needled, or Vaccaria seeds are applied to auricular points.

2. **Electroacupuncture**

   Qihai (CV6), Guanyuan (CV4), Zhongji (CV3), Zusanli (ST36) and Sanyinjiao (SP6) are selected. When inserting the needle into the points on the abdomen, the needling sensation should transmit to the perineum. The disperse and dense wave electricity is attached to the needles for 30 minutes. The treatment is given once or twice a day.

Notes

1. Acupuncture can produce immediate effects for this disease. The combined treatment of the primary disease is needed.

2. The patient should exercise the body to strengthen the constitution.

40. SEMINAL EMISSION

Brief introduction

Seminal emission refers to involuntary discharge of seminal fluid without sexual intercourse. Seminal emission during sleep is referred to as nocturnal emission, while that during dream-disturbed sleep or when being awake is termed as spontaneous emission. It may be considered physiologically normal if it occurs 2–4 times a month. In Western medicine, it may be present in sexual disorder, prostatitis, neurasthenia and seminal vesiculitis.

Aetiology and pathogenesis

It is mainly caused by Kidney deficiency and weakness of the seminal gate. The Kidney Qi must be strong enough in order to store Essence. Deficiency of Kidney Qi is usually closely relevant to indulgence in sexual activities, mental strain, improper diet, and downward flow of Damp Heat, etc.

Syndrome differentiation

Frequent seminal emission of more than twice a weak, accompanied by dizziness, lassitude, fatigue, soreness and weakness of the lower back and knees, etc.

1. **Kidney deficiency**: Frequent nocturnal emission, possibly spermatorrhoea, pale complexion, dizziness, blurred vision, tinnitus, soreness and weakness of the lower back and knees, cold limbs, pale tongue with thin white coating, deep, thready and weak pulse.

2. **Deficiency of the Spleen and Heart**: Seminal emission that occurs when fatigued, palpitations, insomnia, forgetfulness, sallow complexion, weakness of the limbs, poor appetite, loose stools, pale tongue with thin coating, thready and weak pulse.

3. **Hyperactivity of Fire due to Yin deficiency**: Nocturnal emission with erotic dreams, insomnia, dizziness, tinnitus, blurred vision, palpitations, fatigue, lassitude, scanty yellow urine, red tongue with scanty coating, thready and rapid pulse.

4. **Damp Heat infusing downwards**: Frequent seminal emission with erotic dreams, dark turbid urine, burning sensation during urination, bitter taste in the mouth, red tongue with yellow greasy coating, slippery and rapid pulse.

Treatment
Body acupuncture

1. **Principles of treatment**
   - *Kidney deficiency and deficiency of the Spleen and Heart*: Both needling and moxibustion are applied with the reinforcing method to tonify the Spleen and Heart.
   - *Hyperactivity of Fire due to Yin deficiency*: Needling is applied with reinforcing or even method to nourish the Yin.
   - *Damp Heat infusing downwards*: Needling is applied with the reducing method to clear Heat and drain Dampness.

2. **Prescription**

Points of the Conception Vessel and the Bladder Meridian of Foot-Taiyang are selected as principal points. Huiyin (CV1), Guanyuan (CV4), Shenshu (BL23), Ciliao (BL32), Sanyinjiao (SP6).

3. **Explanation**

Huiyin (CV1), the Crossing point of the Governor Vessel and Conception Vessel, is applied to coordinate Yin and Yang. Guanyuan (CV4) is used to nourish Kidney Qi. Ciliao (BL32) and Shenshu (BL23) are applied to tonify the Kidneys and secure the Essence. Sanyinjiao (SP6), the Crossing point of the Spleen, Liver and Kidney Meridians, are used to regulate Qi of the Spleen, Liver and Kidneys.

4. **Modification**

- *Kidney deficiency*: + Zhishi (BL52) and Taixi (KI3) to tonify the Kidneys and secure the Essence.

- *Deficiency of the Spleen and Heart*: + Xinshu (BL15) and Pishu (BL20) to tonify the Heart and Spleen.

- *Hyperactivity of Fire due to Yin deficiency*: + Taixi (KI3) and Shenmen (HT7) to clear Heat and nourish the Yin.

- *Damp Heat infusing downwards*: + Zhongji (CV3) and Yinlingquan (SP9) to clear Heat and drain Dampness.

5. **Manipulation**

Huiyin (CV1) is needled deeply. Ciliao (BL32) should be needled into the posterior sacral foramen. The routine method is used on the rest of the points.

Other therapies

1. **Auricular acupuncture**

Points: Internal Genitalia (TF2), Endocrine (CO18), Ear-Shenmen (TF4), Liver (CO12) and Kidney (CO10). Each time 2–4 points are selected and needled with medium stimulation, or embedded with needles, or Vaccaria seeds are applied to auricular points.

2. **Cutaneous needle**

Guanyuan (CV4), Zhongji (CV3), Sanyinjiao (SP6), Taixi (KI3), Xinshu (BL15), Shenshu (BL23) and Zhishi (BL52), or Jiaji (EX-B2) on the lumbosacral region, and points of the Spleen, Liver and Kidney Meridians below the knee joint are selected. Tap on these points until the skin becomes slightly red. The treatment is given once every night.

3. **Point injection**

   Guanyuan (CV4), Zhongji (CV3) and Zhishi (BL52) are selected. The injection of Danggui (当归 *Radix Angelicae Sinensis*) and the injection of vitamin B$_1$ are used. Each point is injected with 0.5–1ml of liquid. The needling sensation should transmit to the perineum.

4. **Catgut implantation**

   Guanyuan (CV4), Zhongji (CV3), Shenshu (BL23) and Sanyinjiao (SP6) are selected. Each time 2 points are selected. Embed with surgical catgut. The treatment is given once or twice every month.

Notes

1. Acupuncture can produce satisfactory effects for this disease. The combined treatment of the primary disease is needed.

2. Mostly it is a kind of functional disease.

3. Avoidance of too much sexual activity is effective in treating the disease.

4. The patient who suffers from this disease should sleep on his side.

41. IMPOTENCE

Brief introduction

Impotence is a disease manifesting with the inability to achieve or maintain an erection. It is one of the major reasons for sexual dissatisfaction. In Western medicine, impotence can occur in male sexual disorders or in some chronic diseases.

Aetiology and pathogenesis

The disease is usually attributive to excessive sexual activities and masturbation. It may also be caused by anxiety, fear, worry and fright. In some cases, it is due to the downward movement of Damp Heat. The Damp Heat drives downward to make the penis unable to become erect, resulting in impotence.

Syndrome differentiation

Inability to achieve or maintain an erection.

1. **Failure of the Fire in the gate of vitality**: Impotence, pale complexion, soreness and weakness of the lower back and knees, dizziness, blurred vision, lassitude, cold intolerance, cold limbs, tinnitus, pale tongue with white coating, deep and thready pulse.

2. **Deficiency of the Heart and Spleen**: Impotence, sallow complexion, poor appetite, lassitude, insomnia, forgetfulness, timidity, being suspicious, palpitations, pale tongue with thin white coating, thready and weak pulse.

3. **Shock and fear injuring the Kidneys**: Impotence, depression, anxiety, palpitations, timidity, insomnia, red tongue with thin white coating, thready and wiry pulse.

4. **Downward flow of Damp Heat**: Impotence, Damp and smelly scrotum, yellow urine, red tongue with yellow greasy coating, slippery and rapid pulse.

Treatment

Body acupuncture

1. **Principles of treatment**

    - *Failure of the Fire in the gate of vitality*: Both needling and moxibustion are applied with the reinforcing method to tonify the Kidneys and fortify the Yang.

    - *Deficiency of the Heart and Spleen*: Both needling and moxibustion are applied with the reinforcing method to tonify the Heart and Spleen.

    - *Shock and fear injuring the Kidneys*: Needling is applied with reinforcing or even method to augment the Kidney and quiet the Mind.

    - *Damp Heat infusing downwards*: Needling is applied with the reducing method to clear Heat and drain Dampness.

2. **Prescription**

    The points of the Conception Vessel are selected as the principal points. Guanyuan (CV4), Zhongji (CV3), Shenshu (BL23), Sanyinjiao (SP6).

3. **Explanation**

    Guanyuan (CV4) is the meeting point of the Conception Vessel and the Spleen, Liver and Kidney Meridians. It is used to promote the primary Qi and invigorate the Kidney function. Shenshu (BL23) is applied to strengthen the Kidney Yang. Sanyinjiao (SP6) is good for activating the Qi of the Spleen and eliminating the Damp Heat.

4. **Modification**

- *Failure of the Fire in the gate of vitality:* + Mingmen (GV4), Zhishi (BL52) and Qihai (CV6) to tonify the Kidneys and fortify the Yang.

- *Deficiency of the Heart and Spleen:* + Xinshu (BL15), Pishu (BL20) and Zusanli (ST36) to tonify the Heart and Spleen.

- *Shock and fear injuring the Kidneys:* + Mingmen (GV4), Baihui (GV20) and Shenmen (HT7) to augment the Kidneys and quieten the Mind.

- *Damp Heat infusing downwards:* + Yinlingquan (SP9), Yanglingquan (GB34) and Qugu (CV2) to clear Heat and drain Dampness.

5. **Manipulation**

Zhongji (CV3) and Guanyuan (CV4) are needled obliquely with the pinpoint downward. The needling sensation should transmit to the perineum. Moxibustion on Fuzi (附子 *Radix Aconiti Lateralis Preparata*) cake is applied on Qihai (GV4), Mingmen (GV4) and Zhishi (BL52). The routine method is used on the rest of the points.

Other therapies

1. **Auricular acupuncture**

   Points: External Genitalia (HX4), Internal Genitalia (TF2), Endocrine (CO18), Shenmen (TF4) and Kidney (CO10). Each time 2–4 points are selected and needled with medium stimulation, or embedded with needles, or Vaccaria seeds are applied to auricular points.

2. **Electroacupuncture**

   The selected points are Ciliao (BL32) and Zhibian (BL54) or Guanyuan (CV4) and Sanyinjiao (SP6). The disperse and dense wave electricity is attached to the needles for 20–30 minutes.

3. **Point injection**

   Guanyuan (CV4), Zhongji (CV3) and Shenshu (BL23) are selected. Each time 2 points are selected and injected with 150mg of the injection of vitamin B_1 with 0.1mg of vitamin B_{12} added in. The treatment is given once a day.

4. **Catgut implantation**

Guanyuan (CV4), Zhongji (CV3), Shenshu (BL23) and Sanyinjiao (SP6) are selected. Each time 1–3 points are selected. Embed with size zero surgical catgut. The treatment is given once or twice every month.

Notes

1. Acupuncture and moxibustion can produce satisfactory effects for this disease. The combined treatment of the primary disease is needed.

2. Mostly it is a type of functional disease. Massage is effective in treating this disease.

42. PROSPERMIA

Brief introduction

Prospermia refers to early ejaculation of semen at the beginning of sexual intercourse. In Western medicine, it can occur in male sexual disorder.

Aetiology and pathogenesis

The disease is usually attributive to excessive sexual activity and masturbation. It is due to the downward movement of Damp Heat. It may also be caused by Liver Qi stagnation, or mental strain impairs the Heart, Spleen and Kidneys.

Syndrome differentiation

Premature ejaculation at the beginning of sexual intercourse.

1. **Kidney deficiency**: Fatigue after ejaculation, soreness and weakness of the lower back and knees, hyposexuality, frequent urination, pale tongue with thin coating and weak pulse.

2. **Deficiency of the Spleen and Heart**: Sensation fatigue in the limbs, pale complexion, palpitations, insomnia, pale tongue with scanty coating, thready and weak pulse.

3. **Hyperactivity of Fire due to Yin deficiency**: Seminal emission, soreness and weakness of the lower back and knees, feverish sensation in the chest, palms and soles, hectic fever, night sweat, red tongue with scanty coating, thready and rapid pulse.

4. **Damp Heat in the Liver Meridian**: Damp pudendum, bitter taste in the mouth, distension and pain in the lower abdomen, yellow urine, red tongue with yellow greasy coating, wiry and rapid pulse.

5. **Liver Qi stagnation**: Depression, anxiety, discomfort in the lower abdomen, testes, chest stuffiness, sighing, insomnia, dream-disturbed sleep, red tongue with thin white coating and wiry pulse.

Treatment
Body acupuncture

1. **Principles of treatment**
   - *Kidney deficiency*: Both needling and moxibustion are applied with the reinforcing method to tonify the Kidneys and secure the Essence.
   - *Deficiency of the Spleen and Heart*: Both needling and moxibustion are applied with the reinforcing method to tonify the Heart and Spleen.
   - *Hyperactivity of Fire due to Yin deficiency*: Needling is applied with mild reinforcing and the reducing method to clear Heat and nourish the Yin.
   - *Damp Heat in the Liver Meridian and Liver Qi stagnation*: Needling is applied with the reducing method to clear Heat and spread constrained Liver Qi.

2. **Prescription**

   Guanyuan (CV4), Sanyinjiao (SP6), Shenshu (BL23), Jinggong (Extra).

3. **Explanation**

   Guanyuan (CV4) and Sanyinjiao (SP6) are both meeting points of the Spleen, Liver and Kidney Meridians. They are used to tonify the Liver, Spleen and Kidneys, and secure the Essence. Shenshu (BL23), the Back-Shu point of the Kidney Meridian, is applied to tonify the Kidneys and secure the Essence.

4. **Modification**
   - *Kidney deficiency*: + Mingmen (GV4) and Taixi (KI3) to tonify the Kidneys and secure the Essence.
   - *Deficiency of the Spleen and Heart*: + Xinshu (BL15) and Pishu (BL20) to tonify the Heart and Spleen.
   - *Hyperactivity of Fire due to Yin deficiency*: + Taixi (KI3) and Zhaohai (KI6) to clear Heat and nourish the Yin.

- *Damp Heat in the Liver meridian*: + Yinlingquan (SP9) and Xingjian (LR2) to clear Heat and drain Dampness.

- *Liver Qi stagnation*: + Taichong (LR3) and Xingjian (LR2) to spread constrained Liver Qi.

5. **Manipulation**

The routine method is used on all the points. For Kidney deficiency, moxibustion is applied on Guanyuan (CV4), Shenshu (BL23) and Mingmen (GV4).

Other therapies

1. **Auricular acupuncture**

Points: External Genitalia (HX4), Internal Genitalia (TF2), Endocrine (CO18), Ear-Shenmen (TF4) and Heart (CO15). Each time 2–4 points are selected and needled with medium stimulation, or embedded with needles, or Vaccaria seeds are applied to auricular points.

2. **Cutaneous needle**

Tap on Jiaji (EX-B2) on the neck and lumbosacral region, lower abdomen, inguinal region and root of penis with mild or medium stimulation (strong stimulation on the root of penis), until the skin becomes slightly red.

3. **Point application**

Grind 10g Lufengfang (露蜂房 *Nidus Vespae*) and 10g Baizhi (白芷 *Radix Angelicae Dahuricae*) into powder, mix it with vinegar to make paste, put the paste into umbilicus, fix it with adhesive tape before sleep. Remove it next morning. The treatment is given once a day.

Notes

1. The effect of acupuncture and moxibustion on this disease is certain.

2. Avoidance of excessive sexual activity is essential.

3. Being confident is effective in treating this disease.

43. STERILITY

Brief introduction

Sterility refers to the inability to conceive more than 2 years after marriage with a normal sexual life and without contraception. This section refers only to male sterility.

Aetiology and pathogenesis

Sterility is related to the Kidneys, Heart, Liver and Spleen. The main causes of this disease are insufficiency of Kidney Essence, Qi and Blood deficiency, Qi stagnation and Blood stasis and downward flow of Damp Heat.

Syndrome differentiation

Inability to conceive more than 2 years after marriage with normal sexual life and without contraception.

1. **Insufficiency of Kidney Essence**: Oligospermia, asthenospermia, lassitude, soreness and weakness of the lower back and knees, dizziness, tinnitus, thready and weak pulse.

2. **Kidney Yang deficiency**: Soreness of the lower back, cold intolerance, cold limbs, pale complexion, pale tongue with white coating, deep and thready pulse.

3. **Qi and Blood deficiency**: Sallow complexion, shortness of breath, lassitude, fatigue, palpitations, insomnia, dizziness, vertigo, poor appetite, and loose stools, and pale tongue, deep, thready and weak pulse.

4. **Qi stagnation and Blood stasis**: Testicular distension, varicocele, chest distress, purple tongue, deep and wiry pulse.

5. **Damp Heat infusing downwards**: Asthenospermia, may be accompanied by seminal emission, scanty urine, bitter taste in the mouth, dry throat, red tongue with yellow greasy coating, slippery and rapid pulse.

Treatment

Body acupuncture

1. **Principles of treatment**

    - *Insufficiency of Kidney Essence, Kidney Yang deficiency and Qi and Blood deficiency*: Both needling and moxibustion are applied with the reinforcing method to tonify Qi and replenish Blood, tonify the Kidneys.

    - *Qi stagnation and Blood stasis and Damp Heat infusing downwards*: Needling is applied with the reducing method to activate Blood and move Qi, clear Heat and drain Dampness.

2. **Prescription**

    The points of the Conception Vessel and the Bladder Meridian of Foot-Shaoyang are selected as the principal points. Guanyuan (CV4), Qihai (CV6), Sanyinjiao (SP6), Shenshu (BL23), Ciliao (BL32), Zhibian (BL54), Zusanli (ST36).

3. **Explanation**

    Qihai (CV6), Guanyuan (CV4) and Sanyinjiao (SP6) are the meeting points of the Spleen, Liver and Kidney Meridians. They are used to tonify the Liver, Spleen and Kidneys. Shenshu (BL23), Ciliao (BL32) and Zhibian (BL54) are applied to tonify the Kidneys. Zusanli (ST36) is applied to tonify the Spleen and Stomach.

4. **Modification**

    - *Insufficiency of Kidney Essence*: + Taixi (KI3) to tonify the Kidneys.

    - *Kidney Yang deficiency*: + Guanyuan (CV4) and Shenque (CV8) to tonify the Yang.

    - *Qi and Blood deficiency*: + Pishu (BL20) and Weishu (BL21) to tonify Qi and Blood.

    - *Palpitations and insomnia*: + Shenmen (HT7) and Neiguan (PC6) to nourish the Heart to tranquillize.

    - *Qi stagnation and Blood stasis*: + Taichong (LR3) and Geshu (BL17) to activate Blood and move Qi.

    - *Damp Heat infusing downwards*: + Yinlingquan (SP9) and Zhongji (CV3) to clear Heat and drain Dampness.

5. **Manipulation**

Ciliao (BL32) and Zhibian (BL54) are needled deeply with the pinpoint towards the perineum. The needling sensation should transmit to the perineum. For insufficiency of Kidney Essence, Kidney Yang deficiency, as well as Qi and Blood deficiency, moxibustion is applied on Qihai (GV4), Guanyuan (CV4) and Shenshu (BL23). The routine method is used on the rest of the points.

Other therapies

1. **Intradermal needle**

   Guanyuan (CV4) and Sanyinjiao (SP6) are selected. Embed the thumbtack-type needle into the points, then fix it with a piece of adhesive tape. The treatment is given once every 1–2 days.

2. **Auricular acupuncture**

   Points: External Genitalia (HX4), Internal Genitalia (TF2), Endocrine (CO18) and Kidney (CO10) are selected and needled with medium stimulation, or Vaccaria seeds are applied to auricular points.

3. **Point injection**

   Zusanli (ST36), Guanyuan (CV4), Shenshu (BL23) and Sanyinjiao (SP6) are selected. Each time 2 points are selected and injected with 500 units of Choriogonadotropin. The treatment is given once a day.

Notes

1. Acupuncture and moxibustion can produce satisfactory effects for this disease.

2. Avoidance of smoking and alcohol is effective in treating the disease.

3. Avoidance of excessive sexual activity is essential.

44. DIABETES

Brief introduction

Diabetes is a common endocrinal metabolic disease. In TCM, diabetes is known as Xiao Ke, which means loss of weight and thirst. Clinically, polydipsia, polyphagia, polyuria, emaciation, glycosuria and increase of blood sugar concentration are the main manifestations. The pathological changes are caused by the absolute or relative insufficiency of insulin secretion, leading to metabolic disturbance of protein and fat imbalance. Patients with this condition are mostly of middle and old age. It is more common in males than females.

Aetiology and pathogenesis

Diabetes has a principal pathogenesis of Yin deficiency as the root, and Heat Dryness as the branch. The major affected organs include the Lungs, Stomach and Kidneys. Lung Yin deficiency with Heat Dryness will lead to polydipsia and increased fluid intake. Excess Stomach Heat will lead to excessive hunger and polyphagia. Kidney Yin deficiency will lead to increased fluid intake and polyuria. Yin deficiency and Heat Dryness influence and aggravate each other.

Syndrome differentiation

There are no symptoms in the early stage. Clinically, polydipsia, polyphagia, polyuria, emaciation are the main manifestations at the later stage. There are some complications and concomitant diseases, such as cerebral arteriosclerosis, hypertension, coronary heart disease, infection of the urinary tract, retinitis, cataract, skin itching, numbness of limbs, infection, tuberculosis, etc. Ketoacidosis and hyperosmotic nonketotic coma will occur in severe cases.

1. **Consumption of fluid by Lung Heat**: Dry mouth and tongue, irritability, frequent drinking, red edge to the tongue with thin yellow coating, flooding and rapid pulse.

2. **Excess Stomach Heat**: Polyphagia, propensity to hunger, restlessness, fever, profuse sweating, emaciation, dry stools, profuse urine, dry yellow tongue coating, slippery and rapid pulse.

3. **Kidney Yin deficiency**: Profuse and frequent urination, turbid urine, thirst and polydipsia, dizziness, blurred vision, red cheeks, vexation, seminal emission, soreness and weakness of the lower back and knees, dry skin, general pruritus, red tongue with scanty coating, thready and rapid pulse.

4. **Deficiency of both the Yin and Yang**: Polyuria, turbid urine, Dryness of earlobe, soreness and weakness of the lower back and knees, cold limbs, sexual hypoaesthesia, dry tongue with white coating, deep, thready and weak pulse.

Treatment

Body acupuncture

1. **Principles of treatment**

   - *Consumption of fluid by Lung Heat*: Needling is applied with reducing or even method to clear Heat, moisten the Lungs, generate fluid and alleviate thirst.

   - *Excess Stomach Heat*: Needling is applied with reducing or even method to clear Heat from the Stomach, and nourish the Yin.

   - *Kidney Yin deficiency*: Needling and moxibustion are applied with the reinforcing method to nourish the Yin and consolidate the Kidneys.

   - *Deficiency of both Yin and Yang*: Needling and moxibustion are applied with the reinforcing method to warm the Yang, nourish the Yin and consolidate the Kidneys.

2. **Prescription**

   Back-Shu points are selected as principal points. Feishu (BL13), Pishu (BL20), Weishu (BL21), Shenshu (BL23), Weiwanxiashu (EX-B3), Zusanli (ST36), Sanyinjiao (SP6), Taixi (KI3).

3. **Explanation**

   Feishu (BL13) is applied to clear Heat, moisten the Lungs, generate fluid and alleviate thirst. Pishu (BL20), Weishu (BL21), Zusanli (ST36) and Sanyinjiao (SP6) are applied to clear Heat from the Stomach, and nourish the Yin. Shenshu (BL23) and Taixi (KI3) are applied to nourish the Yin and consolidate the Kidneys. Weiwanxiashu (EX-B3) is a well-established point for treating this disease.

4. **Modification**

   - *Lung Heat injuring the fluid*: + Taiyuan (LU9) and Shaofu (HT8) to clear Heat.

   - *Excess Stomach Heat*: + Zhongwan (CV12) and Neiting (LR2) to clear Heat from the Stomach.

   - *Kidney Yin deficiency*: + Taichong (LR3) and Zhaohai (KI6) to nourish the Yin and consolidate the Kidneys.

   - *Deficiency of both the Yin and Yang*: + Yingu (KI10), Qihai (CV6) and Mingmen (GV4) to warm the Yang, nourish the Yin and consolidate the Kidneys.

- *Palpitations*: + Neiguan (PC6) and Xinshu (BL15) to nourish the Heart to tranquillize.

- *Insomnia*: + Shenmen (HT7) and Baihui (GV20) to nourish the Heart to tranquillize.

- *Blurred vision*: + Taichong (LR3) and Guangming (GB37) to clear Liver Heat and improve vision.

- *Skin itching*: + Fengshi (GB31), Xuehai (SP10) and Ligou (LR5) to cool the Blood and moisten Dryness.

- *Numbness of the limbs*: + Baxie (EX-UE9) and Bafeng (EX-LE10) to unblock the meridians and activate collaterals.

5. **Manipulation**

   Feishu (BL13), Xinshu (BL15), Pishu (BL20), Weishu (BL21), Shenshu (BL23), and Weiwanxiashu (EX-B3) should not be needled perpendicularly and deeply to avoid pricking the organs. The routine method is used on the rest of the points.

Other therapies

1. **Auricular acupuncture**

   Points: Pancreas and Gallbladder (CO11), Endocrine (CO18), Kidney (CO10), Triple Burner (CO17), Heart (CO15), Liver (CO12), Ear-Shenmen (TF4) and Groove of the Back Auricle (PS) are selected. Each time 2–4 points are selected and needled with mild stimulation. Or the electricity is attached to the needles. Or Vaccaria seeds are applied to auricular points.

2. **Cutaneous needle**

   Tap on the back, from T3 to L2 with mild or medium stimulation. The treatment is given once every other day.

3. **Point injection**

   Feishu (BL13), Xinshu (BL15), Pishu (BL20), Weishu (BL21), Shenshu (BL23), Weiwanxiashu (EX-B3), Zusanli (ST36) and Sanyinjiao (SP6) are selected. Each time 2–4 points are selected. Each point is injected with 0.5–2ml of the Danggui (当归 *Radix Angelicae Sinensis*) injection, Huangqi (黄芪 *Radix Astragali seu Hedysari*) injection or insulin. The treatment is given once every other day.

Notes

1. In the early stage of this disease, acupuncture and moxibustion can produce satisfactory results. For chronic cases, combined treatment will be needed.

2. Patients who suffer from this disease are more likely to have infection, so strict disinfection measures should be taken during treatment.

3. Proper diet is effective in treating the disease.

4. If ketoacidosis and hyperosmotic nonketotic coma occur in severe cases, combined treatment with Western medicine is necessary.

45. GOITRE

Brief introduction

Goitre is manifested as swelling bilateral to the Adam's Apple in the neck, with neither pain nor ulceration, which gets large gradually and is difficult to remove. It is a common disease in the plateau and mountain regions and predominates in females of middle and young age. Simple goitre, thyroiditis, thyroid adenoma and hyperthyroidism in Western medicine, can be treated in reference to this disease.

Aetiology and pathogenesis

Low quality of the Water in the living conditions injures the Spleen and Stomach, leading to retention of Damp and Phlegm. Emotional dysfunction results in depression and stagnation of Qi and Phlegm. Constitutional Yin deficiency steams Body Fluids into Phlegm, Qi and Phlegm stagnation forms Blood stagnation gradually. The stagnation of Qi, Phlegm and stasis in the neck region results in this disease. The disease is localized bilaterally in the anterior part of the neck, which is related to the Liver, Heart, Spleen, Stomach and Kidneys, especially to the Liver.

Syndrome differentiation

Slow onset, gradual thickening, swelling or mass forming in the neck, normal skin colour, neither pain nor ulceration, being movable when swallowing, difficulty in removing the growth. General symptoms do not present in the early stages and excessive Fire due to Yin deficiency or deficiency of Qi and Yin is commonly seen in later stages.

1. **Stagnation of Qi and Phlegm**: Swelling of the neck with unclear borders, normal skin colour, and swelling alleviated by joy and worsened by anger; thin and sticky tongue coating, string-taut and rolling pulse.

2. **Excessive Fire due to Yin deficiency**: Mild or moderate swelling of the neck, irritability, hot temper, feverish sensation in palms, soles and chest, swelling of eyes, exophthalmos; red tongue with little coating, string-taut, thready and rapid pulse.

3. **Deficiency of Qi and Yin**: Chronic goitre, aggravation of swelling, apparent thickening or mass forming in the neck, lassitude, chest distress, shortness of breath, dyspnoea, hoarse voice; thin and sticky tongue coating, thready and string-taut pulse.

Treatment

Body acupuncture

1. **Principles of treatment**

    - *Stagnation of Qi and Phlegm*: Smooth Liver Qi, remove stagnation and resolve Phlegm. Acupuncture is applied only with reducing technique.

    - *Excessive Fire due to Yin deficiency*: Nourish Yin and reduce Fire, regulate Qi circulation to resolve Phlegm. Acupuncture is the chief therapy with even-needling technique.

2. **Prescription**

    Main points are selected from the neck region and acupoints of the Conception Vessel and Bladder Meridian of Foot-Yangming. Local points of the affected area: Tiantu (CV22), Tanzhong (CV17), Hegu (LI4), Zusanli (ST36), Sanyinjiao (SP6), Fenglong (ST40).

3. **Explanation**

    Tiantu (CV22) is the local point of goitre in the throat region to promote local Qi circulation, reduce the reversed Qi, resolve Phlegm and shrink swelling. Tanzhong (CV17) and Hegu (LI4) are for promoting Qi and Blood circulation, resolving Phlegm and removing mass and swelling. Zusanli (ST36), Sanyinjiao (SP6) and Fenglong (ST40) are for strengthening the Spleen in transportation to resolve Phlegm and remove goitre.

4. **Modification**

    - *Stagnation of Qi and Phlegm*: + Taichong (LR3) and Neiguan (PC6) to pacify Liver Qi and resolve Phlegm.

- *Excessive Fire due to Yin deficiency*: + Taixi (KI3), Fuliu (KI7) and Yinxi (HT6) to nourish Yin and reduce Fire.

- *Deficiency of Qi and Yin*: + Guanyuan (CV4) and Zhaohai (KI6) to benefit Qi and nourish Blood.

- *Hoarse voice*: + Futu (LI18) and Lianquan (CV23) are added to nourish Yin and benefit the throat.

5. **Manipulation**

Perpendicular insertion is applied to Tiantu (CV22), 0.2–0.3 cun at first, then, the needle tip is downward and the needle is inserted along the posterior of the sternum, about 1–1.5 cun in depth. Surrounding acupuncture is applied in the affected area based on the size of goitre. 4 filiform needles of 1 cun are inserted around the cyst at 45 and 1 needle is inserted from the top to the base of the cyst. Needles are rotated, lifted and thrust in small amplitude, avoiding injury of the common carotid artery and recurrent laryngeal nerve. Futu (LI18) is punctured perpendicularly, 0.5–0.8 cun. For deficiency of Qi and Yin, moxibustion is applicable on Dazhui (GV14) and Guanyuan (CV4). Routine acupuncture technique is applied to other acupoints.

Other therapies

1. **Auricular acupuncture**

Points: Ear-Shenmen, Endocrine, Subcortex, Sympathetic, Antitragic apex, Neck. In each treatment, 2 or 3 points are selected and punctured by filiform needle. Needles are retained for 30 minutes. Needle-embedding or Vaccaria seeds can be applied to auricular points.

2. **Electroacupuncture**

Four Ashi points are selected in the local affected area. After the arrival of Qi, positive and negative electrodes of the apparatus are attached to the same sides respectively. Dense-disperse wave and moderate stimulation are applied for 20 to 30 minutes. The treatment is given once every 2 days.

3. **Cutaneous needle**

Repeated gentle tapping is applied to the locality of the goitre, bilateral sides from T5–11, bilateral Bladder Meridian of the spine as well as Yifeng (TE17), Jianjing (GB21), Quchi (LI11), Hegu (LI4), Zusanli (ST36) until the skin turns slightly red. The treatment is applied once every 2 days.

Notes

1. Acupuncture and moxibustion have good efficacy on simple goitre. The efficacy will be even better if iodine is administered in combination.

2. In areas where this disease is epidemic, apart from improving the quality of drinking water, it is advisable to provide iodinated table salt for group prevention until puberty. It is advised that patients eat iodine-containing food, such as kelp and seaweed. Iodine supplementation is especially important for teenagers at puberty and for women during pregnancy and lactation.

3. An operation should be considered if the thyroid glands are obviously swelling and there are symptoms of compression.

4. If the patient with hyperthyroidism has a high fever, vomiting and delirium, the probability of a hyperthyroidism crisis should be considered and comprehensive emergency measures must be taken, such as first aid treatment.

46. SIMPLE OBESITY

Brief introduction

Simple obesity is a condition in which actual body mass is over standard body mass by over 20% without any apparent endocrinal-metabolic reason, and with protein increase due to retention of water and sodium or muscular body excluded.

Aetiology and pathogenesis

This disease is related to the dysfunction of the Spleen, Stomach and Kidneys. Dysfunction of the Spleen and Stomach and deficiency of the Kidneys lead to excess or deficiency of Qi and Blood, and imbalance of Yin and Yang, resulting in obesity. Weakness of the Spleen and Stomach develops failure of transformation of Water and Damp, and thus Phlegm and turbidity are produced. Heat of the Stomach leads to excessive appetite, thus turbid fat is formed from essential parts of water and food. Insufficiency of primary Qi results in failure of Qi to promote water circulation, thus Body Fluids are stagnant and Phlegm is formed. Gradually, retention of Phlegm, Damp and turbid fat in the muscles and skin develops into obesity.

Syndrome differentiation

Simple obesity is manifested as even distribution of fat, fatty face and neck, thick nape region, big abdomen and lumbar region, big muscles in the buttocks and legs. Moderate obesity is commonly manifested as aversion to Heat, profuse sweating, susceptibility to fatigue, shortness of breath, dizziness, palpitations. Severe obesity is manifested as slow movement, chest distress, shortness of breath, even orthopnoea. Moderate and severe obesity are commonly complicated by hypertension, coronary heart disease, diabetes, gout, cholelithiasis, degenerative changes in joints, etc.

1. **Heat in the Stomach and intestine**: Constitutional obesity, solid muscle, excessive appetite and easy hunger, dry mouth, desire for drinks, aversion to Heat, profuse sweating, abdominal distension, constipation, scanty and yellow urine; red tongue, rolling and forceful pulse.

2. **Deficiency of the Spleen and Stomach**: Obesity of the face and neck, loose muscles, poor appetite, palpitations, shortness of breath, somnolence, dislike of speaking, loose stools, normal or scanty urine, general oedema; pale tongue with teeth marks on the border, thin and white coating; thready, retarded or deep slow pulse.

3. **Insufficiency of the Kidneys**: Obesity in the buttock region, lassitude, sweating after activity, aversion to cold, dizziness, soreness of lumbar region, irregular menstruation or impotence, premature ejaculation; pale and delicate tongue with teeth marks, thin and white coating; deep, thready and retarded pulse.

Treatment
Body acupuncture

1. **Principles of treatment**

   - *Heat in the Stomach and intestines*: Clear away Stomach Heat, promote circulation in the intestines. Only acupuncture is applied; reducing technique is used.

   - *Deficiency of the Spleen and Stomach*: Benefit Spleen Qi, resolve Phlegm and Damp.

   - *Insufficiency of genuine Yuan Qi*: Warm the Kidneys, strengthen Yang, and enhance the Spleen to resolve Damp. Acupuncture and moxibustion are applied together and reinforcing technique is used.

2. **Prescription**

Acupoints are selected chiefly from the Spleen Meridian of Foot-Taiyin and the Stomach Meridian of Foot-Yangming. Zhongwan (CV12), Tianshu (ST25), Daheng (SP15), Quchi (LI11), Zhigou (TE6), Neiting (ST44), Fenglong (ST40), Shangjuxu (ST37), Yinlingquan (SP9).

3. **Explanation**

Obesity is commonly related to dysfunction of the Spleen, Stomach and intestines. Zhongwan (CV12) is the Front-Mu point of the Stomach and the Influential point of the Fu organ. Quchi (LI11) is He-Sea point of the Large Intestine Meridian. Tianshu (ST25) is the Front-Mu point of the Large Intestine Meridian of Hand-Yangming. Shangjuxu (ST37) is the Inferior He-Sea point of the Large Intestine Meridian. All of these can promote circulation in the intestines, reduce the turbidity and fats. Daheng (SP15) can strengthen the Spleen to enhance transportation. Fenglong (ST40) and Yinlingquan (SP9) can benefit removal of Damp and resolve Phlegm. Zhigou (TE6) regulates the functions of the Triple Burner. Neiguan (ST44) can clear away Heat from the Stomach. All of these used in combination can strengthen the Spleen and Stomach, benefit the intestines, resolve Phlegm and remove fat.

4. **Modification**

- *Heat in the Stomach and intestines*: + Hegu (LI11) to reduce Heat from the Stomach and intestines.

- *Deficiency of the Spleen and Stomach*: + Pishu (BL20), Zusanli (ST36) to benefit the Spleen to resolve Damp.

- *Insufficiency of genuine Yuan*: + Shenshu (BL23), Guanyuan (CV4) to benefit the Kidneys and cultivate primary Yang.

- *Shortness of breath and dislike of speaking*: + Taibai (SP3) and Qihai (CV6) to tonify Qi in the Middle Burner.

- *Palpitations*: + Shenmen (HT7) and Xinshu (BL15) to tranquillize the Mind.

- *Chest distress*: + Tanzhong (CV17) and Neiguan (PC6) to relax the chest and regulate Qi.

- *Somnolence*: + Zhaohai (KI6) and Shenmai (BL62) to regulate Yin and Yang.

5. **Manipulation**

Perpendicular and deep puncture is avoided on Xinshu (BL15), Pishu (BL20), Sanjiaoshu (BL22) and Shenshu (BL23) to prevent the injury of internal organs. Moxibustion is supplemented for deficiency of the Spleen and Stomach and insufficiency of the Kidneys on Tianshu (ST25), Shangjuxu (ST37), Yinlingquan (SP9), Sanyinjiao (SP6), Qihai (CV6), Guanyuan (CV4), Pishu (BL20), Zusanli (ST36), Shenshu (BL23), etc. Deeper puncturing, 0.5–1.5 cun is applicable compared with the routine depth of insertion on other acupoints of the Fu organs in light of the severity of obesity in individual patients.

Other therapies

1. **Auricular acupuncture**

Points: Mouth, Stomach, Spleen, Lung, Triple Burner, Hunger Point, Endocrine, Subcortex; in each treatment, 3 to 5 points are selected and punctured shallowly by filiform needle with moderate stimulation. Needles are retained for 30 minutes. The therapy is applied once every day or every other day. In addition, embedding needles and the Vaccaria seed compress method are applicable on the points. The time of retention and replacement is determined in accordance with the seasons. During treatment, the patients are advised to press the points for 2–3 minutes before meals or when feeling hungry to enhance the stimulation of points.

2. **Electroacupuncture**

The points are selected in accordance with the main prescription and its modification. Electroacupuncture is applied after the arrival of Qi, with dense-disperse wave, strong stimulation for 30 to 40 minutes.

3. **Cutaneous needle**

The points are selected in accordance with the main prescription and its modification, or local Ashi points. The tapping method is applied by cutaneous needle. Forceful tapping is used for an excess syndrome to induce Blood exudation on the skin, and moderate stimulation is used for a deficiency syndrome until the skin turns slightly red. The treatment is given once every 2 days.

Notes

1. Acupuncture and moxibustion have good efficacy on simple obesity. One to two more courses of treatment should be applied to consolidate the efficacy when the effectiveness is achieved so that weight regain can be prevented.

2. Guide the patient to change any adverse diet and life habits, suggest to them that they take light food, with less greasy, sweet and fried food, chew every meal slowly, have few snacks; avoid excessive sleep, keep to a proper schedule of work and physical exercise.

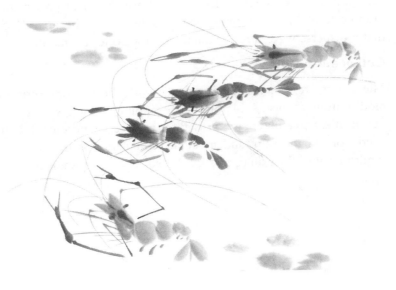

II. GYNAECOLOGICAL DISEASES

1. PREMENSTRUAL SYNDROME
Brief introduction

Premenstrual syndrome consists of a series of mental and physical symptoms appearing before menstruation and disappearing during menstruation. Clinically, these symptoms are in the category of 'menstrual headache', 'menstrual dizziness', 'menstrual diarrhoea' in Chinese medicine.

Aetiology and pathogenesis

This disease is associated with insufficiency of Blood flow in the Thoroughfare Vessel and Conception Vessel, Blood deficiency in the whole body, imbalance of Yin and Yang and disturbance of Zang Fu functions. The Liver, Spleen and Kidneys are involved in the disease, manifested as disorders of two organs or three organs in combination, or a disorder of both Qi and Blood.

Syndrome differentiation

The main symptoms are premenstrual mental stress, neurotic behaviour, irritability, hot temper, distending pain of the breasts, which attacks periodically and is associated with headache, dizziness (even the inability to stand up), or diarrhoea, fever, haematemesis, etc.

1. **Insufficiency of Qi and Blood**: Palpitations, shortness of breath, insomnia, dream-disturbed sleep, mental and physical fatigue, scanty menstrual flow, which is of light colour, and thin in quality; pale tongue with thin coating; thready and weak pulse.

2. **Yin deficiency of the Liver and Kidney**: Distension of the breasts, soreness and weakness of lumbar region and knee joints, dry eyes, throat and mouth, feverish sensation in the palms, soles and chest; red tongue, lack of moisture; thready and rapid pulse.

3. **Upward-disturbance of Phlegm and turbidity**: Dizziness, heaviness of the head, chest distress, nausea, poor appetite, abdominal distension, even an unclear Mind; profuse vaginal discharge in general, of white colour, and sticky in quality; scanty menstrual flow, a light colour; flabby and pale tongue with thick and sticky coating; soft and rolling pulse.

4. **Stagnation of Qi and Blood**: Distending pain of breasts, radiating to the hypochondriac regions; pain aggravated by pressure, menses of purplish and dark colour or with clots; dark tongue, or with stagnated spots; deep, string-taut and forceful pulse.

Treatment
Body acupuncture

1. **Principles of treatment**

   - *Insufficiency of Qi and Blood*: Benefit Qi and nourish Blood. Acupuncture and moxibustion are applied with reinforcing technique.

   - *Yin deficiency of the Liver and Kidney*: Nourish the Liver and Kidney. Acupuncture is the chief therapy with even-needling technique.

   - *Upward-disturbance of Phlegm and turbidity*: Resolve Phlegm and promote circulation in collaterals. Acupuncture is the chief therapy and the reducing technique is applied.

   - *Stagnation of Qi and Blood*: Promote Qi circulation and activate the Blood. Acupuncture is the chief therapy and reducing technique is applied.

2. **Prescription**

   Shenmen (HT7), Baihui (GV20), Tanzhong (CV17), Taichong (LR3), Sanyinjiao (SP6).

3. **Explanation**

   Shenmen (HT7) is the Yuan-Primary point of the Heart Meridian to tranquillize the Mind. Baihui (GV20) is located on the vertex, in which the Governor Vessel enters the brain. It calms down the Mind. Tanzhong (CV17) is the Influential point of Qi and has significant efficacy in regulating Qi activity. Taichong (LR3) is the Yuan-Primary point of the Liver Meridian, acting by smoothing Liver Qi, removing stagnation, clearing away Liver Fire and nourishing Blood. Sanyinjiao (SP6) is the Crossing point of the Spleen, Liver and Kidney Meridians, acting by strengthening the Spleen to control Blood, tonifying the Liver and benefiting the Kidneys. It is the major point for gynaecologic diseases.

4. **Modification**

   - *Insufficiency of Qi and Blood*: + Zusanli (ST36) and Pishu (BL20) to cultivate acquired foundation.

- *Yin deficiency of the Liver and Kidney*: + Taixi (KI3) and Ganshu (BL18) to tonify the Liver and Kidney and benefit Essence and Blood.

- *Upward-disturbance of Phlegm and turbidity*: + Pishu (BL20) and Fenglong (ST40) to remove Damp and resolve Phlegm.

- *Stagnation of Qi and Blood*: + Hegu (LI4) and Geshu (BL17) to promote Qi circulation and activate Blood.

- *Headache and dizziness*: + Yintang (EX-HN3) and Taiyang (EX-HN5) to regulate the Mind and stop pain.

- *Distending pain of the breasts*: + Neiguan (PC6) and Qimen (LR14) to promote Qi circulation and stop pain.

- *Emotional abnormality, irritability and hot temper*: + Shuigou (GV26) and Shenting (GV24) to calm down the Mind.

5. **Manipulation**

The routine needling technique is applied mainly to the points. Oblique puncture is applied to Pishu (BL20), Ganshu (BL18) and Geshu (BL17) with the needle tip downward or toward the spine to avoid injury to the internal organs. Treatment starts 5 to 7 days before menstruation.

Other therapies

1. **Auricular acupuncture**

Points: Liver, Kidney, Uterus, Subcortex, Endocrine. Moderate stimulation is achieved by filiform needle. Needles remain for 15 to 30 minutes. Embedding needles or Vaccaria seeds may also be applied to the points.

2. **Cutaneous needle**

Gentle tapping is applied to the lower abdominal region of the Conception Vessel, Spleen Meridian, Liver Meridian and three Yin meridians of foot in the groin groove and the lower limb until the local skin turns slightly red.

Notes

1. Acupuncture and moxibustion treatment of this disease focuses on holistic regulation of neurological endocrinal balance. Effective prevention will be achieved if the treatment starts 5 to 7 days before the occurrence of premenstrual syndrome.

2. The disease is greatly impacted by psychological factors. It is necessary to release the emotional tension of the patient. The patient should have stable lifestyle and maintain an even mood.

2. IRREGULAR MENSTRUATION

Brief introduction

Irregular menstruation refers to menstrual disorder mainly manifested as menstrual cycle abnormality. In clinical terms, the disease includes advanced menstruation, delayed menstruation and irregular menstruation. In Western medicine uterine bleeding due to ovulation dysfunction, reproductive inflammation or abnormal vaginal haemorrhage due to tumour could be treated in reference to this disease.

Aetiology and pathogenesis

Advanced menstruation is mainly due to Qi deficiency leading to dysfunction of control or Heat disturbing the Thoroughfare Vessel and Conception Vessel. Blood Heat leads to extravasations; hence, menstrual flow appears early. Delayed menstruation is divided into excess and deficiency types. *Excess type* is related to either Cold and Blood stagnation retarding the circulation in the Thoroughfare Vessel and Conception Vessel or stagnation of Qi and Blood blocking the Thoroughfare Vessel and Conception Vessel. Hence, menstrual flow appears in postpone. *Deficiency type* is due to either insufficiency of nutrient Blood or deficiency and declining of Yang Qi that delays the filling-up of the sea of Blood. Irregular menstruation is attributed to the disarrangement of Qi and Blood in the Thoroughfare Vessel and Conception Vessel and abnormal filling-up of the Sea of Blood, which is commonly caused by Liver Qi stagnation or the decline of Kidney Qi. This disease is closely related to the Kidneys, Liver and Spleen as well as the Thoroughfare Vessel and Conception Vessel.

Syndrome differentiation

Abnormal changes in menstrual cycle includes advanced menstruation, delayed menstruation and irregular menstruation, associated with abnormality in the quantity, colour and quality of the menstrual flow.

1. **Qi deficiency**: Advanced menstrual flow, of light colour, and thin in quality; lassitude, empty and bearing-down feeling in the lower abdomen, poor appetite, loose stools; pale tongue with white coating; thready and weak pulse.

2. **Blood deficiency**: Delayed menstruation, scanty menstrual flow, of light colour and thin in quality; dull pain in the lower abdomen, dizziness, blurred vision, palpitations, insomnia, pale or sallow complexion; little tongue coating, thready and weak pulse.

3. **Kidney deficiency**: Irregular menstruation, scanty menstrual flow, of light colour, thin in quality; dizziness, tinnitus, soreness and weakness of lumbar region and knee joints; pale tongue with thin coating, deep and thready pulse.

4. **Qi stagnation**: Retarded menstrual flow, either advanced or delayed menstruation, either profuse or scanty menstrual flow, purplish in colour, clots; distending pain in the chest, hypochondriac regions and breasts, sighing; thin white or thin yellow tongue coating, string-taut pulse.

5. **Blood Heat**: Excess Heat syndrome is differentiated in light of advanced menstruation, profuse menses, deep red or purplish in colour, thick in quality; feverish sensation in the chest, red face, dry mouth, constipation; red tongue with yellow coating, rolling and rapid pulse. Deficiency Heat syndrome is differentiated in light of advanced menstruation, scanty menses, red in colour and thick in quality, feverish sensation in the palms, soles and chest, soreness and weakness of the lumbar region and knee joints; red tongue with little coating, thready and weak pulse.

6. **Blood Cold**: Delayed menstruation, scanty menses, dark red in colour, clots, cold pain in the lower abdomen that is alleviated by Heat, chills, cold limbs; white tongue coating, deep and tense pulse.

Treatment
Body acupuncture

1. **Principles of treatment**

    - *Qi deficiency, Blood deficiency and Kidney deficiency*: Benefit Qi, nourish Blood, tonify the Kidneys to regulate menstruation. Acupuncture and moxibustion are applied in combination. Reinforcing technique is used.

    - *Blood Cold*: Warm meridians to expel Cold, and regulate the Thoroughfare Vessel and Conception Vessel. Acupuncture and moxibustion are applied in combination. Even-needling technique is used.

    - *Qi stagnation and Blood Heat*: Regulate Liver Qi, clear away Heat to regulate menstruation. Acupuncture alone is applied with reducing technique.

2. **Prescription**

Guanyuan (CV4), Xuehai (SP10), Sanyinjiao (SP6).

3. **Explanation**

Dysfunction of the Thoroughfare Vessel and Conception Vessel is the major pathogenesis of the disease. Guanyuan (CV4) is the key point of the meridian and crosses with the three Yin meridians of foot. The Thoroughfare Vessel and Conception Vessel share the same source, thus Guanyuan (CV4) is also the major point of the Thoroughfare Vessel. Xuehai (SP10) and Sanyinjiao (SP6) are located in the same meridian. Sanyinjiao (SP6) crosses with the Liver and Kidney Meridians and is the major point in Blood and menstrual regulation of gynaecology.

4. **Modification**

- *Qi deficiency:* + Zusanli (ST36) and Pishu (BL20) to strengthen the Spleen and Stomach and benefit Qi and Blood.
- *Blood deficiency:* + Pishu (BL20) and Geshu (BL17) to enhance the source of Blood production.
- *Kidney deficiency:* + Shenshu (BL23) and Taixi (KI3) to regulate and tonify Kidney Qi.
- *Qi stagnation:* + Taichong (LR3) and Qimen (LR14) to smooth Liver Qi and remove stagnation.
- *Blood Heat:* + Xingjian (LR2) and Diji (SP8) to reduce Heat from the Blood system.
- *Blood Cold:* + Moxibustion is applied to Guilai (ST29) and Mingmen (GV4) to warm and promote circulation of the meridians, activate Blood and regulate menstruation.

5. **Manipulation**

Routine manipulation is applied mainly to the points. Oblique puncture is applied to Pishu (BL20) and Geshu (BL17) with the needle tip downward or toward the spine. Perpendicular and deep puncture should be avoided. Moxibustion is applied to the points on the abdomen for Qi deficiency or Blood Cold. Treatment starts 5 to 7 days before menstruation and discontinues during menstruation. If it is not possible to be sure of the menstrual time, acupuncture and moxibustion can start on the day when menstrual flow ends. Treatment is given once every 2 days until menstrual flow appears and continues for 3 to 5 menstrual cycles.

Other therapies

1. **Auricular acupuncture**

   Points: Liver, Spleen, Kidney, Uterus, Subcortex, Endocrine. Moderate stimulation is applied by filiform needle. Needles remain for 15 to 30 minutes. Vaccaria seed can also be applied to the points.

2. **Cutaneous needle**

   Gentle tapping is given from the lumbar vertebrae to the coccyx, on the running courses of the Conception Vessel, Spleen and Liver Meridians in the lower abdomen, groin groove and the running courses of three Yin meridians of foot in the lower limbs until the local skin turns slightly red.

Notes

1. Acupuncture and moxibustion have good efficacy in treating functional irregular menstruation. Comprehensive measurements should be provided if the case is induced by organic disorder in the reproductive system.

2. The treatment at the proper time increases the efficacy. In general, the treatment starts 5 to 7 days before menstruation and discontinues during menstruation.

3. Attention is paid to having a regular lifestyle and menstrual health, such as maintain an even mood, dressing appropriately for the weather, having plenty of rest, avoiding cold, raw and spicy food.

3. DYSMENORRHOEA

Brief introduction

Dysmenorrhoea is also known as 'abdominal pain during menstruation'. It is a kind of periodic pain in the lower abdomen during, before and after menstruation and is commonly seen in young females. Western medicine divides it into primary and secondary types. The primary type refers to no apparent abnormality of the reproductive organs. The secondary type is mostly induced by an organic disorder in the reproductive organs, such as endometriosis, adenomyosis, chronic pelvic inflammation and myoma of the uterus.

Aetiology and pathogenesis

Dysmenorrhoea is closely related to the Thoroughfare Vessel and Conception Vessel as well as periodic physiological change of the uterus; and it also has a connection with the Liver and Kidneys. Disharmony of Qi and Blood in the Thoroughfare Vessel and Conception Vessel before menstruation and blockage of the meridians leads to retarded Qi and Blood circulation in the uterus, thus 'pain results from obstruction'. Malnutrition of the uterus may also result in pain. In addition, emotional disorder leads to Liver Qi stagnation and blockage of Blood circulation. Cold and Damp attack the uterus, leading to retarded circulation of Qi and Blood; deficiency of Qi and Blood and insufficiency of the Liver and Kidneys may all result in obstruction of the uterus and malnutrition of the uterus. Hence, dysmenorrhoeal is induced.

Syndrome differentiation

Pain in the lower abdomen appears periodically during, before or after menstruation. Pain may radiate to the hypochondriac regions, breasts, lumbar sacrum, medial aspect of the femur, vaginal region or anus, etc. In general, pain starts several hours before menstruation and is taken as the pre-sign of menstruation. In severe cases, the patient has intolerable pain, blue complexion, cold limbs, vomiting, sweating, general weakness, even coma.

1. **Stagnation of Cold and Damp**: Cold pain in the lower abdomen before or during menstruation, which is alleviated by warmth; scanty menstrual flow, purplish and dark in colour, clots; associated with chills, cold limbs, profuse urine; white tongue coating, thready or deep tense pulse.

2. **Qi and Blood stagnation**: Distending pain in the lower abdomen before or after menstruation, which is aggravated by pressure, distending pain in the chest, hypochondriac region and breasts, retarded menstrual flow, purplish and dark in colour, clots; purplish dark tongue or with stagnated spots, deep, string-taut or hesitant pulse.

3. **Insufficiency of Qi and Blood**: Dull pain in the lower abdomen during or after menstruation, which is alleviated by pressure, empty and bearing-down feeling in the abdomen, scanty menstrual flow, pale colour, lassitude, dizziness, blurred vision, palpitations, shortness of breath; pale tongue with thin coating, thready and string-taut pulse.

Treatment

Body acupuncture

1. **Principles of treatment**

   - *Stagnation of Cold and Damp, stagnation of Qi and Blood*: Warm meridians to expel Cold, remove stasis to stop pain. Acupuncture and moxibustion are applied in combination, with reducing technique.

   - *Insufficiency of Qi and Blood*: Benefit Qi, nourish Blood and regulate and tonify the Thoroughfare and Conception Vessels. Acupuncture and moxibustion are applied in combination with reinforcing technique.

2. **Prescription**

   Acupoints are mainly selected from the Spleen Meridian of Foot-Taiyin. Guanyuan (CV4), Sanyinjiao (SP6), Diji (SP8), Shiqizhui (EX-B8).

3. **Explanation**

   Guanyuan (CV4) connects with the uterus and meets with three Yin meridians of foot. Acupuncture on this point can promote Qi and Blood circulation, and remove stasis to stop pain. Moxibustion on the point can warm the meridians to expel Cold and regulate the Thoroughfare and Conception Vessels. Sanyinjiao (SP6) is the Crossing point of the three Yin meridians of foot and can regulate the Spleen, Liver and Kidneys. Diji (SP8) is the Xi-Cleft point of the Spleen Meridian of Foot-Taiyin. The Spleen Meridian of Foot-Taiyin runs on the bilateral sides of the abdomen. The points located in Yin meridians can treat Blood syndrome, regulate Blood and promote menstruation to stop pain. Shiqizhui (EX-B8) is well established as the effective point for dysmenorrhoea.

4. **Modification**

   - *Stagnation of Cold and Damp*: + Moxibustion on Shuidao (ST28) to warm meridians and stop pain.

   - *Stagnation of Qi and Blood*: + Hegu (LI4), Taichong (LR3) and Ciliao (BL32) to regulate Qi and activate Blood circulation.

   - *Insufficiency of Qi and Blood*: + Xuehai (SP10), Pishu (BL20) and Zusanli (ST36) to nourish Qi and stop pain.

5. **Manipulation**

   Continuous rotating technique is applied to Guanyuan (CV4) to conduct the needling sensations downward. Moxibustion is applied to the lower abdomen after acupuncture for stagnation of Cold and Blood. During an attack, the treatment is applied 1 to 2 times a day. In the recovery stage, the treatment is applied once every 2 days. Treatment starts 3 days before menstruation.

Other therapies

1. **Application method**

   Zhongji (CV3), Guanyuan (CV4), Sanyinjiao (SP6), Shenshu (BL23) and Ashi points are selected. Tong Shu Ning Tian Gao (plaster for relieving pain) of 1cm in size is applied before or during menstruation. It is replaced once every day.

2. **Auricular acupuncture**

   Points: Endocrine, Internal Reproductive Organ, Liver, Kidney, Subcortex, Ear-Shenmen. 3–5 points are selected each treatment and moderately stimulated by filiform needles. Needles remain for 30 minutes. Embedding needles or Vaccaria seed is also used.

3. **Cutaneous needle**

   Tapping Jiaji (EX-B2) in the lumbar sacral region and the relevant acupoints in the lower abdomen. Moderate stimulation is applied until the skin turns slightly red.

4. **Point injection**

   Ganshu (BL18), Shenshu (BL23), Pishu (BL20), Qihai (CV6), Guanyuan (CV4), Guilai (ST29), Zusanli (ST36) and Sanyinjiao (SP6) are used. Two or three acupoints are selected each time and injected with herbal preparations, such as, injections of Huangqi (黄芪 *Astraglus*), Danggui (当归 *Radix Angelicae Sinensis*), or Honghua (红花 *Carthami Flos*) or placenta tissue, vitamin B$_{12}$ injection, 1–2ml in each point.

Notes

1. Acupuncture and moxibustion have significant efficacy on primary dysmenorrhoea. The treatment should start 3 to 5 days before menstruation until the end of menstruation, continuously for 2 to 3 menstrual cycles. Generally, the disease can be largely cured after 2 to 4 menstrual cycle treatments.

2. For secondary dysmenorrhoea, acupuncture and moxibustion can alleviate the symptoms of it. It is necessary to receive a definite diagnosis of the primary disease so as to provide the appropriate corresponding treatment.

3. Patients should avoid emotional stimuli and excessive stress, Cold attack or excessive cold and raw food during menstruation.

4. AMENORRHOEA

Brief introduction

Amenorrhoea is diagnosed if the female has no menarche after the age of 18 years or has menstrual discontinuity for 3 cycles. Western medicine divides the disease into primary amenorrhoea and secondary amenorrhoea. Absence of menstruation before puberty, during pregnancy or lactation refers to physiological phenomena and cannot be described as disease.

Aetiology and pathogenesis

Deficiency and excess are included in the aetiology of the disease. Deficiency refers to insufficiency of the Liver and Kidneys, deficiency of Qi and Blood, emptiness of the Sea of Blood, which leads to amenorrhoea due to absence of Blood. Excess refers to Qi and Blood stagnation and stagnation of Cold blocking the Thoroughfare and Conception Vessels, resulting in blockage of menstrual flow. The disease is localized in the Liver and connects with the Spleen and Kidneys.

Syndrome differentiation

Menstruation discontinuity for more than 3 cycles, delayed menarche, and delayed menstruation, associated with maldevelopment of the female reproductive organs, menopause symptoms, obesity, hirsutism, tuberculosis, etc. Clinical manifestations may be various due to different aetiologies. Generally, delayed menarche, or a prolonged cycle of menstruation, or scanty menstrual flow may gradually result in amenorrhoea.

1. **Deficiency of the Liver and Kidneys**: Delayed menarche, or delayed menstruation, scanty menstrual flow, which develops gradually into amenorrhoea; dizziness, tinnitus, soreness and weakness of lumbar region and knee joints; red tongue with little coating, deep weak or thready and hesitant pulse.

2. **Insufficiency of Qi and Blood**: Gradual postponing of menstrual cycle, scanty menstrual flow, pale colour, no lustre on the face, dizziness, vertigo, palpitations, shortness of breath, poor appetite; pale tongue with thin and white coating, deep retarded or thready and weak pulse.

3. **Qi and Blood stagnation**: Absence of menstruation for months, pain in the lower abdomen that is worse on pressure, mental depression, irritability, hot temper, distension and fullness in the chest and hypochondriac region; purplish tongue or with stagnated spots, deep string-taut and forceful pulse.

4. **Stagnation of Cold and Damp**: Absence of menstruation for months, Cold pain in the lower abdomen that is worse on pressure and aggravated by warmth, chills, Cold limbs, blue and pale complexion; purplish tongue with white coating, deep and slow pulse.

Treatment
Body acupuncture

1. **Principles of treatment**

   - *Deficiency of the Liver and Kidney, insufficiency of Qi and Blood*: Tonify the Liver and Kidney, nourish Qi and Blood. Acupuncture and moxibustion are applied in combination with reinforcing technique.

   - *Stagnation of Qi and Blood and stagnation of Cold and Damp*: Activate Blood circulation to remove stasis, warm meridians to expel Cold. Acupuncture and moxibustion are applied in combination with reducing technique.

2. **Prescription**

   Tianshu (ST25), Guanyuan (CV4), Hegu (LI4), Sanyinjiao (SP6), Shenshu (BL23).

3. **Explanation**

   Tianshu (ST25) is located in the abdomen. Acupuncture on the point can activate Blood circulation and remove stasis and moxibustion on it can warm the meridian to promote circulation. Guanyuan (CV4) and Sanyinjiao (SP6) regulate the Spleen, Liver and Kidneys and the Thoroughfare and Conception Vessels. Hegu (LI4) and Sanyinjiao (SP6) together regulate the Thoroughfare and Conception Vessels and Qi and Blood of the uterus. Shenshu (BL23) is the Back-Shu point of the Kidneys, and acts on tonifying Kidney Qi. Excessive Kidney Qi results in abundant menstrual flow.

4. **Modification**

   - *Deficiency of the Liver and Kidney*: + Ganshu (BL18) and Taixi (KI3) to benefit the Liver and Kidney and regulate the Thoroughfare and Conception Vessels.

- *Insufficiency of Qi and Blood*: + Qihai (CV6), Xuehai (SP10), Pishu (BL20) and Zusanli (ST36) to strengthen the Spleen and Stomach to promote the transformation of Qi and Blood.

- *Stagnation of Qi and Blood*: + Taichong (LR3), Qimen (LR14) and Ganshu (BL18) to promote Qi and activate Blood circulation, remove stasis and promote circulation in meridians.

- *Stagnation of Cold and Damp*: + Mingmen (GV4) and Dazhui (GV14) to warm meridian, expel Cold and remove Damp so as to promote menstrual flow.

5. **Manipulation**

Oblique needling is applied to Geshu (BL17) and Pishu (BL20) with the tip downward or toward the spine. Perpendicular and deep insertion is avoided. For insufficiency of Qi and Blood, and stagnation of Cold and Damp, moxibustion is added on the points of the back and abdominal region. For stagnation of Qi and Blood, Blood-letting puncturing and cupping is applied in combination.

Other therapies

1. **Auricular acupuncture**

Points: Kidney, Liver, Spleen, Heart, Endocrine, Internal Reproductive Organ and Subcortex. In each treatment, 3 to 5 points are selected and stimulated moderately by filiform needle. Needles are retained for 15 to 30 minutes. Embedding needle or Vaccaria seed is also applicable.

2. **Cutaneous needle**

Tap corresponding Back-Shu points and Jiaji (EX-B2) in lumbar sacral region, as well as relevant meridian points in the lower abdomen.

3. **Point injection**

Points: Ganshu (BL18), Shenshu (BL23), Pishu (BL20), Qihai (CV6), Guanyuan (CV4), Guilai (ST29), Qichong (ST32) and Sanyinjiao (SP6). In each treatment, 2 or 3 points are selected and injected with herbal preparations, such as, injections of Huangqi (黄芪 *Radix Astragali seu Hedysari*), Danggui (当归 *Radix Angelicae Sinensis*), Honghua (红花 *Carthami Flos*) or placenta tissue, vitamin B$_{12}$ injection, 1–2ml in each point.

Notes

1. Due to the complicated aetiology of amenorrhoea, the treatment is quite hard. The efficacies of acupuncture and moxibustion for the disease vary according to the different causative factors. Comparatively, the efficacy is better for cases caused by invasion of Cold, stagnation of Qi and Blood, insufficiency of Qi and Blood and emotional factors; and the efficacy is poor in cases induced by severe malnutrition, tuberculosis, Kidney disorder, incomplete development of uterus, etc.

2. It is necessary to undertake careful examination to determine the aetiology and apply the corresponding treatment. Amenorrhoea induced by congenital reproductive organ or acquired organic injury is not discussed in the category of acupuncture and moxibustion in treatment.

3. A long course of treatment with acupuncture and moxibustion is required for amenorrhoea. Hence, the patient is advised to coordinate her efforts with the treatment and maintain regular treatment, keep to a regular lifestyle, avoid Cold attack or excessive cold food and drinks during menstruation, pay attention to her emotion regulation and maintain an optimistic mood.

5. UTERINE BLEEDING

Brief introduction

Uterine bleeding refers to sudden profuse vaginal bleeding or dribbling that does not happen during menstruation, known as 'Beng Lou' in Chinese medicine. 'Beng' or 'Bengzhong' refers to sudden, drastic and profuse vaginal bleeding. 'Lou' or 'Louxia' refers to dribbling, slow onset and scanty menstrual flow. The two conditions of the disease happen alternately. Hence the disease is termed 'Beng Lou'. The disease is commonly seen in puberty, during the menopause stage or after delivery. Irregular vaginal bleeding induced by anovulatory dysfunctional uterine bleeding (DUB), inflammation of the reproductive organs and carcinoma of some reproductive organs as described in Western medicine can be treated in reference to this disease.

Aetiology and pathogenesis

- *The main pathogenesis of the disease:* Injury of the Thoroughfare and Conception Vessels fails to control Blood, thus leading to irregular menstrual bleeding from the uterus.

- *Common aetiology*: Blood Heat, Blood stasis, Kidney deficiency, Spleen deficiency, etc. Heat injures the Thoroughfare and Conception Vessels and forces Blood running abnormally. Spleen Qi deficiency fails to control Blood. Kidney Yang deficiency fails to store Blood. Retention of Phlegm and Blood and abnormal Blood running may all result in dysfunction of the Thoroughfare and Conception Vessels. Hence, the disease is related to the Thoroughfare and Conception Vessels as well as the Liver, Spleen and Kidneys.

Syndrome differentiation

Disturbed menstrual cycle, irregular duration of bleeding time that can be several days or up to 10 days, profuse menstrual flow or dribbling, associated commonly with profuse leucorrhoea, infertility, etc.

1. **Internal disturbance of Blood Heat**: Profuse bleeding or dribbling, deep red or purplish red in colour, thick in quality, little clots, irritability, hot temper, preference for cold drinks, constipation, deep yellow urine; red tongue with yellow coating, rapid or rolling rapid pulse.

2. **Stagnation of Qi and Blood**: Dribbling vaginal bleeding or sudden drastic bleeding, dark or black in colour, pain in the lower abdomen that is alleviated after bleeding; purplish and dark tongue, deep hesitant or string-taut and tense pulse.

3. **Deficiency of Kidney Yang**: Profuse or dribbling vaginal bleeding, light colour, thin in quality, low spirits, chills, cold limbs, soreness and weakness of lumbar region and knee joints, profuse clear urine; pale tongue with thin coating, deep, thready and forceful pulse.

4. **Insufficiency of Qi and Blood**: Scanty menstrual flow, dribbling, light colour, thin in quality, sallow complexion, poor appetite, loose stools; flabby, pale tongue, or with teeth marks, thin and white coating; thready and weak pulse.

Treatment
Body acupuncture

1. **Principles of treatment**

   - *Internal disturbance of Blood Heat, stagnation of Qi and Blood*: Clear away Heat, cool Blood, and promote Qi circulation to remove stasis. Acupuncture is applied only with reducing technique.

- *Deficiency of Kidney Yang and insufficiency of Qi and Blood*: Warm and strength Kidney Yang, tonify Qi to control Blood. Acupuncture and moxibustion are applied in combination with reinforcing technique.

2. **Prescription**

   Points are mainly from the Spleen Meridian of Foot-Taiyin. Guanyuan (CV4), Sanyinjiao (SP6), Xuehai (SP10) and Geshu (BL17).

3. **Explanation**

   Guanyuan (CV4) is the Crossing points of the Conception Vessel with the three Yin meridians of foot, and it regulates the Thoroughfare and Conception Vessels and manages Essence and Blood. Sanyinjiao (SP6) is the Crossing point of the three Yin meridians of foot and it smoothes the Qi of the three Yin meridians to strengthen the Spleen and Stomach, benefit the Liver and Kidneys, tonify Qi and Blood and adjust menstrual flow. Xuehai (SP10) is the key point of the meridian to stop bleeding and regulate menstruation. Geshu (BL17) is the Influential point of Blood and it adjusts menstrual flow effectively.

4. **Modification**
   - *Internal disturbance of Blood Heat*: + Dadun (LR1), Xingjian (LR2) and Qimen (LR14) to reduce Heat from Blood.
   - *Stagnation of Qi and Blood*: + Hegu (LI4) and Taichong (LR3) to regulate Qi circulation to remove stasis and regulate menstrual flow.
   - *Deficiency of Kidney Yang*: + moxibustion on Qihai (CV6) and Mingmen (GV4) to warm and tonify Kidney Yang.
   - *Insufficiency of Qi and Blood*: + Yinbai (SP1), Pishu (BL20) and Zusanli (ST36) to tonify Qi to control Blood and nourish Blood to regulate menstrual flow.

5. **Manipulation**

   Oblique puncture with tip downward is applied to Guanyuan (CV4) and Qihai (CV6) and the needle sensations are conducted to the pubic symphysis. Oblique puncture is applied to Geshu (BL17) and Pishu (BL20), with needle tip downward or toward the spine; perpendicular and deep needling is avoided. For stagnation of Qi and Blood, the bleeding method is applied in combination. For deficiency of Kidney Yang and insufficiency of Qi and Blood, moxibustion is applicable on the abdomen and back.

Other therapies

1. **Auricular acupuncture**

   Points: Uterus, Ovary, Endocrine, Subcortex, Liver, Spleen and Ear-Shenmen. 3 or 4 points are selected each time. *Excess syndrome:* Acupuncture is applied and needles are retained for 15 to 30 minutes. *Deficiency syndrome:* Seed compress is used on the points with Semen Vaccariae. The treatment is applied once every other day.

2. **Cutaneous needle**

   Tapping along the Governor Vessel and the Bladder Meridian of Foot-Taiyang in the lumbar sacral region, the Conception Vessel, and the Kidney Meridian of Foot-Shaoyin, Stomach Meridian of Foot-Yangming, Spleen Meridian of Foot-Taiyin in the lower abdomen, and the three Yin meridians of foot in the lower limbs, repeated 3 times up to down, moderate stimulation, once or twice a day.

3. **Pricking**

   Red pimple-like reaction spots are detected in the Governor Vessel or the Bladder Meridian of Foot-Taiyang in lumbar sacral region. Select 2 to 4 spots and prick with three-edged needle, 0.2cm–0.3cm long and 0.1cm deep to break the white fibre. The treatment is applied once a month, for 3 treatments without a break.

4. **Scalp acupuncture**

   Bilateral reproductive area (MS4) is stimulated by filiform needles. Needles are retained for 30 to 60 minutes and manipulated repeatedly.

5. **Point injection**

   Points: Qihai (CV6), Xuehai (SP10), Sanyinjiao (SP6), Geshu (BL17), Zusanli (ST36). In each treatment, 2 or 3 points are selected and injected with vitamin B_{12} or injections of Huangqi (黄芪 *Radix Astragali seu Hedysari*), Danggui (当归 *Radix Angelicae Sinensis*), 2ml in each point. The treatment is applied once a day.

Notes

1. Acupuncture and moxibustion are certainly effective in treating the disease. But comprehensive therapy should be administered for profuse bleeding and critical cases.

2. If repeated bleeding appears in menopausal women, gynaecological examination is required to exclude the pathogen of carcinoma.

3. The patient should pay attention to regulation of their diet, enhance their nutrition, avoid spicy, cold and raw food and avoid overstress.

6. MORBID LEUCORRHOEA

Brief introduction

Colourless, thick and non-smelly vaginal discharge or slightly increased leucorrhoea during or before menstruation and during pregnancy is a normal physiological sign. If vaginal discharge is increased apparently in amount and abnormal in colour, quality and smell or associated with general or local symptoms, it is known as morbid leucorrhoea. Such a disease is seen as leukorrhagia induced by vaginitis, cervicitis, pelvic inflammatory disease, endocrinal disorder, cervical and uterus carcinoma, etc.

Aetiology and pathogenesis

The disease is commonly induced by dysfunction of the Thoroughfare and Conception Vessels in controlling, and dysfunction of the Belt Vessel, which leads to the downward flow of Damp and turbid fluids. Improper diet and overstress injure the Spleen and Stomach in their transportation and transformation. Hence, Damp is accumulated and flows downward to injure the Conception Vessel, thus morbid leucorrhoea occurs. Constitutional Kidney Qi insufficiency and Kidney Yang deficiency may also lead to dysfunction of the Belt Vessel and Conception Vessel, thus morbid leucorrhoea happens. Yellow discharge is mostly due to Damp Heat in the Spleen meridian and white discharge is due to deficiency and Cold. Emotional disorder leads to Liver Qi stagnation, and Heat is transformed after long-term stagnation. Struggling between Blood and Heat and the downward movement of Damp Heat results in red and white discharge. Dysfunction of the Spleen and Kidneys is an internal factor of the disease. Injury of the Conception Vessel and dysfunction of the Belt Vessel are the keys of pathogenesis.

Syndrome differentiation

Constant fishy and thick vaginal discharge like nasal discharge or pus is the chief symptom of the disease.

There are profuse vaginal discharges, which may be white, light yellow or mixed red and white in colour, or yellow green like pus, or turbid like washed-rice water, clear in quality like water, or sticky like pus, or granular or frothy; no smell, or fishy, even an intolerable smell; associated with burning, itching, bearing-down feeling or pain in external genitalia and vagina.

1. **Downward of Damp Heat**: Profuse vaginal discharge, yellow, sticky and stinking, or itching in external genitalia, chest distress, irritability, bitter taste in the mouth, dry throat, poor appetite, pain in bilateral sides or lower abdomen, scanty and deep yellow urine; red tongue with yellow sticky coating, soft and rapid pulse.

2. **Retention of Damp due to Spleen deficiency**: Profuse vaginal discharge, white or light yellow in colour, thin in quality, no smell, lassitude, cold limbs, poor appetite, loose stools; pale tongue with white or sticky coating, retarded and weak pulse.

3. **Deficiency of Kidney Yin**: Profuse vaginal discharge, yellow or reddish white in colour, thick in quality or smelly, Dryness of vaginal region or burning sensation, soreness and weakness of lumbar region and knee joints, dizziness, tinnitus, flushed cheeks, red lips, feverish sensation in palms, soles and chest, insomnia, dream-disturbed sleep; red tongue with little or yellow sticky coating, thready and rapid pulse.

4. **Insufficiency of Kidney Yang**: Profuse vaginal discharge, white, clear and thin like water, dribbling, severe lumbar pain, chills, cold limbs, cold sensation in the lower abdomen, frequent urination especially at night, loose stools; pale tongue with thin and white coating, deep thready and slow pulse.

Treatment

Body acupuncture

1. **Principles of treatment**

   - *Downward flow of Damp Heat*: Clear away Heat and remove Damp. Acupuncture alone is applied with reducing technique.

   - *Retention of Damp due to Spleen deficiency and insufficiency of Kidney Yang*: Strengthen the Spleen, benefit the Kidneys. Acupuncture and moxibustion are used in combination with reinforcing technique.

   - *Deficiency of Kidney Yin*: Nourish Yin and clear away Heat. Acupuncture is the chief therapy using the even technique.

2. **Prescription**

   Daimai (GB26), Guanyuan (CV4), Sanyinjiao (SP6), Baihuanshu (BL30).

3. **Explanation**

Daimai (GB26) is the Crossing point of the Gallbladder Meridian of Foot-Shaoyang and Belt Vessel and is the site where Qi of the Belt Vessel passes. It acts on coordinating the Thoroughfare and Conception Vessels, regulating the Lower Burner, adjusting menstruation and stopping leucorrhoea. Guanyuan (CV4) and Sanyinjiao (SP6) regulate the Spleen, Liver and Kidneys. Baihuanshu (BL30) can regulate Qi of the Lower Burner to resolve Damp from the Lower Burner and stop leucorrhoea.

4. **Modification**

- *Downward flow of Damp Heat:* + Zhongji (CV3) and Ciliao (BL32) to reduce Damp Heat of the Lower Burner.

- *Retention of Damp due to Spleen deficiency:* + Pishu (BL20) and Zusanli (ST36) to strengthen the Spleen and resolve Damp.

- *Deficiency of Kidney Yin and insufficiency of Kidney Yang:* + Shenshu (BL23), Taixi (KI3) and Mingmen (GV4) to tonify the Kidneys, and adjust Yin and Yang.

5. **Manipulation**

Routine needling is mainly applied to all the points. Oblique needling is applied to Guanyuan (CV4) and Qihai (CV6) with the tip downward and needling sensations are conducted to the pubic symphysis. Daimai (GB26) is punctured obliquely to the anterior, deep puncturing is avoided. Baihuanshu (BL30) is punctured perpendicularly to induce strong soreness and distension in the sacral region.

Other therapies

1. **Blood-letting puncturing and cupping**

A three-edged needle is used to bleed Shiqizhui (EX-B8), Yaoyan (EX-B7) and points around the sacral foramen and cupping follows and is retained for 5 to 10 minutes. Blood volume is about 3 to 5ml, maximal volume can be up to 60ml. The treatment is given once every 3 to 5 days. The therapy is applicable for the downward flow of Damp Heat.

2. **Auricular acupuncture**

Points: Internal Reproductive Organ, Adrenal, Ear-Shenmen, Spleen, Kidney, Liver, Triple Burner. 3 or 4 points are selected in one treatment and stimulated moderately by filiform needle. Needles are retained for 15 to 30 minutes. The treatment is given every day or once every other day. Points on the two ears are selected alternately.

3. **Electroacupuncture**

   Points: Daimai (GB26), Sanyinjiao (SP6). Electroacupuncture is applied after the arrival of Qi, with dense-disperse wave, lasting 15 to 20 minutes.

4. **Point injection**

   Point: Bilateral Sanyinjiao (SP6), Berberine injection, 1 to 3ml on each point.

Notes

1. Acupuncture and moxibustion is efficacious for morbid leucorrhoea. For quite severe cases, the internal application of medicine, and medical bathing of the external genitalia is applied in combination to enhance the efficacy.

2. The patient should be advised to maintain good sanitary habits, wear clean underwear, pay attention to hygiene during menstruation, and of the nursing and regulation during pregnancy and delivery, and make sure the perineum is kept clean.

3. Pay attention to a healthy lifestyle, follow a light diet with little greasy and sweet food, appropriate sexual activity, avoid overstress, do more out-of-doors activities.

7. PRURITUS VULVAE

Brief introduction

Pruritus vulvae refers to itching in external genitalia or intravaginal itching, commonly in females of menopause age. It is mainly caused by various forms of vaginitis and can be induced by emotional factors. In Western medicine this is commonly seen in external genitalia pruritus, vulvitis, trichomonal vaginitis, vaginal thrust, senile vaginitis, vulval leukoplakia, vulvar dystrophy.

Aetiology and pathogenesis

The disease is related to the Liver, Spleen and Kidneys, the Conception and Governor Vessels. It can be caused by the downward flow of Damp Heat and impregnation of leucorrhoea in the vaginal region, or deficiency of Liver and Kidney Yin resulting in malnutrition of the external genitalia. Pruritus vulvae is commonly mixed with morbid leucorrhoea, and the cause of vaginal pain may be complicated in severe cases.

Syndrome differentiation

Intolerable prutritus or burning pain in the external genitalia or vulvae, even around the anus; irritability, poor sleep and restlessness; some cases may present whitening, thickening, drying and ulceration in the skin of the vulvae and anus. Gynaecologic examination may find skin depigmentation, whitening, thickening, atrophy or ulceration in the vulvae. A large amount of purulent discharge, or yellow frothy, bean dregs-like or milk curd-like discharge may be found in the vulvae.

1. **Damp Heat in the Liver Meridian**: Vaginal prutritus, even acute pain, restlessness, profuse vaginal discharge which is white or yellow in colour, frothy or washed-rice water like discharge, stinking in smell, irritability, chest distress, bitter taste and stickiness in the mouth, epigastric fullness, poor appetite; yellow and sticky tongue coating, string-taut and rapid pulse.

2. **Deficiency of Liver and Kidney Yin**: Dry vulvae, with burning sensation and pruritus, profuse vaginal discharge, yellow in colour; feverish sensations in the palms, soles and chest, dizziness, vertigo; feverish feeling and occasional sweating, soreness of lumbar region, tinnitus; red tongue with little coating; thready and rapid pulse.

Treatment
Body acupuncture

1. **Principles of treatment**

   - *Damp Heat of Liver Meridian*: Clear away Heat and remove Damp, kill bacteria and relieve itching. Acupuncture alone is used with reducing technique.

   - *Deficiency of Liver and Kidney Yin*: Regulate and tonify the Liver and Kidneys, nourish Yin to stop itching. Acupuncture is the main therapy with even-needling technique.

2. **Prescription**

   Acupoints are mainly from the Liver Meridian of Foot-Jueyin. Dadun (LR1), Ligou (LR5), Taichong (LR3), Zhongji (CV3) and Sanyinjiao (SP6).

3. **Explanation**

Dadun (LR1) is the Jing-Well point of the Liver Meridian, acting on reducing Liver Heat and stopping vaginal itching. Ligou (LR5) is the Luo-Connecting point of the Liver Meridian of Foot-Jueyin, acting on removing Damp Heat of the Liver and Gallbladder, killing bacteria and stopping itching. It is the key point in pruritus vulvae. Taichong (LR3) is Yuan-Primary point of the Liver Meridian, acting to clear away Damp Heat from the Liver Meridian and tonifying Liver and Kidney Yin in deficiency cases. Zhongji (CV3) acts on reducing the Damp Heat of the Lower Burner, regulating vaginal discharge to stop itching. Sanyinjiao (SP6) can regulate the functions of the Spleen, Liver and Kidneys and remove Damp Heat from the Lower Burner so as to relieve pruritus vulvae.

4. **Modification**

- *Damp Heat of Liver Meridian*: + Xingjian (LR2) and Qugu (CV2) to clear away Damp Heat and stop turbid discharge and vaginal itching.

- *Deficiency of Liver and Kidney Yin*: + Ququan (LR8), Taixi (KI3) and Zhaohai (KI6) to nourish Yin, clear away Heat, and regulate vaginal discharge to stop itching.

5. **Manipulation**

Ligou (LR5) is punctured obliquely with the tip upward. The needling sensation should be conducted to the media of the thigh. Zhongji (CV3) is punctured obliquely with the tip slightly downward and the needling sensation is spread to the external genitalia. Routine acupuncture technique is applied to other acupoints.

Other therapies

1. **Auricular acupuncture**

Points: Ear-Shemen, Ovary, External Genitalia Organ, Spleen, Liver, Kidney, Adrenal. 3 to 5 points are selected in each treatment with moderate stimulation. Needles are retained for 15 to 30 minutes. Embedding needles or Vaccaria seed is applicable to the points.

2. **Point injection**

Points: Changqiang (GV1), Qugu (CV2), Huantiao (GB30), Sanyinjiao (SP6). 2 to 3 points are selected in each treatment and injected with vitamin B_{12} injection, 0.5–1ml in each point. injection is applied once every other day.

Notes

Acupuncture and moxibustion are certainly effective in treating the disease. Drastic and intolerable itching or lingering sickness can be treated with local application of medicines in combination with acupuncture and moxibustion. But strong irritating and corroding drugs are prohibited. Topical medication should be applied with great caution in cases with excessive scratching and local skin mucosal lesion.

8. MORNING SICKNESS

Brief introduction

Morning sickness refers to repeated nausea, vomiting, dizziness, anorexia, even vomiting after eating, due to reversed Qi of Thoroughfare Vessel in the early stage of pregnancy (about 6 weeks). Western medicine describes it as vomiting during pregnancy, or drastic vomiting of pregnancy. It is commonly seen in young women during the first pregnancy, with emotional disturbance and excessive mental stress.

Aetiology and pathogenesis

The main pathogenesis is related to the failure of Stomach Qi to descend and the disturbance of Qi ascending and descending the Liver and Spleen Meridians, as well as the Thoroughfare Vessel and Conception Vessel. In pregnancy, Blood is stored rather than leaked so that Yin Blood flows down to the Thoroughfare Vessel and Conception Vessel to foster the foetus. Thus, the Qi and Blood of the Thoroughfare Vessel and Conception Vessel are abundant and the Qi of the Spleen and Stomach Meridians are relatively insufficient. Therefore, for pregnant women with a weak constitution, deficiency and weakness of the Spleen and Stomach is commonly seen, and insufficiency of Yang of the Middle Burner; thus turbid Qi fails to descend, and then ascends in the reverse direction with Qi of the Thoroughfare Vessel to attack the Stomach. For those with a strong constitution, excessive Damp in the Spleen is commonly seen, and internal production of Phlegm; thus, Phlegm attacks in the reverse direction the Stomach, together with the Qi of the Thoroughfare Vessel. For those with constitutional Liver hyperactivity, emotional disturbance or mental stress, Liver Qi stagnation may occur and Liver Qi may attack the Stomach transversely, which results in failure of the Stomach Qi to descend, and vomiting occurs.

Syndrome differentiation

Main symptoms: repeated nausea, vomiting, dizziness and anorexia in the early stage of pregnancy, even feeling nausea and vomiting after eating, unable to eat and drink. In mild cases, the symptoms are vomiting, especially after eating, associated with anorexia, lassitude, somnolence, insomnia, urinary ketone negative. In moderate cases, the symptoms are frequent vomiting, vomiting whenever smelling food, severe general dehydration, slightly increased body temperature, accelerative pulse, blood pressure decreasing, urinary ketone positive. Severe vomiting is seldom seen in clinic. The main symptoms are continuous vomiting, inability to eat and drink, vomiting of thick fluids, biles or coffee-colour bloody residue, scanty urine or no urine, body temperature increasing, urinary ketone positive, accelerative pulse, blood pressure decreasing, even somnolence, shock, severe dehydration and electrolytic disturbance, urinary ketone positive, urea nitrogen increases and hyperbilirubinemia

1. **Disharmony between the Liver and Stomach**: Abdominal distension, nausea, vomiting of acid or bitter fluid after eating, mental stress or depression, belching, sighing, distending pain of hypochondriac region and breasts, thirst, bitter taste in the mouth, distension of the head, vertigo; thin and yellow tongue coating, string-taut and rolling pulse.

2. **Deficiency of the Spleen and Stomach**: Poor appetite, vomiting of saliva or clear liquid after eating, dizziness, lassitude, somnolence, pale tongue with thin and white coating, rolling and forceless pulse.

3. **Retention of Phlegm and Damp**: Distension and fullness in epigastrium, nausea, vomiting of saliva or sticky liquid when smelling food (or continuous vomiting), unable to eat and drink (especially after getting up in the morning), severe lassitude; flabby and pale tongue with white and sticky coating, rolling pulse.

Treatment
Body acupuncture

1. **Principles of treatment**

   Strengthen the Spleen to resolve Phlegm, smooth the Liver and harmonize the Stomach, reduce reversed Qi and stop vomiting. For deficiency of the Spleen and Stomach and retention of Phlegm, acupuncture and moxibustion are applied in combination. For disharmony of the Liver and Stomach, acupuncture alone is applied with even-needling technique.

2. **Prescription**

   Zhongwan (CV12), Neiguan (PC6), Gongsun (SP4), Zusanli (ST36).

3. **Explanation**

Zhongwan (CV12) is the Front-Mu and Influential point of Fu of the Stomach Meridian, acting on regulating Qi of the Fu organs, harmonizing the Stomach and reducing the reversed Qi. Neiguan (PC6) is Luo-Connecting point of the Pericardium Meridian and it communicates between the three Burners up and down, harmonizes the interior and adjusts the exterior. Gongsun (SP4) is the Luo-Connecting point of the Spleen Meridian, communicating with the Stomach and making the pair point with Neiguan (PC6) as the Confluent point. The pair points not only strengthen the Spleen to resolve Damp and benefit the Stomach to reduce turbidity, but also regulate the Thoroughfare Vessel and Conception Vessel and reduce reversed. Zusanli (ST36) is the Inferior He-Sea point of the Stomach Meridian and it not only strengthens the Spleen and Stomach, transforms Qi and Blood, but also smoothes the Liver, harmonizes the Stomach, regulates Qi and reduces reversed Qi.

4. **Modification**

- *Deficiency of the Spleen and Stomach*: Moxibustion is supplemented on Pishu (BL20) and Weishu (BL21) to strengthen Yang of the Middle Burner and the Spleen to stop vomiting.

- *Disharmony between the Liver and Stomach*: + Qimen (LR14) and Taichong (LR3) to smooth Liver Qi and reduce reversed Qi.

- *Retention of Phlegm*: + Sanyinjiao (SP6) and Fenglong (ST40) to strength the Spleen to resolve Damp and Phlegm and reduce the turbid.

- *Dizziness*: + Baihui (GV20) and Fengchi (GB20) to calm the Mind.

- *Lassitude and somnolence*: Moxibustion is applied to Baihui (GV20) and Qihai (CV6) to benefit Qi and nourish the Blood.

- *Anorexia*: Moxibustion is applied to Zhongwan (CV12) and Tianshu (ST25) and acupuncture to Neiting (ST44) to smooth the intestines and Stomach and promote appetite.

- *Insomnia, dream-disturbed sleep and palpitations*: + Xinshu (BL15) and Shenmen (HT7) for sedation.

5. **Manipulation**

Shallow and gentle puncturing is applied to Neiguan (PC6). Deep puncturing, 1–1.5 cun, is applied to the points in the abdomen and the lifting and thrusting technique is applied cautiously. Warming needling is applied for deficiency of the Spleen and Stomach and retention of Phlegm. All of the points are stimulated with the even-needling method. Tonifying technique is not used for the deficiency because it may worsen reversed turbid Qi. Reducing technique is not used for the excess because it may damage the foetus and induce it by accident.

Other therapies

1. **Auricular acupuncture**

   Points: Liver, Stomach, Ear-Shenmen, Endocrine, Subcortex. In each treatment, 2 or 3 points are selected and stimulated by needle, Vaccaria seeds or magnetic seeds.

2. **Electroacupuncture**

   One or two pairs of main points are selected in the light of the acupuncture prescription. Disperse-dense wave, slow frequency and weak stimulation are applied for about 30 minutes each time.

3. **Cutaneous needle**

   In light of the acupuncture prescription, tapping is applied locally or to Jiaji (EX-B2) from T4 to L5 and Back-Shu points from up to down with gentle stimulation until local skin turns slightly red.

4. **Point injection**

   Points: Geshu (BL17), Ganshu (BL18), Pishu (BL20), Weishu (BL21), Zusanli (ST36), etc. In each treatment, 2 points are selected and injected with 10% Glucose injection or 2% Lidocarine Hydrochloride injection, 1–2ml in each point.

Notes

1. Acupuncture and moxibustion have apparent efficacy in morning sickness. But at the early stage of pregnancy, the foetus is not yet strong enough, so, fewer points should be selected in acupuncture treatment and deep insertion and strong manipulation should be avoided to prevent the foetus from being injured.

2. Easily digested and light food is selected. Eating less but more frequently is suggested. Irritating food of offensive flavour should be avoided.

3. For critical cases of drastic vomiting, the intake and output volume should be recorded and intravenous infusion applied to prevent dehydration and electrolytic disturbance.

4. This disease needs to be differentiated from vomiting induced by acute gastroenteritis, digestive ulceration, viral hepatitis, gastric carcinoma, etc.

9. MALPOSITION OF FOETUS

Brief introduction

The occipital anterior position is commonly seen in most malposition of the foetus. At 30 weeks of pregnancy, a pre-labour examination discovers occipital posterior, buttock position or occipital transverse of foetus, thus, a malposition of foetus is determined, which is commonly seen in multipara or pregnant women with loose abdominal wall.

Aetiology and pathogenesis

Cold stagnation due to Kidney deficiency, retention of Damp due to Spleen deficiency and Liver Qi stagnation are relevant with the disease. The Kidney dominates reproduction and development and connects with the uterus internally. Kidney Qi deficiency results in Cold stagnation and weakness of the foetus turning position. Spleen deficiency results in retention of Damp and the foetus being overweight and the limited turning of the foetus. Liver Qi stagnation results in retarded Qi activity, which develops a failure of the foetus to turn its position. Eventually, malposition of foetus occurs.

Syndrome differentiation

At 30 weeks of pregnancy, pre-delivery examination discovers occipital posterior, oblique position, transverse position, buttock position or foot position of foetus, etc.

1. **Cold stagnation due to Kidney deficiency**: Emaciation, pallid complexion, lassitude, soreness of lumbar region and cold abdomen; pale tongue with thin and white coating, rolling and weak pulse.

2. **Damp retention due to Spleen deficiency**: Overweight body, lassitude, somnolence, weakness of four limbs; flabby and pale tongue with white and sticky coating; soft and rolling pulse.

3. **Liver Qi stagnation**: Mental depression or irritability, hot temper, distension in hypochondriac region, belching, irregular defecation; red tongue with slightly yellow coating; string-taut and rolling pulse.

Treatment

Body acupuncture

1. **Principles of treatment**

   Benefit the Kidneys, warm the uterus, strengthen the Spleen to resolve Damp, smooth Liver Qi and regulate Qi and Blood of the uterus. Acupuncture and moxibustion are used in combination for Cold stagnation due to Kidney deficiency, and retention of Damp due to Spleen deficiency, with reinforcing technique. For Liver Qi stagnation, acupuncture alone is used with even technique.

2. **Prescription**

   Zhiyin (BL67), Taixi (KI3), Sanyinjiao (SP6).

3. **Explanation**

   Zhiyin (BL67) is Jing-Well point of the Bladder Meridian of Foot-Taiyang and pertains to Metal in Five Elements. The Qi of the meridian communicates with the Kidney Meridian of Foot-Taiyin. The point benefits Kidney Water, and regulates Kidney Qi and is well known as an effective point for foetus position correction. Taixi (KI3) is the Yuan-Primary point of the Kidney Meridian of Foot-Taiyin and it tonifies the Kidneys and regulates the uterus. Sanyinjiao (SP6) is the Crossing point. It strengthens the Spleen, smoothes Liver Qi, benefits the Kidneys, removes stagnation and regulates the uterus. The point is the key in gynaecologic disorders and assists to the correction of foetus position.

4. **Modification**

   - *Cold stagnation due to Kidney deficiency*: + Qihai (CV6) and Shenshu (BL23) with moxibustion to benefit the Kidneys and warm the uterus so as to strengthen the foetus.

   - *Damp retention due to Spleen deficiency*: + Yinlingquan (SP9), Fenglong (ST40) and Zusanli (ST36) to strengthen the Spleen, resolve turbidity so as to remove Damp.

   - *Liver Qi stagnation*: + Taichong (LR3) and Qimen (LR14) to smooth Liver Qi and remove depression and stagnation.

5. **Manipulation**

   The pregnant woman is placed in half-lying position or sitting with the back against the chair, being sure the Bladder is empty and belting loosened. Moxa stick, warming moxibustion or sparrow-pecking moxibustion is applied to Zhiyin (BL67) bilaterally, for 15–20 minutes, or small moxa cone is used, 7–10 cones each time. Even-needling technique is applied to Taixi (KI3) and Sanyinjiao (SP6) (warming needling is supplemented for Cold stagnation due to Kidney deficiency and Damp retention due to Spleen deficiency), 1 to 2 times a day until the position of foetus is corrected.

Other therapies

1. **Electroacupuncture**

   Electroacupuncture is applied bilaterally to Zhiyin (BL67) and Taixi (KI3), with disperse-dense wave for 10 to 15 minutes.

Notes

1. Acupuncture and moxibustion have definite efficacy for the malposition of foetus. The success rate in the majority of statistics is up to 80%. The position of the foetus is corrected in about 3 treatments generally. The key to efficacy is the right time for treatment. It is indicated in clinical data that the successful rate is up to 90% in acupuncture and moxibustion for malposition of the foetus of 28 to 32 weeks. The efficacy is slightly poorer if the treatment is applied after pregnancy of 32 weeks. Before 28 weeks of pregnancy, the size of foetus is small and there is more amniotic fluid. Hence, there is quite a large space for the foetus to move in the uterus and the position and posture of the foetus can be altered easily. But, after 32 weeks of pregnancy, the foetus grows fast and the aminotic fluid is relatively less. The more closely the foetus is attached to the uterus wall, the more the posture and position of it is relatively fixed. Hence, the efficacy is poor in this stage.

2. After acupuncture and moxibustion treatment, the patient is guided to keep a knee-chest position for 10 to 15 minutes so that the efficacy can be improved.

3. Malposition of foetus caused by uterus deformity, pelvic stenosis or pelvic carcinoma is not suitable for treatment with acupuncture and moxibustion. Management by the obstetric and gynaecological department should be provided as early as possible to avoid accidents.

10. PROLONGED LABOUR

Brief introduction

Prolonged labour, also known as a difficult delivery. It refers to difficulty in the delivery of a fully matured foetus, in which the duration of delivery is over 24 hours. It is commonly seen in abnormal contraction of the uterus, abnormal development of pelvic cavity, cervix and vulvae, foetus abnormality or abnormal development of foetus. Acupuncture and moxibustion is applied in the case of obstructed labour due to abnormal uterine action.

Aetiology and pathogenesis

Deficiency and excess are involved in the aetiology. Deficiency refers to Qi and Blood deficiency. Excess refers to Qi and Blood stagnation. No matter which are the factors involved, they all result in weak contractions of the uterus and unsmooth labour.

Syndrome differentiation

Weak contraction of the uterus, short duration of contraction, prolonged and irregular intervals; no abdominal bulging and hardness at the peak of uterus contraction, or no coordinating contraction of the uterus, no feeling subjectively strong contraction by parturient, persistent abdominal pain that is worse on pressure, irritability, intolerable pain, but still no strong fundus contraction (strong contraction at the middle or lower section of the uterus is determined as an invalid contraction); prolonged duration of delivery, over 24 hours in total.

1. **Deficiency of Qi and Blood**: No apparent bulging of abdomen or short-term bulging, bearing-down sensation, distension, dull paroxysmal pain, pale complexion, lassitude, shortness of breath; deep, thready, weak pulse or large but deficiency pulse.

2. **Stagnation of Qi and Blood**: Persistent bulging of the abdomen, not soft; drastic pain in lumbar region and abdomen, which is worse on pressure, dark complexion, irritability, restlessness, mental tension, terror; deep pulse of excess type or string-taut and tense pulse.

Treatment

Body acupuncture

1. **Principles of treatment**

   Regulate Qi and Blood to promote labour. Acupuncture and moxibustion are used together for deficiency of Qi and Blood mainly with reinforcing technique and coordination of reinforcing and reducing techniques. For stagnation of Qi and Blood, acupuncture alone is used mainly with reducing technique and coordination of reinforcing and reducing techniques.

2. **Prescription**

   Tanzhong (CV17), Hegu (LI4), Sanyinjiao (SP6), Zhiyin (BL67), Duyin (EX-LE11).

3. **Explanation**

   Tanzhong (CV17) is the Influential point of Qi in the Conception Vessel, and acts on regulating the Qi activity of the uterus, benefiting labour strength and reducing Qi to promote labour. Hegu (LI4) is Yuan-Primary point of the Large Intestine Meridian of Hand-Yangming and acts on regulating the Qi system. Sanyinjiao (SP6) is the Crossing point of the three Yin meridians of foot, and acts on regulating the Blood system. In the combination of the 2 points, reinforcing Hegu (LI4) can benefit Qi circulation and reducing Sanyinjiao (SP6) can promote Qi circulation and remove stasis so that the delivery is promoted. Zhiyin (BL67) is the Jing-Well point of the Bladder Meridian of Foot-Taiyin. Duyin (EX-LE11) is the Extra point. 2 points are used together to benefit Kidney Qi, and regulate the uterus. They are the established effective points for prolonged labour.

4. **Modification**

   - *Deficiency of Qi and Blood*: + Zusanli (ST36) to tonify Qi and Blood, increase contraction strength to promote labour.

   - *Stagnation of Qi and Blood*: + Taichong (LR3) to regulate Qi circulation and remove stasis so as to promote labour.

   - *Lassitude and palpitations*: + Qihai (CV6) with moxibustion and Neiguan (PC6) with acupuncture are supplemented to benefit Qi and sedate the Heart.

   - *Drastic abdominal pain*: + Qichong (ST30) with moxibustion and Diji (SP8) with acupuncture are supplemented to promote circulations in collaterals and stop pain.

5. **Manipulation**

Transverse puncture is applied to Tanzhong (CV17) with needle tip downward, 1 to 1.5 cun; the lifting-thrusting and rotating technique is used to achieve reinforcing or even-needling technique is used. Perpendicular puncture is applied to Hegu (LI4), about 1 cun and manipulated with reinforcing technique. Perpendicular puncture is applied to Sanyinjiao (SP6), about 1.2 cun and manipulated with reducing technique. Zhiyin (BL67) and Duyin (EX-LE11) are punctured obliquely, about 0.3 cun. Moxibustion alone is applied to the acupoints on the abdomen. Needles are retained for 1hr or until uterine contractions become regular and forceful. While the needles are retained, needles are manipulated about once every 5 minutes.

Other therapies

1. **Electroacupuncture**

Zhiyin (BL67) and Duyin (EX-LE11) are selected and punctured about 0.3 cun in depth respectively. Electroacupuncture is used to the points, with disperse-dense wave for 60 minutes until uterine contractions are regular and forceful.

2. **Auricular acupuncture**

Points: Uterus, Ear-Shenmen, Subcortex, Endocrine, Kidney. The points are stimulated moderately by filiform needle and manipulated about once every 5 minutes; or stimulated by electroacupuncture, with disperse-dense wave for 60 minutes until uterine contractions become regular and forceful.

Notes

1. Acupuncture and moxibustion have apparent efficacy on prolonged labour due to abnormal uterine action.

2. Prolonged labour is extremely hazardous to the health of parturient and foetus. Therefore, comprehensive measurements should be adopted for critical cases. An operation is required promptly if it becomes necessary.

3. If prolonged labour is induced by uterine deformity, pelvic stenosis, other managements methods should be applied to prevent accidents.

11. LOCHIORRHOEA

Brief introduction

For 1–3 weeks after labour, uterine residues are discharge from the vulvae, which is a normal phenomenon, known as postpartum haemorrhage. If vaginal haemorrhage continues over 3 weeks after labour, lochiorrhoea is diagnosed. In Western medicine this disease is the equivalent of postpartum haemorrhage of a late stage, incomplete involution of uterus, partial residue of placenta, residue of decidua and puerperal infection.

Aetiology and pathogenesis

Essentially, the disease is related to dysfunction of the Conception Vessel and Thoroughfare Vessel, dysfunction of Qi and Blood circulation which leads to abnormal bleeding. It is induced commonly by a failure of control due to Qi deficiency, internal disturbance of Blood Heat and stagnation of Qi and Blood.

Syndrome differentiation

Vaginal haemorrhage and discharge over 3 weeks after labour as the main symptoms, or sudden bleeding or repeated bleeding within about 20 days of labour, dribbling afterward; smelly odour in the discharge, associated with low fever and general discomfort.

1. **Failure of control due to Qi deficiency**: Persistent postpartum haemorrhage, heavy amount or dribbling, light red in colour, thin in quality, no smell, empty and bearing-down sensation in lower abdomen, lassitude, dislike of speaking, pallid complexion, pale tongue with thin coating, retarded and weak pulse.

2. **Internal disturbance of Blood Heat**: Persistent postpartum haemorrhage, heavy amount, fresh red or deep red in colour, thick in quality, stinking smell, red face, dry mouth and throat; red tongue with thin and yellow coating, thready and rapid pulse of deficiency type.

3. **Stagnation of Qi and Blood**: Dribbling postpartum haemorrhage, small amount, purplish and dark colour with clots, pain in lower abdomen that is worse on pressure, or something hard is felt on palpation; purplish dark tongue or with stagnated spots, thin and white coating; string-taut and hesitant or deep forceful pulse.

Treatment

Body acupuncture

1. **Principles of treatment**

   Consolidate the Thoroughfare Vessel and Conception Vessel, clear away Heat, cool the Blood, remove stasis and stop bleeding. Acupuncture and moxibustion are used together for Qi deficiency with reinforcing technique. Acupuncture alone is used for Blood Heat and stagnation of Qi and Blood with reducing technique.

2. **Prescription**

   Points are mainly selected from the Conception Vessel and the Spleen Meridian of Foot-Taiyin. Guanyuan (CV4), Qihai (CV6), Xuehai (SP10), Sanyinjiao (SP6).

3. **Explanation**

   The reinforcing method is used on Guanyuan (CV4) and Qihai (CV6) to benefit primary Qi to consolidate the Thoroughfare Vessel and Conception Vessel, regulate the uterus, conduct regular Blood circulation, benefit Qi to control and manufacture Blood. Xuehai (SP10) and Sanyinjiao (SP10) are the key points in regulating Blood and meridians. The reinforcing method is used on the points to regulate and tonify Blood so as to generate fresh Blood. The reducing method is used on the points to promote circulation of the collaterals and activate Blood circulation to remove stasis, and even-needling technique is used to nourish Yin, cool Blood and clear away Heat of deficiency type.

4. **Modification**

   - *Qi deficiency*: + Zusanli (ST36) and Pishu (BL20) to strengthen the Spleen, benefit Qi, control Blood and produce Blood.

   - *Internal disturbance of Blood Heat*: + Zhongji (CV3), Xingjian (LR2) and Rangu (KI2) to disperse pathogenic Heat and clear Heat of deficiency type.

   - *Stagnation of Qi and Blood*: + Diji (SP8) and Geshu (BL17) to regulate Qi circulation and activate Blood circulation to remove stasis.

   - *Empty and bearing-down sensation of lower abdomen*: + Baihui (BV20) with moxibustion to elevate Yang.

   - *Abdominal pain that is worse on pressure*: + Guilai (ST29) with moxibustion to warm meridians, remove stasis and stop pain.

5. **Manipulation**

   Perpendicular needling is applied to Guanyuan (CV4) and Qihai (CV6) for about 1 cun; deep puncturing is unsuitable because of the need to prevent injury of unrecovered uterus. Reinforcing technique or warming needling is applied. For failure to control due to Qi deficiency, reinforcing technique is used on Xuehai (SP10) and Sanyinjiao (SP6), after reducing technique to benefit Qi, control Blood and avoid retention of remained pathogens. For stagnation of Qi and Blood and internal disturbance of Blood Heat, coordination of reinforcing and reducing technique is used.

Other therapies

1. **Auricular acupuncture**

   Points: Internal Reproductive Organ, Subcortex, Sympathetic Nerve, Endocrine. Weak stimulation is applied, 15–20 minutes in each treatment. Embedding needle, Vaccaria seeds or magnetic seeds may be applied to the points.

2. **Electroacupuncture**

   Main points in acupuncture prescription are selected. After the arrival of Qi, electroacupuncture is used, with disperse-dense wave and tolerable stimulation, 20–30 minutes in each treatment.

Notes

1. Acupuncture and moxibustion are quite effective for postpartum lochiorrhoea.

2. Because the patient after labour is mostly deficient, reinforcing for deficiency syndrome must be applied while reducing technique is used for excess syndrome. Hence coordination of reinforcing and deficiency technique is commonly applied in clinical situations.

3. The patient should rest in a lying position, keep her emotions stable, eat food that is light and rich in nutrients, avoid raw and cold food; pay attention to climatic change, avoid overheat and Cold attack; not become overtired and sexual activity is prohibited.

12. POSTPARTUM HYPOGALACTIA

Brief introduction

This refers to lactation deficiency or no lactation at early lactating stage after labour.

Aetiology and pathogenesis

Deficiency and excess are divided in this disease. Deficiency refers to constitutional deficiency or lack of nutrition after labour, which leads to deficiency of Qi and Blood, and insufficiency of milk production. Excess refers to Liver Qi stagnation that leads to retarded Qi activity and blockage of lactation, thus hypogalactia or no lactation happens.

Syndrome differentiation

Less secretion of milk or no lactation at early lactating stage after labour, normal breast development, no apparent organic changes.

1. **Deficiency of Qi and Blood**: Hypogalactia after labour, no breast distension, no lustre of the face, poor appetite, lassitude; pale tongue with little coating, thready pulse of deficiency type.

2. **Liver Qi stagnation**: Hypogalactia after labour, distending pain of the breasts, mental depression, poor appetite; thin tongue coating, string-taut pulse.

Treatment

Body acupuncture

1. **Principles of treatment**

   - *Deficiency of Qi and Blood*: Benefit Qi and tonify Blood. Acupuncture and moxibustion are applied together with reinforcing technique.

   - *Liver Qi stagnation*: Smooth Liver Qi and promote circulations of collaterals and lactation. Acupuncture alone is applied with reducing technique.

2. **Prescription**

   Points are mainly selected from Yangming meridians. Rugen (ST18), Tanzhong (CV17), Shaoze (SI1), Zusanli (ST36).

3. **Explanation**

Rugen (ST18) is a point of the Stomach Meridian of Foot-Yangming that contains excessive Qi and Blood. The point is located beneath the breast, acts on tonifying Qi and Blood, and promoting lactation. In addition, it promotes Qi circulation and activates Blood and opens the collaterals of the breasts. Tanzhong (CV17) is an Influential point of Qi. Reinforcing technique is applied to it to benefit Qi and Blood and nourish lactation, and reducing technique is applied to regulate Qi, open depression and promote lactation. Shaoze (SI1) is the Jing-Well point of the Small Intestine Meridian of Hand-Taiyang. It refers to Metal in Five Elements, acts on reducing Liver stagnation and promoting breast vessels. It is the established effective point to produce and promote lactation. Zusanli (ST36) is He-Sea point of the Stomach Meridian of Foot-Yangming. It refers to Earth in Five Elements and is the 'Earth point on Earth Meridian'. It acts on benefiting Qi and Blood, smoothing Liver Qi and removing stagnation.

4. **Modification**

- *Deficiency of Qi and Blood*: + Qihai (CV6), Xuehai (SP10), Pishu (BL20), Weishu (BL21) and Sanyinjiao (SP6) to tonify Qi and Blood and promote lactation.

- *Liver Qi stagnation*: + Qimen (LR14), Neiguan (PC6) and Taichong (LR3) to regulate Liver Qi and promote lactation.

5. **Manipulation**

Tanzhong (CV17) is punctured transversely to the breasts, 1–1.5 cun. Rugan (ST18) is punctured transversely to the base of breast, about 1 cun to obtain slight distension. Moxibustion can be added on the point. Shaoze (SI1) is punctured shallowly, 0.2–0.3 cun. Needles are retained for 20 to 30 minutes.

Other therapies

1. **Auricular acupuncture**

Points: Liver, Spleen, Kidney, Endocrine, Subcortex. Points are stimulated gently by filiform needle or with Vaccaria seeds and magnetic seeds.

2. **Electroacupuncture**

Electroacupuncture is applied to Rugan (ST18) bilaterally after the arrival of Qi, with disperse-dense wave and mild stimulation. It is correct if patient feels a slight needling sensation. The treatment lasts 20–30 minutes each time, once every day.

Notes

1. Acupuncture and moxibustion have apparent efficacy for postpartum hypogalactia.

2. Parturient should have enriched nutrients, have proper rest, regulate her moods and rectify any incorrect method of breastfeeding.

3. For those with retarded lactation and distending pain of the breasts, lactation should be promoted with squeezing to avoid mastitis.

13. PROLAPSE OF UTERUS

Brief introduction

Prolapse of the uterus refers to the downward displacement of the uterus along the vagina, cervix descends beyond the ischial spine or even completely out of the vagina opening or with the vaginal wall protruding.

Aetiology and pathogenesis

The disease is commonly due to over-exertion during labour or early physical work after labour, which results in deficiency of Spleen Qi, injury of Qi in the Middle Burner and sinking of Qi. Or the disease is due to weak constitution, multiple pregnancies and childbirths, injury of Kidneys because of excessive sexual activity, which leads to injury of the uterus. Or chronic sickness produces Damp and Heat, resulting in Damp Heat flowing downward. Hence, mixed deficiency and excess syndrome occurs, in which the root of disease is deficiency and the symptoms are excess.

Syndrome differentiation

The uterus is displaced below or even out of the vagina completely. There are three degrees of this condition. *Mild degree (I degree)*: The uterus is displaced downward and the cervix droops below the ischial spine but is still within the vagina. The uterus protrudes if abdominal pressure is increased and is withdrawn naturally in lying position. *Moderate degree (II degree)*: The cervix and a part of the uterus protrudes out of the opening of the vagina, and cannot be replaced naturally. *Severe degree (III degree)*: The entire uterus is outside the vagina. It is difficult to replace. The protruded uterus membrane may have contact with clothes, thus erosion, ulceration, infection and purulent secretions occur.

1. **Qi deficiency of the Spleen and Stomach**: The uterus droops or protrudes outside the opening of vagina, and this is worse on exertion and alleviated when in a lying position; there is a bearing-down sensation in the lower abdomen, lassitude, weakness of the four limbs, white vaginal discharge, thin in quality and profuse in amount, soreness and weakness of the lumbar regions and knees, dizziness, tinnitus, frequent clear urine; pale tongue with white and rolling coating, deep, thready and weak pulse.

2. **Downward flowing of Damp Heat**: Prolonged uterine protrusion, membrane erosion, yellow discharge, distension and burning pain in external genitalia region, deep yellow urine, dry and bitter taste in the mouth; red tongue with yellow sticky coating, rolling and rapid pulse.

Treatment

Body acupuncture

1. **Principles of treatment**

   - *Qi deficiency of the Spleen and Kidney*: Tonify the Spleen and Kidneys, elevate Yang for the prolapse. Acupuncture and moxibustion are used together with reinforcing technique.

   - *Downward flowing of Damp Heat*: Acupuncture alone is used with even-needling technique.

2. **Prescription**

   Points are mainly selected from the Conception Vessel. Baihui (GV20), Qihai (CV6), Guanyuan (CV4), Weidao (GB28), Sanyinjiao (SP6).

3. **Explanation**

   Baihui (GV20) is located on the vertex and is the meeting point of all of the Yang meridians. It invigorates Yang, elevates Yang and consolidates the uterus. Qihai (CV6) and Guanyuan (CV4) are from the Conception Vessel, act on benefiting Qi, consolidating the uterus and regulating the Thoroughfare Vessel and Conception Vessel. Weidao (GB28) is the Crossing point of the Gallbladder Meridian of Foot-Shaoyang and the Belt Vessel. It maintains the Belt Vessel and consolidates the uterus. Sanyinjiao (SP6) regulates the Spleen, Liver and Kidneys and maintains the uterus.

4. **Modification**

- *Spleen deficiency*: + Guilai (ST29), Pishu (BL20) and Zusanli (ST36) to strengthen the Spleen and benefit Qi, elevate Qi and consolidate the uterus.

- *Kidney deficiency*: + Taixi (KI3) and Shenshu (BL23) to tonify Kidney Qi and elevate the protruded uterus.

- *Downward flowing of Damp Heat*: + Zhongji (CV3), Yinlingquan (SP9) and Ligou (LR5) to clear away Heat, remove Damp and consolidate the uterus.

5. **Manipulation**

If Qi deficiency predominates at early stage, reinforcing technique and moxibustion are used. For downward flowing of Damp Heat at later stages, coordination of reinforcing and reducing technique or even-needling technique is used, and moxibustion is not applied. Transverse needling is used on Baihui (GV20) from the anterior to the posterior, 1 to 1.5 cun. Moxibustion can be applied after needling or at the same time as acupuncture. It is applicable with a single moxa cone.

Other therapies

1. **Auricular acupuncture**

Points: Subcortex, Sympathetic Nerve, Internal Reproductive Organ, Spleen and Kidney. In each treatment, 2 or 3 points are selected and stimulated weakly by filiform needle, lasting 20 minutes, or with the application of Vaccaria seed or magnetic seed.

2. **Electroacupuncture**

One or two pairs of main points are selected alternately, with disperse-dense wave, weak stimulation, lasting 20–30 minutes each treatment, once a day.

3. **Point injection**

Guanyuanshu (BL26), Qihaishu (BL24), Shenshu (BL23), Zusanli (ST36). The 2 points are selected in each injection with vitamin B_1, vitamin B_{12}, Andenosine Disodium Triphosphate injection or Compound Angelica injection. 1–2ml of drug is required in each point in each injection, once a day.

Notes

1. Acupuncture and moxibustion have apparent efficacy on prolapse of uterus of I and II degrees. Comprehensive therapy is required for that of III degree with acupuncture and medication.

2. During treatment, the patient is guided in how to do anus elevation (pelvic floor) exercises.

3. Active therapy may induce disorders of abdominal pressure increasing, such as habitual constipation, chronic bronchitis.

4. During treatment, patient is required to have plenty of rest, avoid overstrain and to squat for long periods and do physical work, such as lifting heavy objects.

14. INFERTILITY

Brief introduction

When women of childbearing age fail to become pregnant at childbearing age, having had normal sexual intercourse with a partner who has normal reproductive function, infertility is diagnosed. Or if the women fails to become pregnant for over 2 years continuously, having been pregnant and childbearing before, infertility is also diagnosed.

Aetiology and pathogenesis

Infertility may be induced by uterine Cold due to congenital Kidney deficiency, Blood deficiency of the Thoroughfare Vessel and Conception Vessel and blockage and retention of Phlegm and Damp.

Syndrome differentiation

Uterine Cold due to Kidney deficiency: irregular menstruation, scanty menstrual flow of light colour; soreness of lumbar region and cold abdomen, clear and thin vaginal discharge, sexual hypoaesthesia; pale tongue with thin and white coating, deep, thready and weak pulse.

1. **Blood deficiency of the Thoroughfare Vessel and Conception Vessel**: Delayed or irregular menstruation, scanty menstrual flow, purplish colour with clots; distending pain in breasts and hypochondriac region before

menstruation, pain of lumbar region and knees that is worse on pressure; purplish dark tongue or with stagnated spots, string-taut and hesitant pulse.

2. **Blockage and retention of Phlegm and Damp**: Delayed menstruation, scanty menstrual flow, light colour, profuse thick leucorrhoea, obesity, pale complexion, stickiness in the mouth, poor appetite, hesitant bowel movement or loose stools; flabby and pale tongue with teeth-marks, white sticky coating; rolling pulse.

Treatment
Body acupuncture

1. **Principles of treatment**

   - *Uterine Cold due to Kidney deficiency and Blood deficiency of the Thoroughfare Vessel and Conception Vessel*: Benefit the Kidney, warm the uterus, and regulate the Thoroughfare Vessel and Conception Vessel. Both acupuncture and moxibustion are used with reinforcing technique.

   - *Qi and Blood stagnation and blockage and retention of Phlegm and Damp*: Promote Qi circulation, activate Blood flow, and resolve Phlegm to remove stagnation. Acupuncture is the chief therapy with reducing technique.

2. **Prescription**

   Guanyuan (CV4), Dahe (KI12), Sanyinjiao (SP6), Ciliao (BL32), Zhibian (BL54).

3. **Explanation**

   Guanyuan (CV4) and Dahe (KI12) are both located below the umbilicus and near to the uterus. Both of them act on tonifying Qi and Blood of the Kidney Meridian, strengthening primary Yin and primary Yang. Acupuncture on the points can regulate the Thoroughfare Vessel and Conception Vessel and moxibustion on them can warm the uterus. Sanyinjiao (SP6) acts to strengthen the Spleen to resolve Damp and remove stagnation. In addition, it can smooth Liver Qi, remove stasis, tonify Kidney Yin and Kidney Yang, as well as regulate Qi and Blood of the Thoroughfare Vessel and Conception Vessel. Ciliao (BL32) and Zhibian (BL54) can promote Blood circulation in the pelvic cavity, regulate menstruation and benefit pregnancy. All of the points used together can tonify the congenital foundation and regulate acquired Qi. Hence the treatment promotes pregnancy.

4. **Modification**

- *Uterine Cold due to Kidney deficiency*: Moxibustion is supplemented on Shenshu (BL23), Mingmen (GV4) and Shenque (CV8) to tonify Kidney Yang and warm the uterus so as to expel Cold.

- *Blood deficiency of the Thoroughfare Vessel and Conception Vessel*: + Qihai (CV6) and Xuehai (SP10) to benefit Qi, nourish Blood and fill up Qi and Blood of the uterus.

- *Qi and Blood stagnation*: + Taichong (LR3) and Geshu (BL18) to promote Qi circulation and activate Blood flow and smooth Liver Qi to remove stagnation.

- *Blockage and retention of Phlegm and Damp*: + Fenglong (ST40) and Yinlingquan (SP9) to resolve Phlegm, promote circulations of collaterals, eliminate Damp and remove blockage.

5. **Manipulation**

Guanyuan (CV4) and Dahe (KI12) are needled with reinforcing technique combined with moxibustion or with even-needling technique. Either reinforcing or reducing technique is applied to Sanyinjiao (SP6) depending on deficiency or excess syndrome respectively, and moxibustion can be supplemented. On Ciliao (BL32) and Zhibian (BL54), it is required that needle tip should be toward the external orifice of the urethra, 2–3 cun in depth of insertion and a better result is obtained if the needling sensations are conducted to that region.

Other therapies

1. **Auricular acupuncture**

   Points: Endocrine, Internal Reproductive Organ, Kidney, Subcortex. The points are stimulated weakly by filiform needle or with use of Vaccaria seeds and magnets, or embedding needle.

2. **Moxibustion isolated with drugs**

   Chinese herbal formulas in the category of warming Kidney Yang, promoting Qi circulation and removing stasis are selected and ground into powder. Shenque (CV8) is filled up with herbal powder and a big moxa cone is placed over the powder, isolated with a slice of ginger (the numbers of moxa cones are determined depending on the patient's age). This therapy is applied once a day.

Notes

1. Acupuncture and moxibustion are certainly effective in treating infertility. But in treatment, infertility should be excluded if it is induced by male factors or self induced physiological factors. The relevant adjuvant examinations should be conducted if necessary so that appropriate corresponding therapies are selected.

2. For the patient with infertility, it is necessary to lay stress on specific situations, such as sexual history, menstruation, miscarriage or abortion, delivery, whether contraceptives have been used, whether the patient has breastfed for long time, whether she is obese, whether she has maldevelopment of the secondary sex characteristics, and other conditions.

15. MENOPAUSE SYNDROME

Brief introduction

Menopause syndrome is due to the declining of Kidney Qi and Taigui and imbalance of Yin and Yang before and after the menopause phase in females, manifested as dribbling menstruation, disturbance of menstrual cycle and quality, associated with mental abnormality (mental restlessness, irritability, hot temper), sudden feverish sensation, sweating, dizziness, tinnitus, insomnia, poor memory, palpitations, paroxysmal flushed cheeks, puffy face, loose stools, etc.

Aetiology and pathogenesis

Declining Kidney Qi, insufficiency of Essence and Blood and deficiency of the Thoroughfare Vessel and Conception Vessel are the root of the disease. The main factors of this disease include disharmony of the Heart and Kidneys, internal disturbance of Heart Fire, Yin deficiency of the Liver and Kidneys, hyperactivity of Liver Yang, Spleen deficiency in transportation, Yang deficiency of the Spleen and Kidneys, etc.

Syndrome differentiation

Changes in menstruation and the reproductive organ: Disturbance of the menstrual cycle happens usually before menopause, which is manifested as prolonged or shortened menstrual cycle, increased menstrual flow, even heavy bleeding; afterwards, irregular menstruation occurs, with gradually reduced menstrual flow and amenorrhoea (menstruation may stop suddenly in a few women). Atrophy occurs gradually in the external genitalia region, vulvae, uterus, ovary duct, mammary glands, etc. The tissues on the base of pelvis and around the vulvae gradually become loose.

1. **Symptoms of the psychological and nervous systems**: Unstable emotions, excitability, mental stress, depression, irritability, hot temper, emotional susceptibility, insomnia, fatigue, declining memory, absent Mind; occasional hyperaesthesia or hypoaesthesia, headache, joint pain or skin numbness, pricking itching, creeping sensation of the skin, etc.

2. **Symptoms of the vegetative nerve and cardiac vascular system**: Paroxysmal feverish sensation in the body, sweating, cold or warm sensations, associated with chest distress, shortness of breath, palpitations, dizziness or temporary increased or decreased blood pressure, etc.

3. **Yin deficiency of the Liver and Kidneys**: Advanced or delayed menstruation, fresh colour, profuse or less menstrual flow, dry vulvae, soreness and weakness of lumbar region and knee joints, dizziness, tinnitus, insomnia, dream-disturbed sleep, tidal fever, sweating, feverish sensation of palms, soles and chest, dry mouth and tongue, dry stools, or skin itching or with a creeping sensation; red tongue with little coating, thready and rapid pulse.

4. **Yang deficiency of the Spleen and Kidney**: Delayed menstruation or amenorrhoea, profuse menstrual flow, of light colour, and thin in quality or dribbling, lassitude, cold limbs, dark complexion, lumbar soreness, frequent urination or poor appetite, loose stools, puffy face, oedema of limbs, or palpitations, poor memory; pale and flabby tongue with white slippery coating, deep, thready and weak pulse.

5. **Disharmony of the Heart and Kidney**: Palpitations, anxiety, insomnia, dream-disturbed sleep, tidal fever, sweating, feverish sensation of the palms, soles and chest, unstable emotions, soreness and weakness of the lumbar region and knee joints, dizziness, tinnitus; red tongue with little coating, deep, thready and rapid pulse.

Treatment
Body acupuncture

1. **Principles of treatment**

   Benefit the Kidney, tranquillize the Mind, regulate the Thoroughfare Vessel and Conception Vessel, smooth the Liver, strengthen the Spleen and have peaceful emotions.

- *Yang deficiency of the Spleen and Kidney*: Acupuncture and moxibustion are used together with reinforcing technique.

- *Disharmony of the Heart and Kidney and Yin deficiency of the Liver and Kidney*: Acupuncture is the chief therapy with even-needling technique or coordination of reinforcing and reducing techniques.

2. **Prescription**

Baihui (GV20), Guanyuan (CV4), Shenshu (BL23), Taixi (KI3), Sanyinjiao (SP6).

3. **Explanation**

Baihui (GV20) can elevate the clear, reduce the turbid, pacify Liver Yang and clarify the head and eyes. Guanyuan (CV4) is the point of the Conception Vessel that can tonify primary Qi and regulate the Thoroughfare Vessel and Conception Vessel. Shenshu (BL23) is the Back-Shu point of the Kidney Meridian. Taixi (KI3) is the Yuan-Primary point of the Kidney Meridian. These 2 points together tonify Kidney Qi, benefit brain marrow, and strengthen the lumbar region and knees. Sanyinjiao (SP6) is the point of the Spleen Meridian that communicates with the Conception Vessel and the three Yin meridians of foot. It can strengthen the Spleen, smooth the Liver, regulate Qi to remove depression and regulate the Thoroughfare Vessel and Conception Vessel.

4. **Modification**

- *Disharmony of the Heart and Kidney and internal disturbance of Heart Fire*: + Xinshu (BL15), Shenmen (HT7), Laogong (PC8) and Neiguan (PC6) to clear wary Fire of deficiency type and nourish Kidney Yin.

- *Yin deficiency of the Liver and Kidney, and hyperactivity of Liver Yang*: + Fengchi (GB20), Taichong (LR3) and Yongquan (KI1) to smooth Liver Qi, nourish Yin and pacify Yang.

- *Yang deficiency of the Spleen and Kidney*: + Qihai (CV6), Pishu (BL21) and Zusanli (ST36) to strengthen the Spleen, benefit Qi and warm and tonify Kidney Yang.

5. **Manipulation**

Routine needling is applied to every point with reinforcing technique first and reducing afterward, or with even-needling technique.

Other therapies

1. **Auricular acupuncture**

   Points: Subcortex, Endocrine, Internal Reproductive Organ, Kidney, Ear-Shenmen, Sympathetic Nerve. 2 or 3 points are selected in each treatment and stimulated by needle or by embedding needle method, or the use of seeds or magnets. The treatment is given once every 2 days in alternative ears.

2. **Electroacupuncture**

   Sanyinjiao (SP6) and Taixi (KI3) are selected. After the arrival of Qi, electroacupuncture is used to the points, with disperse-dense wave and weak stimulation to induce slight irritation, lasting 20–30 minutes. The treatment is given once a day.

Notes

1. Acupuncture and moxibustion are effective for this disease. But, during treatment, it is necessary that the patient should receive mental comfort and maintain even moods, she should be optimistic and open and avoid depression, anxiety and irritability.

2. The patient should keep a good balance between overstress and rest, ensure she gets adequate sleep, pay attention to physical outdoor exercise, such as taking a walk, playing Taiji, enjoying life, etc.

3. Dietetic therapy is an adjuvant treatment to enhance the efficacy. For example, those with hypertension and excessive Fire due to Yin deficiency, should take more celery, kelp, silver fungus, etc.

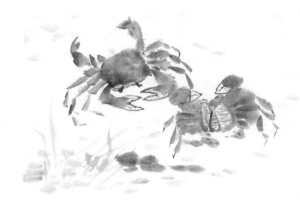

III. PAEDIATRIC DISEASES

1. ACUTE INFANTILE CONVULSIONS

Brief introduction

Acute infantile convulsions is a common critical disease seen in paediatric depart-ments, manifested as convulsions of the four limbs, stiffness of the neck, staring upward, clenched jaws, even loss of consciousness. It corresponds to infantile con-vulsions in Western medicine, commonly seen in many diseases, such as high fever, encephalitis B, epidemic meningitis (or sequela of encephalitis and meningitis), primary epilepsy, etc. The disease is most common in children aged between 1 and 5 years.

Aetiology and pathogenesis

The aetiology of this disease is quite complicated and mainly related to invasion of exogenous pathogenic factors, internal retention of Phlegm and Heat, or sudden fear and fright.

Syndrome differentiation

The main symptoms are convulsions of the four limbs, stiffness of the neck, staring upward, clenched jaws, loss of consciousness, etc.

1. **Invasion of exogenous pathogens**: Sudden onset, high fever, headache, cough, sore throat, red face and lips, shortness of breath, nasal flaring, irri-tability; then loss of consciousness, stiffness of spine, convulsions of the four limbs or trembling, staring upward, clenched jaw; thin and yellow tongue coating, superficial and rapid pulse.

2. **Internal retention of Phlegm and Heat**: Fever, profuse yellow sputum, difficulty in expectoration, shortness of breath, abdominal distension and pain, constipation, staring; sticky tongue coating, rolling pulse.

3. **Sudden fear and fright**: Restless sleep at night, convulsions or somnolence, frequent screaming, crying after waking up, being frightened frequently, blue or red complexion; thin tongue coating, thready and rapid pulse.

Treatment
Body acupuncture

1. **Principles of treatment**

   Clear away Heat, stop Wind, resolve Phlegm, regain consciousness, tranquillize Mind and remove fright. Acupuncture alone is applied with reducing technique.

2. **Prescription**

   Shuigou (GV26), Zhongchong (PC9), Hegu (LI4), Taichong (LR3).

3. **Explanation**

   Shuigou (GV26) is the point of the Governor Vessel that acts on opening the orifices, removing fright and regaining consciousness. Zhongchong (PC9) is Jing-Well point of the Pericardium Meridian and acts on reducing Heat, opening the orifices, removing fright and tranquillizing the Mind. Hegu (LI4) and Taichong (LR3) are 'the Four Gates' points and act on promoting Qi and Blood circulation, stopping Wind and fright.

4. **Modification**

   - *Invasion of exogenous pathogens:* + Waiguan (TE5) and Fengchi (GB20) are added to eliminate the exterior and reduce Heat.
   - *Internal retention of Phlegm and Heat:* + Zhongwan (CV12) and Fenglong (ST40) to remove Phlegm.
   - *Sudden fear and fright:* + Yintang (EX-HN3) and Taiyang (EX-HN5) to remove fright and tranquillize the Mind.
   - *High fever:* + Dazhui (GV14) and Quchi (LI11) to reduce Heat and remove fright.
   - *Headache:* + Yintang (EX-HN3) and Taiyang (EX-HN5) to expel Wind and stop pain.
   - *Clenched jaw:* + Xiaguan (ST7) and Jiache (ST6) to open the orifices and stop spasms.
   - *Opisthotonus:* + Dazhui (GV14) and Jinsuo (GV8) to regulate the Governor Vessel.

5. **Manipulation**

Shuigou (GV26) is needled toward the nasal septum with strong stimulation. Zhongchong (PC9) and Dazhui (GV14) are stimulated by pricking to induce bleeding. Burning rush moxibustion is applied to Yintang (EX-HN3) and Chengjiang (CV24). Routine needling technique is applied to the rest of the points.

Other therapies

1. **Auricular acupuncture**

Points: Heart, Liver, Sympathetic Nerve, Ear-Shenmen, Subcortex. The points are stimulated strongly by filiform needle.

2. **Finger pressure**

Heavy nipping by thumb nail is applied to Shuigou (GV26), Yintang (EX-HN3), Hegu (LI4) and Taichong (LR3) until spasm stops.

3. **Three-edged needle**

Bleeding method is used on Shixuan (EX-UE11) or twelve Jing-Well points.

Notes

1. Acupuncture and moxibustion have definite efficacy in this disease. It is necessary to detect the aetiology so that the appropriate treatment and prevention are provided.

2. If the convulsion is accompanied by profuse sputum and saliva, it is necessary to keep the respiratory tract smooth and ensure quiet in the room to avoid frightening the patient.

2. WHOOPING COUGH

Brief introduction

Whooping cough is characterized clinically as infantile paroxysmal spasmodic cough and special inspiratory croup after cough. It corresponds to pertussis syndrome in Western medicine. This disease commonly occurs in winter and spring in school-age children. The younger the patient is, the more severe the disease and its combined symptoms are. The duration of sickness is quite long, lasting generally 2 to 3 months.

Aetiology and pathogenesis

Invasion of exogenous Wind Cold or Wind Heat and internal disturbance of Phlegm block Qi passage, resulting in dysfunction of Lung Qi in dispersing and Qi reversion to the throat, thus, the disease occurs. Chronic sickness injures the Lungs and Spleen, resulting in insufficiency of Lung Yin and deficiency of the Spleen and Stomach.

Clinical symptoms are paroxysmal cough and special inspiratory croup after cough.

Syndrome differentiation

1. **Early cough phase**: There are symptoms similar to those of common cold, such as cough, nasal discharge, sneezing, mild chills and fever, etc. If Wind Cold predominates, the tongue coating is thin and white and the pulse is superficial and tense. If Wind Heat predominates, there is yellow and sticky sputum, difficulty in expectoration, red throat; thin yellow tongue coating and superficial and rapid pulse. Apart from the cough that is aggravated day by day, most symptoms are relieved in about 2 days. This phase may last 1 to 2 weeks.

2. **Spasmodic cough phase**: There is a paroxysmal cough that is mild during the daytime and worse at night, continuous coughing without inspiratory intervals; red face and ears, tearing, lumbar bending, fisting; afterwards, when the cough discontinues temporarily, deep and long inspiration with croups; right after which, a paroxysmal drastic cough starts. Those symptoms repeat several times until a large amount of sputum, saliva or gastric content is discharged. Thus, the spasmodic cough can be relieved temporarily. Some cases have puffy eyes, subconjunctive bleeding, nasal bleeding, blood-stained sputum, sublingual swelling and ulceration. A minority of critical cases have coma and convulsions. The tongue is red with yellow sticky coating. The pulse is rolling and rapid. This phase may last 2 to 6 weeks.

3. **Recovery phase**: Gradual alleviation of cough, weak coughing. For Spleen Qi deficiency, the constitution is weak, lassitude, pale and puffy face, shortness of breath, speaking in low voice, thin and little sputum, poor appetite, loose stools; pale tongue with little coating, thready and weak pulse. For Lung Yin deficiency, there is a dry cough, no sputum, irritability, insomnia, flushed cheeks, night sweating, feverish sensation in the palms, soles and chest; red tongue with little coating, thready, rapid and weak pulse. This phase may last 2 to 3 weeks.

Treatment
Body acupuncture

1. **Principles of treatment**
   - *Early cough phase*: Disperse Lung Qi, eliminate the exterior influences, stop cough and resolve Phlegm. Acupuncture is applied with reducing technique and moxibustion is added for Wind Cold type.
   - *Spasmodic cough phase*: Clear away Heat, resolve Phlegm, disperse Lung Qi and stop cough. Acupuncture alone is applied with reducing technique.
   - *Recovery phase*: Strengthen the Spleen, benefit the Lungs and manufacture Qi and Blood. Both acupuncture and moxibustion are used with reinforcing technique.

2. **Prescription**

   Lieque (LU7), Feishu (BL13), Fengmen (BL12), Fenglong (ST40).

3. **Explanation**

   Lieque (LU7) is the Luo-Connecting point of the Lung Meridian and acts on dispersing Wind, eliminating the exterior, dispersing Lung Qi and stopping cough. Feishu (BL13) and Fengmen (BL12) act on dispersing Lung Qi, eliminating the exterior and stopping cough. Fenglong (ST40) acts on strengthening the Spleen, removing Damp, resolving Phlegm and stopping cough.

4. **Modification**
   - *Early cough phase*: + Hegu (LI4) and Waiguan (TE5) to disperse Lung Qi and eliminating the exterior.
   - *Spasmodic cough phase*: + Tiantu (CV22) and Kongzui (LU5) to benefit the throat and stop cough.
   - *Recovery phase*: + Taiyuan (LU9), Taibai (SP2), Pishu (BL21) and Zusanli (ST36) to tonify Lung and Spleen Qi.
   - *Blood-stained sputum*: + Yuji (LU10), Kongzui (LU5) and Geshu (BL17) to clear away Heat and stop bleeding.
   - *Frequent coughing*: + Neiguan (PC6) and Neiting (ST44) to stop cough and vomiting.
   - *Weak constitution*: + Qihai (CV6), Gaohuang (BL43) and Zusanli (ST36) to tonify Qi and nourish Blood.

5. **Manipulation**

Oblique and shallow puncturing is suitable on the points on the back to prevent injury of the internal organs. Oblique needling is applied to Tiantu (CV22) along the posterior of the sternum, 1–1.5 cun. Deep puncturing or oblique puncturing laterally is prohibited. Routine needling technique is applied to the other points.

Other therapies

1. **Cutaneous needle**

Tapping is applied to Tiantu (CV22), Tanzhong (CV17), Fengmen (BL12), Feishu (BL13), Fenglong (ST40) and Zusanli (ST36) as well as the meridian section from Taiyuan (LU9) to Chizhe (LU5) and Jiaji (EX-B2) from T1 to T4 until there is slight or mild bleeding in local areas. The treatment is given once a day.

2. **Three-edged needle**

The pricking method is applied to Shenzhu (GV12) by three-edged needle to cause bleeding and a small-gauge cup is placed over it and retained for 5 to 10 minutes. The therapy is applied once every 2 days.

3. **Cupping**

Small cups are retained on Tanzhong (CV17), Shenzhu GV12) Fengmen (BL12), Feishu (BL13), Pishu (BL21), Gaohuang (BL43), etc. The cupping is given once every day.

4. **Auricular acupuncture**

Points: Lung, Trachea, Ear-Shenmen, Sympathetic Nerve, Anti-tragic Apex. In each treatment, 2 or 3 points are selected and stimulated moderately by filiform needle, without retaining. Or the points can be stimulated with the use of Vaccaria seeds.

5. **Point injection**

Points: Feishu (BL13), Shenzhu (GV12), Dashu (BL11). 0.25% Procaine injection is provided, 0.5 to 1ml to each point. The therapy is given once a day.

Notes

1. Acupuncture and moxibustion are quite effective in stopping cough. Integrated Chinese and Western medicine should be provided for critical cases or those complicated by pneumonia.

2. In the spasmodic cough phase, attention should be paid to preventing dyspnoea due to the difficulty of expectoration of sticky sputum.

3. ANOREXIA IN CHILDREN

Brief introduction

Anorexia refers to long-term poor appetite in children.

Aetiology and pathogenesis

The Zang Fu organs are delicate in children and the Spleen function is always deficient. Improper diet or malnutrition after sickness may impair the Spleen and Stomach functions and result in dysfunction in the reception of food, transportation and transformation. The disease occurs as a result.

Syndrome differentiation

Long-term poor appetite, even refusal to eat, emaciation, no lustre on the face, but fair spirits; emaciation, reduced body weight, mental fatigue and poor body resistance in prolonged sickness.

1. **Deficiency of the Spleen and Stomach**: Sallow complexion, lassitude, loose stools or with indigested food; pale tongue with thin and white coating, weak and forceful pulse.

2. **Disharmony of the Spleen and Stomach**: No lustre on the face, dry stools, no specific changes in tongue coating and pulse.

3. **Insufficiency of Stomach Yin**: Sallow complexion, dry mouth, desire to drink more, even having a drink with every meal, irritability, restlessness, dry stools, deep yellow urine; red tongue without coating or peeled coating, thready and weak pulse.

4. **Liver hyperactivity and Spleen deficiency**: Restlessness, crying, irritability, hot temper, bruxism; mirror tongue without coating, string-taut and thready pulse.

Treatment

Body acupuncture

1. Principles of treatment

Harmonize the Stomach, strengthen the Spleen, benefit Qi and nourish Yin. For deficiency of the Spleen and Stomach, acupuncture and moxibustion are used in combination with reinforcing technique. For other syndromes, acupuncture is prescribed as the main therapy with even-needling technique.

2. Prescription

Main points are selected from the Conception Vessel and Stomach Meridian of Foot-Yangming. Zhongwan (CV12), Jianli (CV11), Liangmen (ST21), Zusanli (ST36).

3. Explanation

Zhongwan (CV12), Jianli (CV11) and Liangmen (ST21) regulate meridian Qi in the epigastric and abdominal regions to benefit the Stomach in receiving food, and the Spleen in transportation and transformation. Zusanli (ST36) is the He-Sea point of the Stomach Meridian of Foot-Yangming. It can harmonize the Stomach, strengthen the Spleen and tonify and nourish Qi and Blood.

4. Modification

- *Deficiency of the Spleen and Stomach*: + Pishu (BL20) and Weishu (BL21) to tonify Qi in the Middle Burner.
- *Disharmony of the Spleen and Stomach*: + Neiguan (PC6) and Gongsun (SP4) to harmonize the Stomach and strengthen the Spleen.
- *Insufficiency of Stomach Yin*: + Sanyinjiao (SP6) and Neiting (ST44) to nourish Yin and clear away Heat.
- *Liver hyperactivity and Spleen deficiency*: + Taichong (LR3) and Taibai (SP3) to reduce the Liver and strength the Spleen.

5. Manipulation

The routine operation is applied to all points. But perpendicular and deep puncture is not appropriate on the Back-Shu points. Moxibustion is applicable.

Other therapies

1. **Auricular acupuncture**

   Points: Stomach, Spleen, Large Intestine, Small Intestine, Ear-Shenmen, Subcortex. In each treatment, 2 or 3 points are selected and stimulated with the use of Vaccaria seeds. The points need to be pressed 3 to 5 times each day.

2. **Point injection**

   Zusanli (ST36) is selected bilaterally for injection with vitamin B_1 or B_{12}, 1ml on each point. The injection is provided twice a week.

Notes

1. Acupuncture and moxibustion have satisfactory efficacy for infantile anorexia. It is necessary to find out actively the aetiology of the condition and provide appropriate measures.

2. Correct the adverse diet habits of the patient and maintain a regular life style so as to improve the treatment of anorexia.

4. INFANTILE MALNUTRITION

Brief introduction

Improper feeding leads to damage of the Spleen and Stomach and impacts upon the growth and development of infants. Malnutrition is a chronic disease, corresponding to the relevant disease and an aspect of parasitosis in Western medicine. This disease is commonly seen in children younger than 5 years old.

Aetiology and pathogenesis

Improper infantile feeding, indulgence in milky food or earlier ablactation, desire for and indulgence in specific foods, desire for sweet and greasy food, all of which may impair the Spleen and Stomach and injure Qi and Blood production in the long term, leading to malnutrition.

Syndrome differentiation

Main symptoms are sallow complexion, skinny body, big head, thin neck, loose hair, low spirits, abnormal diet, abdominal distension like a drum or abdominal depression like a boat, skeletal body, etc.

1. **Malnutrition of Qi type**: Poor appetite, or excessive eating and frequent defecation, dry or loose stools, slightly emaciation, slight sallow complexion, low spirits, hot temper; sticky tongue coating, thready and rolling pulse. This syndrome is commonly seen in the early stage of the disease.

2. **Malnutrition due to accumulation**: Declining appetite, or excessive eating but easy hunger, or indulgence in eating something peculiar, such as raw rice, mud, defecation with worms; apparent emaciation, sallow complexion, loose hair and hair loss, abdominal distension, skeletal body, irritability or rubbing of the eyebrows, digging in the nose, sucking fingers, gnashing of teeth; pale tongue with light yellow and sticky coating, soft, thready and rolling pulse. This type is commonly seen in the middle stage of the disease.

3. **Malnutrition of Dryness type**: Low spirits, extreme emaciation, skeletal body, dry skin with wrinkles like old person, weak crying, hopelessness, abdominal depression like a boat, or oedema of the limbs, or purpura, nasal depression, bleeding of gums; pale tongue or mirror red tongue without moisture, weak pulse. This type is commonly seen in the late stage of the disease.

Treatment
Body acupuncture

1. **Principles of treatment**

   Strengthen the Spleen and Stomach, tonify Qi and Blood, promote digestion and remove food accumulation. Acupuncture and moxibustion are used in combination with even-needling technique.

2. **Prescription**

   Sifeng (EX-UE10), Zhongwan (CV12), Zusanli (ST36), Pishu (BL20).

3. **Explanation**

   Sifeng (EX-UE10) is the established effective point for infantile malnutrition. Modern study indicates that acupuncture on this point can enhance the activity of various kinds of digestive enzymes. Zhongwan (CV12) is the Front-Mu point of the Stomach and Influential point of the Fu organs.

Zusanli (ST36) is the He-Sea point of the Stomach. Pishu (BL20) is the Back-Shu point of the Spleen. All 3 points used together can strength the Spleen and Stomach, benefit Qi and nourish Blood, regulate Qi in the Fu organs and promote digestion, which benefits the development of the infant.

4. **Modification**

   - *Malnutrition of Qi type:* + Zhangmen (LR13) and Weishu (BL21) to strengthen the Spleen and Stomach.

   - *Malnutrition due to accumulation:* + Jianli (CV11), Tianshu (ST25) and Sanyinjiao (SP6) to promote digestion and remove accumulation.

   - *Malnutrition of Dryness type:* + Ganshu (BL18) and Geshu (BL18) to regulate and nourish Qi and Blood.

   - *Parasitosis:* + Baichongwu (EX-LE3) to kill parasites and promote digestion.

5. **Manipulation**

   The pricking method is used on Sifeng (EX-UE10) by three-edged needle after strict sterilization, to squeeze a little yellow fluid or milky white mucus. Perpendicular and deep puncturing is prohibited on the Back-Shu points and Zhangmen (LR13) to prevent from injury to the internal organs. Routine operation is applied to the remaining points. Generally, quick needling should be given.

Other therapies

1. **Chiropractic method**

   The rolling and nipping method is applied to the bilateral Huatuojiaji (EX-B2) on the back by thumb and index finger 3 to 5 times.

2. **Cutaneous needle**

   Tapping on the Governor Vessel and bilateral Huatuojiaji (EX-B2) and points of the Bladder Meridian of Foot-Taiyang until skin turns slightly red. The treatment is given once every other day.

3. **Acupoint incision**

   After strict sterilization, surgical knife is used to incise the skin of the large thenar, about 0.5cm in length; then, some yellow-white milky-like substance is squeezed and cut off. Afterwards, the incision is bandaged for 5 days.

Notes

1. Acupuncture and moxibustion have quite good efficacy for infantile malnutrition of Qi type and that due to accumulation. If the case is related to parasitosis infection, medication should be provided in combination.

2. Breastfeeding should be provided if possible for infants. It is necessary not to stop lactation too early. The adjunct food should be supplemented gradually with easily digested and rich-nutrient food. Indulgence in specific foods must be avoided.

3. Maintain outdoor activities, plenty of fresh air, enjoy more sunshine and generally strengthen the constitution of the child.

5. ENURESIS

Brief introduction

Enuresis, also named 'bed wetting' and 'sleeping urination syndrome', refers to a disease in which children over 3 years old involuntarily urinate during sleep. 'Bed wetting' appearing in the children younger than 3 years old cannot be diagnosed as enuresis, since the brain marrow is still insufficient, they are weak in the central nervous system, and the normal urination habits have not yet been built up. The disease will not be diagnosed for those with occasional involuntary urination due to over-playing, lack of sleep, fatigue and drinking too much before sleep in older children.

Aetiology and pathogenesis

Western medicine holds that the disease is caused by dysfunction of the cortex and subcortical centre of the brain. In Traditional Chinese Medicine, it is believed to be caused by failure of the Bladder to control urine due to deficiency of the Kidney Qi, insufficiency of the Lower Burner, or deficiency of both Spleen and Lungs and Damp Heat of the Lower Burner.

Syndrome differentiation

Bed wetting during sleep, once every night or every few nights, or even several times one night.

1. **Deficiency of Kidney Qi**: Pale complexion, lassitude, dull response, frequent urination during the day, or even cold limbs and weakness of the lumbus and legs, pale tongue, deep, thready and weak pulse.

2. **Deficiency of both Spleen and Lung Qi**: Enuresis during sleep, aggravated when fatigued, pale complexion, fatigue, loose stools, pale tongue, thready and weak pulse.

3. **Damp Heat of the Lower Burner**: Frequent urination, scanty urine, deep yellow in colour and fishy in smell, pruritus of the external genitalia, dream-disturbed sleep, teeth grinding, anxiety and irritability, dry mouth, red tongue with yellow coating, wiry and rapid pulse.

Treatment

Body acupuncture

1. **Principles of treatment**

   - *Deficiency of the Kidney Qi, deficiency of both Spleen and Lung*: To warm and tonify Kidney Yang, tonify and benefit Lung and Spleen; both acupuncture and moxibustion are applied, the reinforcing method.

   - *Damp Heat of the Lower Burner*: To clear Heat, eliminate Dampness, and regulate Bladder; acupuncture alone is applied with the reducing method.

2. **Prescription**

   Select Back-Shu and Front-Mu points of Spleen as the principal points. Zhongji (CV3), Pangguangshu (BL28), Sanyinjiao (SP6).

3. **Explanation**

   Zhongji (CV3) and Pangguangshu (BL28), the Back-Shu and the Front-Mu points, can promote the Bladder to control urine; Sanyinjiao (SP6) is the Crossing point of the three Yin Meridians of Foot and works to relieve enuresis by regulating the Spleen, Liver and Kidneys.

4. **Modification**

   - *Deficiency of Kidney Qi*: + Guanyuan (CV4) and Shenshu (BL23) to reinforce Kidney Qi.

   - *Deficiency of Lung and Spleen Qi*: + Feishu (BL13), Pishu (BL20) and Zusanli (ST36) to tonify the Qi of the Lungs and Spleen so as to increase the abilities of promoting astringency and stopping collapse.

   - *Damp Heat of the Lower Burner*: + Qugu (CV2) and Yinlingquan (SP9) to clear Heat, eliminate Dampness and regulate the Bladder.

5. **Manipulation**

Puncture Zhongji (CV3) and Guanyuan (CV4) perpendicularly or obliquely and it is better to let the needling sensation arrive at the genitalia. Warming needling or herbal monkshood cake is applied to Shenshu (BL23) and Guanyuan (CV4). Routine acupuncture technique is applied to other acupoints.

Other therapies

1. **Auricular acupuncture**

   Points: Kidney, Bladder, Liver, Endocrine, Uterus. 3 to 4 points are selected each time and punctured shallowly with filiform needles. Needle-embedding or pills can be applied.

2. **Scalp acupuncture**

   Lateral Line 3 of the Forehead: Middle Line of Vertex. Manipulate needles for 5–10 minutes after inserting slowly.

3. **Cutaneous needle**

   Select Jiaji points from T4 to L2, Guanyuan (CV 4), Qihai (CV6), Qugu (CV2), Shenshu (BL23) and Sanyinjiao (SP6). Tap with cutaneous needle until the skin turns red.

4. **Point injection**

   Apply Strychnine Nitrate injection 2ml at Huiyin (CV1), once a day.

Notes

1. Acupuncture and moxibustion are effective for this condition.

2. The affected children should be encouraged to develop good habits of on-time urination and waking up to urinate regularly at night.

3. Pay attention to proper nutrition and avoid over fatigue and drinking too much before sleep.

4. Be patient in educating the children, compliment them and increase their self-confidence, and do not laugh at and discriminate against them so as to prevent them from being afraid, nervous, or having feelings of inferiority.

6. CEREBRAL PARALYSIS

Brief introduction

Cerebral paralysis is a non-progressive central motor dysfunction due to cerebral injuries, and is part of the range of 'five kinds of maldevelopment', 'five kinds of flaccidity', 'five kinds of stiffness' and 'Wei syndrome' in Chinese medicine.* In the perinatal or prenatal period, it is mainly caused by intracranial anoxia or haemorrhage, etc., such as foetal distress due to infection in gestational period, neonatal asphyxia, premature birth, cerebrovascular disease or general haemorrhagic disease, etc.

Aetiology and pathogenesis

This disease is mainly due to deficiency of congenital Essence, injuries of both Liver and Kidney, impaired nourishment of acquired Essence or deficiency of both Qi and Blood.

Syndrome differentiation

The main syndromes are motor dysfunctions of the extremities. The motor disturbance type is mainly manifested as athetoid movement or choreiform movement, etc.; the spastic type is manifested as muscular tension increasing strained muscles, hyperfunction of the tendon reflex and pyramidal sign positive, leading to monoplegia, hemiplegia, paraplegia, triplegia or quadriplegia, etc. The ataxic type is manifested as having an unsteady gait due to injury of the cerebellum, failure in the finger–nose test, and muscular tension reduction, etc. The mixed type includes the syndromes of the two types above or more than two types. It is often followed by intellectual disturbance, epilepsy, abnormal vision, dysacusis and language disorders, etc.

1. **Deficiency of both Liver and Kidneys**: Paralysis of the extremities, mental retardation, slow physical growth, contraction of tendons, impairment of extremities, irritability, or hyperactivity with profanity; red tongue, wiry pulse, or wiry and thready pulse.

2. **Weakness and deficiency of both Spleen and Stomach**: Flaccidity and weakness of the extremities, impairment of the hands and feet, weakness in chewing, mouth opening, extension of tongue, salivation, sallow

---

*   'Five kinds of maldevelopment' refers to delayed development in standing, walking, hair growth, tooth eruption and speech. 'Five kinds of flaccidity' refers to flaccidity of head and neck, mouth, hands, feet and muscles. 'Five kinds of stiffness' refers to stiffness of the head and neck, hands, feet, chest and waist and muscles.

complexion, sluggishness, slow response, lack of Qi, reluctance to speak, emaciation, coldness of extremities; pale tongue, deep and thready pulse.

Treatment

Body acupuncture

1. **Principles of treatment**

   To tonify and benefit the Liver and the Kidneys, benefit Qi and nourish Blood, open meridians and collaterals, strengthen tendon and bones; both acupuncture and moxibustion are applied, the reinforcing method.

2. **Prescription**

   The acupoints of the Governor Vessel are selected as the principal ones. Dazhui (GV14), Shenzhu (GV12), Fengfu (GV16), Sishencong (EX-HN1), Xuanzhong (GB39), Yanglingquan (GB34).

3. **Explanation**

   Dazhui (GV14) and Shenzhu (GV12) are used for opening Qi of the Governor Vessel; Fengfu (GV16) and Sishencong (EX-HN1) are used to benefit the brain and promote intelligence; Xuanzhong (GB39) is the one of the Eight Influential Points dominating the marrow and used for nourishing the marrow, strengthening the brain and filling up the bone; Yanglingquan (GB34), the one of the Eight Influential Points dominating the tendons, and is used for relaxing tendons and collaterals, and strengthening tendons and bones.

4. **Modification**

   - *Deficiency of Liver and Kidneys*: + Ganshu (BL18), Shenshu (BL23), Taixi (KI3) and Sanyinjiao (SP6) to tonify Liver and Kidneys.

   - *Deficiency of Spleen and Stomach*: + Zhongwan (CV12), Pishu (BL20) and Zusanli (ST36) to strengthen Spleen and Stomach.

   - *Facial paralysis*: + Quchi (LI11), Shousanli (LI10), Hegu (LI4), Waiguan (TE5), Futu (ST32), Huantiao (GB30), Fengshi (GB31), Weizhong (BL40), Chengshan (BL57) and Fenglong (ST40) to promote Qi of the meridians distributed in limbs.

5. **Manipulation**

   Puncture Fengfu (GV16) with the needle tip towards the tip of nose for about 1 cun in depth. Upward and deep insertion is prohibited so as to avoid inserting into the great occipital foramen; puncture 4 points of Sishencong

(EX-HN1) toward Baihui (GV20) successively; needling obliquely or superficially on Back-Shu points is required. Routine acupuncture technique is applied to other acupoints.

Other therapies

1. **Auricular acupuncture**

   Points: Subcortex, Sympathetic Nerve, Ear-Shenmen, Brain Stem, Adrenal, Heart, Liver, Kidney and Small Intestine. Paralysis of upper limbs: shoulder, elbow and wrist; paralysis of lower limbs: hip, knee and ankle. Select 4–6 points in every treatment; puncture, or apply Vaccaria seeds to auricular points, pressing 2–3 times every day.

2. **Scalp acupuncture**

   Anterior Oblique Line of Vertex-Temporal, Lateral Line 1 of Vertex, Lateral Line 2 of Vertex, Anterior Temporal Line, Lower-Lateral Line of Occiput. Puncturing by filiform; retaining for 1–4 hours. Treatment once a day.

3. **Point injection**

   Select Fengchi (GB20), Dazhui (GV14), Shenshu (BL23), Quchi (LI11), Shousanli (LI10), Zusanli (ST36), Yanglingquan (GB34) and Chengshan (BL57), etc. Select 2–3 points in every treatment; injecting with placenta tissue fluid, Dengzhanhua (灯盏花 *Erigeron Breviscapus Hand Mazz*) injection, vitamin B_1 injection and vitamin B_{12} injection on the points using 0.5–1ml. Once a day.

Notes

1. Acupuncture and moxibustion have good efficacy for this disease, especially for younger children with short-term course of the disease.

2. During the treatment period, parents are advised to help their children to train the functions of the extremities, language and intelligence.

7. ATTENTION DEFICIT HYPERACTIVITY DISORDER

Brief introduction

Attention deficit hyperactivity disorder is one of the common neuropsychosis syndromes of childhood. It is characterized by hyperactivity, difficultly in concentrating the Mind, poor ability in participating despite essentially normal intelligence.

It is in the range of 'hysteria' and 'restlessness' in Chinese medicine, and related to poor memory and deafness. It is commonly seen in school-age children with a male predominance. Most of the cases improve and are cured in puberty with a favourable prognosis.

Aetiology and pathogenesis

This disease is mainly due to deficiency of congenital Essence. deficiency of both Heart and Spleen, failure of filling-up of the brain marrow, hyperactivity of Liver Yang and disturbance of the primary Mind.

Syndrome differentiation

The symptoms are hyperactivity, restlessness, difficulty in long-time mental concentration and carrying tasks through to the end, excitable temperaments, excessive and unmanageable activities and speaking, lack of discipline, capriciousness, emotional lability, poor ability to participate, despite nearly or completely normal intelligence.

1. **Deficiency of Kidneys and hyperactivity of Liver**: Hyperactivity of both hands and feet, wooden movements, explosive personality, difficulty in sitting quietly, feverish sensation in the chest, palms and soles, constipation, red tongue with thin coating, thready and wiry pulse.

2. **Deficiency of both Heart and Spleen**: Unease, lassitude, thin or puffy appearance, hyperactivity without irritability, beginning well but falling off towards the close, poor sleeping, poor memory, spontaneous perspiration, night sweating, pale complex, pale and delicate tongue with scanty or thin and white coating, weak pulse of deficiency type.

Treatment
Body acupuncture

1. **Principles of treatment**
   - *Hyperactivity of Liver Yang and deficiency of Kidney Yin*: Regulating the Liver and the Kidneys, nourishing Yin and suppressing Liver Yang; acupuncture is applied with even method.
   - *Deficiency of both Heart and Spleen*: Tonifying and benefiting Heart and Spleen, calming down the spirit; both acupuncture and moxibustion are applied, the reinforcing method.

2. **Prescription**

   Shenmen (HT7), Neiguan (PC6), Sanyinjiao (SP6), Taixi (KI3), Taichong (LR3), Sishencong (EX-HN1).

3. **Explanation**

   Shenmen (HT7) is the Yuan-Primary point of the Heart Meridian of Hand-Shaoyin; Neiguan (PC6) is the Luo-Connecting point of the Pericardium Meridian of Hand-Jueyin, and the combination of the points above can calm down Heart and spirit; Sanyinjiao (SP6) is the Crossing point of the Spleen, Liver and Kidney Meridians; combining with Taixi (KI3) which is the Yuan-Primary point of the Heart Meridian of Hand-Shaoyin; and Taichong (LR3) which is the Yuan-Primary point of the Liver Meridian of Foot-Jueyin, can regulate Liver, Spleen and Kidneys, nourish Yin and suppress Liver Yang; Sishencong (EX-HN1) located on the head can calm the spirit, benefit the brain and promote intelligence.

4. **Modification**

   - *Hyperactivity of Liver Yang and deficiency of Kidney Yin*: + Shenshu (BL23) and Xingjian (LR3) to tonify the Kidneys, replenish Essence, calm and suppress Liver Yang.

   - *Deficiency of both Heart and Spleen*: + Xinshu (BL15), Pishu (BL20) and Zusanli (ST36) to benefit the Heart and nourish the Spleen.

5. **Manipulation**

   Insert 4 points of Sishencong (EX-HN1) towards Baihui (GV20) successively; in order to avoid injury of internal organs, perpendicular and deep needling on the Back-Shu points is not applicable. Routine acupuncture technique is applied to other acupoints.

Other therapies

1. **Auricular acupuncture**

   Points: Subcortex, Heart, Kidney and Ear-Shenmen. Puncture, needle-embed or apply Vaccaria seeds to auricular points, twice a week.

2. **Electroacupuncture**

   Anterior Oblique Line of Vertex-Temporal, Middle Line of Forehead, Middle Line of Vertex, Lateral Line 1 of Vertex, Lateral Line 2 of Vertex, Anterior Temporal Line. Stimulate with disperse and dense wave for 20 minutes after puncturing by filiform needle. Once every other day.

Notes

1. The treatment of acupuncture and moxibustion has good efficacy for this disease.

2. During the treatment, help the patients cultivate good life habits, educate them patiently, give them more care and attentions, make sure they are not maltreated, discriminated against, and that people are not impatient with them, so as to prevent them from loss of self-confidence. Patients who have difficulty in learning should be guided and supported to finish homework step by step; and praised and encouraged to increase their confidence when they improve.

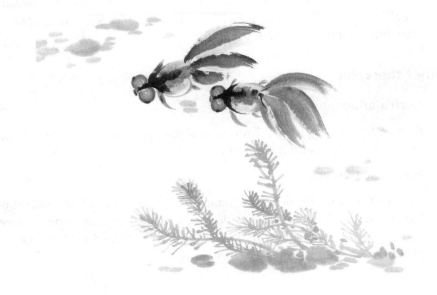

IV. EXTERNAL DISEASES

1. FURUNCLES

Brief introduction

Furuncles is a kind of surgical disease which is mainly manifested on the face, hands and feet. It is characterized by millet-shaped furuncles at the initial stage with a deep and hard root like a nail, with fast onset. This section can serve as a reference to boils, carbuncles, acute whitlow, and acute lymphangitis in the face, hands and feet in Western medicine.

Aetiology and pathogenesis

The disease is mainly due to dirty skin, wrongly squeezing and pricking the affected part with a needle, which leads to an attack of Fire toxin and accumulation of pathogenic Heat on the skin; or maybe due to overeating, a rich fatty diet and excessive drinking, leading to the accumulation of Heat in the Zang Fu organs which develops into an internal toxin; if the toxic Heat is excessive inside the body, it will affect the meridians and collaterals and attack the Zang Fu organs internally, leading to a critical case.

Syndrome differentiation

In the early stage, a cone-shaped inflamed hard lump appears at a hair follicle, like a grain of millet with yellow or purple colours, involving symptoms of redness, swelling, Heat and pain; the lump grows in size within a few days and the pain develops; it then forms a pustule and becomes soft, with alleviation of the pain; after festering, the pustule will gradually heal. The furuncle is called 'red-thread furuncle' if manifested on the four limbs with red thread going upward in the affected parts. General purulent infection involves symptoms of trembling, high fever, unconsciousness, delirious speech, headache and vomiting, known as 'Furuncle Complicated by Septicaemia' in Traditional Chinese Medicine.

Treatment
Body acupuncture

1. **Principles of treatment**

   Clear away Heat and toxin, relieve swelling and pain; acupuncture is mainly applied with the reducing method.

2. **Prescription**

Select acupoints of the Governor Meridian as the principal points. Shenzhu (GV12), Lingtai (GV10), Hegu (LI4), Weizhong (BL40).

3. **Explanation**

Shenzhu (GV12) and Lingtai (GV10) are the points of the Governor Vessel; the Governor Vessel governs all the Yang meridians, and therefore they are applied to clear away pathogenic stagnated Heat and Fire of the Yang meridians. Both of them are established points for treating carbuncles. Because there is plenty of Qi and Blood in the Yangming meridians, Hegu (LI4) is selected to clear away Fire and toxin of Yangming meridians, especially for facial carbuncles. Weizhong (BL40) is the He-Sea point of the Bladder Meridian of Foot-Taiyang, named as 'Xi-Cleft of Blood' also, and it is pricked to cause bleeding to clear Blood Heat, relieve swelling and pain.

4. **Modification**

- *Excessive of Fire and toxin*: + Quchi (LI11), Dazhui (GV16), and Quze (PC3) to remove Fire and clear toxin.

- *Invasion of Ying-nutrient stage by toxic Fire*: Bleeding on the Xi-Cleft point of affected meridian to cool and activate Blood and relieve swelling.

- *Points are applied according to affected meridians*: For example, Yinbai (SP1), Shangyang (LI1) and Neiting (ST44) are added for lip furuncle; Neiguan (PC6), Ximen (PC4) and Yinxi (HT6) are added for palm furuncle; Erjian (LI2) is added for finger furuncle.

- *Modifying points by head-tail combination of same meridian*: For example, selecting contralateral Yingxiang (LI20) for those occurring from Shangyang (LI1) in index finger; pricking to cause bleed at the end of the red thread for red-thread furuncles.

- *Furuncles complicated by septicaemia*: + Shuigou (GV26), twelve Jing-Well points, Baihui (GV20) and Neiguan (PC6) for furuncle complicated by septicaemia to restore the Mind, open the orifices, stop contracture and calm down the Mind.

5. **Manipulation**

Prick to bleed for 3–5 drops on every acupoint by three-edged needle; or cup to promote bleeding; apply indirect moxibustion with garlic, 3–5 cones for every carbuncle.

Other therapies

1. **Auricular acupuncture**

   Points: Ear-Shenmen, Adrenal, Occiput, Furuncle, etc. Choose 2–4 points for one treatment, and puncture with filiform needle with moderate stimulation, or apply Vaccaria seeds to auricular points.

2. **Pricking therapy**

   Select 3–5 papuloid sensitive spots, puncture epidermis with three-edged needle, breaking the white fibre to bleed for 3–4 drops.

Notes

1. The treatment of acupuncture and moxibustion for this disease has a definite effect.

2. Avoid squeezing red, swollen and hard furuncles at the initial stage (especially dangerous with trigonum on the face). Needling manipulation in the affected area should also be avoided to prevent spreading the infection.

3. Patients suffering from furuncles complicated by septicaemia are in an extremely dangerous position and need immediate medical rescue. If the furuncle has suppurated, surgical treatment should be consulted.

4. People who are prone to furuncles are strongly advised to quit smoking and avoid spicy and stimulating food, such as fish, shrimps, etc.

2. MUMPS

Brief introduction

Mumps is an acute epidemic disease characterized by fever, swelling and pain in the parotid. It attacks all year long, especially during winter and spring. Children between the ages of 5 and 9 are vulnerable to the disease and the symptoms in adults are more severe than in children if they are affected. Most cases do not recur all life long, but in a few cases this does happen. It is similar to epidemic parotitis in Western medicine.

Aetiology and pathogenesis

The disease is caused by exogenous invasion of pathogenic toxin of Wind Heat, entering the body through the mouth and nostrils, Fire transformation from accumulated Phlegm leading to obstruction of Shaoyang and Yangming meridians, and failure in maintaining the flow of Qi and accumulation of Qi in the parotid. The Shaoyang and Jueyin meridians are internally–externally related to each other, and the Liver Meridian of Foot-Jueyin curves around the lower abdomen and external genitalia. The condition is often accompanied by lower abdominal pain and swelling in the testicles in severe cases. High fever, unconsciousness and eclampsia can be complicated by excessive pathogenic Heat, and pathogenic Wind caused by excessive Heat toxin, internal production due to extreme Heat and internal interruption of the Heart and Liver.

Syndrome differentiation

The disease has an incubation period of 2 weeks or so. The symptoms in the early stages are fever, headache, dry mouth, poor appetite, vomiting and general fatigue; afterwards swelling and pain in one side of the parotid, dysmasesia, with unclear margins, moderate hardness, elasticity and tenderness; disappearance of the swelling or general symptoms in 4–6 days. Generally, it happens unilaterally although occasionally it is bilateral. For some patients, meningitis, testitis and ovaritis can be complicated if the treatment is not applied in time.

1. **Heat toxin attacking the exterior**: Effusive pain in cheeks in which the ear lobe is taken as the centre beneath the ear unilaterally or bilaterally, normal skin colour, elasticity on pressure, difficulty in opening the mouth, dysmasesia, accompanied by aversion to coldness, fever, red throat, mild discomfort in the whole body, red tongue with thin and yellow coating, superficial and rapid pulse.

2. **Accumulation of Fire toxin**: Heat, pain and hardness in the lower part of the cheeks, dysmasesia, high fever, upset, headache, dry stools, yellow urine, sore throat, swelling and pain in the testicles, red tongue with thick and yellow coating, rolling and rapid pulse.

3. **Heat toxin attacking the Heart**: Swelling in the lower part of cheeks, high fever, headache, upset, fatigue, somnolence, stiffness in the neck, vomiting, even unconsciousness, convulsions of the limbs, dark red tongue with yellow and dry coating, wiry and rapid pulse.

4. **Pathogenic factors attacking the Lower Burner**: Swelling in the lower part of the cheeks, fever, upset, bitter mouth and dry throat, swelling and pain in the testicles in males, lower abdominal pain in females, red tongue with yellow coating, wiry and rapid pulse.

Treatment

Body acupuncture

1. **Principles of treatment**

   To remove Heat and toxin, eliminate swelling and mass; apply acupuncture only with the reducing method.

2. **Prescription**

   Select acupoints of the Triple Burner Meridian of Hand-Shaoyang, the Gallbladder Meridian of Foot-Shaoyang, the Large Intestine Meridian of Hand-Yangming and the Stomach Meridian of Foot-Yangming as the principal ones. Yifeng (TE17), Jiache (ST6), Waiguan (TE5), Hegu (LI4), Neiting (ST44), Zulinqi (GB41).

3. **Explanation**

   Select Jiache (ST6) and Yifeng (TE17) to dispel local stagnation of Qi and Blood, regulate Qi of the Triple Burner Meridian of Hand-Shaoyang, the Gallbladder Meridian of Foot-Shaoyang, the Large Intestine Meridian of Hand-Yangming and The Stomach Meridian of Foot-Yangming; Waiguan (TE5), Hegu (LI4), Neiting (ST44) and Zulinqi (GB41) are the distant points of the Triple Burner Meridian of Hand-Shaoyang, the Gallbladder Meridian of Foot-Shaoyang, the Large Intestine Meridian of Hand-Yangming and the Stomach Meridian of Foot-Yangming, and can remove Heat stagnation, conduct Heat downwards, open collaterals and relieve swelling.

4. **Modification**

   - *Invasion of Heat toxin to the exterior*: + Zhongzhu (TE3) and Guanchong (TE1) to clear away Heat and expel superficial pathogenic factors, disperse Wind and remove toxin.

   - *Retention of Fire and toxins*: + Dazhui (GV14) and Quchi (LI11) to eliminate Fire, clear away toxins, soften and resolve the hard mass.

   - *Attack of the Heart by Heat and toxins*: + Baihui (GV20) and Shuigou (GV26) to restore the Mind and open the orifices, dispel Wind and stop spasms.

- *Attack of the Lower Burner by Damp Heat:* + Taichong (LI3), Dadun (LR1) and Guilai (ST29) to disperse stagnated Qi of the Pericardium Meridian of Hand-Jueyin and the Liver Meridian of Foot-Jueyin, eliminate stasis and relieve pain.

5. **Manipulation**

The routine needling technique is applied to all the acupoints. Prick on Dazhui (GV14), Guanchong (TE1) and Baihui (GV20) to cause bleeding.

Other therapies

1. **Burning rush moxibustion**

   Select Jiaosun (TE20) on affected sides. Cut off the hair where the points are located, and after routine disinfection, burn vegetable oil-stained rush, quickly touching the acupoints and lifting the rush immediately when hearing the sound of beep. Generally, swelling can be relieved after using moxibustion once; one more treatment can be given the next day if the swelling is not relieved completely. This method can be used for prevention from mumps.

2. **Auricular acupuncture**

   Points: Parotid Gland, Cheek, Subcortex, tender points of the corresponding region. Puncture with filiform needle with strong stimulation, apply needle-embedding or the herbal pill to auricular points.

3. **Cutaneous needle**

   Hegu (LI4), Ermen (TE21), Jiache (ST6), Yifeng (TE17), Waiguan (TE5), the Jiaji points of T1–T4. Tap from Ermen (TE21) to Yifeng (TE17), passing through Jiache (ST6) first, and then tap on Hegu (LI4), Waiguan (TE5) and the Jiaji points of T1–T4 to cause redness or slight bleeding on skin.

4. **Point injection**

   Apply 2% Lidocaine or Procaine injection to 1–2 points, 0.5–1ml for each acupoint.

Notes

1. The treatment of acupuncture for mumps has quite a good effect. Patients with complications should be treated in time.

2. The disease is highly infectious and it is necessary to isolate child patients.

3. The patient should follow a light diet, drink more water and maintain smooth defecation during the treatment.

3. MASTITIS

Brief introduction

Mastitis refers to an acute purulent disease manifested as redness, swelling and pain in the breast, and unsmooth lactation, leading to purulence and carbuncle. This disease is often seen in women who are breastfeeding, especially in primipara, usually occurring 2–4 weeks after delivery. It also can be occasionally seen in women before labour, at the late stage of pregnancy or non-breastfeeding women.

Aetiology and pathogenesis

This disease is closely related with the Stomach Meridian of Foot-Yangming as well as the Liver Meridian of Foot-Jueyin. It is usually caused by melancholy, anxiety and irritability, leading to failure of the Liver in maintaining the free flow of Qi; or as a result of a rich fatty diet and accumulation of stagnated Heat in the Stomach, resulting in stagnation of Liver Qi and Stomach Heat, retention of Heat and obstruction of Blood and Qi in the meridians and collaterals, which help develop into carbuncles; or because of ruptured nipples and stagnancy of milk due to failure in sucking out all the milk; or by invasion of exopathogenic factors due to weakness after giving birth; or by retention of milk; or by obstructed lactation, or by hyperactive foetus Qi, fullness of chest, and failure of the Liver in maintaining the free flow of Qi.

Syndrome differentiation

The main clinical manifestations are redness, swelling and pain in the breast, accompanied by aversion to cold, high fever, thirst and constipation; palpable tough mass in the affected breast, tenderness and swelling of subaxillary lymph nodes in the affected side.

1. **Period of lactation stagnation**: Swelling and pain in the breast, stagnation of milk, unsmooth lactation, with slightly red or normal skin, with or without hard mass, accompanied by chill, high fever, thirst and poor appetite; yellow tongue coating and rapid pulse.

2. **Period of pus**: Progressively enlarged mass in the breast, with redness, swelling and pain, lingering fever, continuously throbbing pain, accompanied by high fever, thirst, scanty and deep yellow urine, constipation, red tongue with yellow and sticky coating, surge and rapid pulse.

3. **Period of ulceration**: Formation of purulence, fluctuation sensation, redness and purple in the local area, profuse pus after being cut or its spontaneous collapse. 'Cyst-transferring breast carbuncle' could be complicated by involvement of other breast collaterals due to unsmooth flow of pus, continuous swelling and lingering fever, accompanied by general fatigue, pale complexion and poor appetite; pale tongue with thin coating and weak pulse.

Treatment
Body acupuncture

1. **Principles of treatment**

   To clear away Heat, eliminate mass, promote lactation and relieve swelling in early stage; to expel Heat, clear away toxin, promote lactation and eliminate ulceration in the period of pus; puncture with the reducing method. To tonify and benefit Qi and Blood and regulate Ying-nutrient and Wei-defensive stages in the period of ulceration; apply both acupuncture and moxibustion, reducing or even method.

2. **Prescription**

   Tanzhong (CV17), Rugen (ST18), Qimen (LR14), Jianjing (GB21).

3. **Explanation**

   Tanzhong (CV17) and Rugen (ST18) locate at the breast; Tanzhong (CV17) is the one Eight Influential Point that dominates Qi, and Rugen (ST18) belongs to the Stomach Meridian. Both of the points are applied to soothe chest disorders, regulate Qi and disperse obstruction of Qi and Blood in the affected region. Qimen (LR14) locates near the breast, is the Front-Mu point of Liver, and functions to regulate Liver Qi, eliminating stagnation and relieving swelling. For treating breast swelling, Jianjing (GB21) is the established point to disperse Fire of both the Liver and the Gallbladder.

4. **Modification**
   - *Period of lactation stagnation*: + Hegu (LI4), Taichong (LR3) and Quchi (LI11) to disperse stagnated Liver Qi, soothe chest disorder, regulate Qi, and dispel Heat and toxin of the Large Intestine Meridian of Hand-Yangming and the Stomach Meridian of Foot-Yangming.
   - *Period of pus*: + Neiting (ST44) and Dazhui (GV14) to dispel Heat and toxin stagnation of the Large Intestine Meridian of Hand-Yangming and the Stomach Meridian of Foot-Yangming.

- *Period of ulceration*: + Weishu (BL21), Zusanli (ST36) and Sanyinjiao (SP6) to tonify and benefit Qi and Blood of both the Spleen and the Stomach.

- *Distension and ache of breast*: + Shaoze (SI1) and Zulinqi (GB41) to promote lactation and stop pain.

- *Fever and aversion to cold*: + Hegu (LI4), Waiguan (TE5) and Quchi (LI11) to dispel Wind and Heat.

- *Irritability with bitter mouth*: + Xingjian (LR2) and Neiguan (PC6) to clear away Heart Heat and relieve irritability.

5. **Manipulation**

Puncture Tanzhong (CV17) transversely to the affected breast; puncture Rugen (ST18) upwards to the base of breast, avoiding needling perpendicularly or deeply so as not to hurt the internal organs; puncture Qimen (LR14) outwardly along spatia intercostalia or towards breast, avoiding needling perpendicularly or deeply so as not to hurt the internal organs; puncture Jianjing (GB21) forwardly or posterior-inferiorly so as not to hurt the apex of the Lung, avoiding deep insertion; routine acupuncture technique is applied to other acupoints. Twice a day for severe cases.

Other therapies

1. **Auricular acupuncture**

Points: Mammary Gland, Endocrine, Adrenal, Thoracic Vertebrae. Puncture with filiform needle superficially. Twirl for a few minutes and retain for 20–30 minutes; once a day.

2. **Pricking therapy**

Locate the stasis spots whose colour is not reduced when pressing below the scapula or on bilateral sides of the vertebral column; prick to cause bleeding with three-edged needle. Prick the point located two fingers width above Gaomang (BL43) on the affected side when the stasis spots of the back are not obvious.

3. **Blood-letting puncturing and cupping**

Dazhui (GV14), Jiaji points of T4, Rugen (ST18) (affected side). Prick to cause bleeding with a three-edged needle and then cup on the points, once a day.

4. **Point injection**

Apply vitamin B$_{12}$ injection 4ml and vitamin B$_6$ injection 2ml to 3–5 points in the prescription in each treatment, 1ml for each point.

Notes

1. The treatment of acupuncture and moxibuation for this disease has a good effect in the early stage and is more effective in combination with Tuina and hot compression.

2. In the period of ulceration, it should be treated comprehensively by pus drainage.

3. The patient should be advised to have a light diet and avoid pungent and greasy food.

4. She should pay attention to breast hygiene and maintain a happy mood.

4. HYPERPLASIA OF MAMMARY GLANDS

Brief introduction

Hyperplasia of the mammary glands is a benign hyperplasia of mammary tissue which features palpable mass and pain in the breast and is also related to the menstrual circle. The disease is often seen in middle-aged women.

Aetiology and pathogenesis

This is frequently caused by emotional depression, anxiety, dysfunction of the Liver in maintaining the free flow of Qi, stagnation of the Heart and the Spleen, disorder of Qi and Blood and obstruction of the collaterals in the breast by Phlegm Dampness; or by dysfunction of the Thoroughfare Vessel and the Conception Vessel, deficiency of the Liver and Kidney Yin and malnutrition of meridians.

Syndrome differentiation

Movable mass of different sizes and shapes are palpable in one or both breasts, with unclear margins, accompanied by distending pain or tenderness and closely related to the menstrual circle as well as emotional changes. The pain is usually aggravated before menstruation and reduced or dissolved after menstruation.

1. **Stagnation of Liver Qi**: Breast lump changing with emotions, accompanied by oppression in the chest, distension in sides, depression and irritability, dreaminess, insomnia, vexation, bitter taste in the mouth; thin and yellow tongue coating, wiry and rolling pulse.

2. **Obstruction of Phlegm Damp in collaterals**: Tough breast mass, oppression and discomfort in the chest, nausea, vomiting, heaviness in the head and sleepiness; sticky tongue coating and rolling pulse.

3. **Disorder of the Thoroughfare Vessel and the Conception Vessel**: Often seen in middle-aged women, aggravation of breast mass before menstruation and reduction after it, accompanied by soreness and weakness in the lumbus, lassitude and fatigue, irregular menstruation of scanty volume and light in colour, or amenorrhoea; pale tongue with white coating, deep and thready pulse.

Treatment
Body acupuncture

1. **Principles of treatment**

    *   *Stagnation of Liver Qi, retention of pathogenic Phlegm Damp in the collaterals*: To dispel and regulate stagnant Liver Qi, eliminate Phlegm and mass; puncture with the reducing method.

    *   *Disorder of the Conception Vessel and the Thoroughfare Vessel*: To regulate the Conception Vessel and the Thoroughfare Vessel, soften and resolve the hard mass; puncture with even method.

2. **Prescription**

    Tanzhong (CV17), Rugen (ST18), Wuyi (ST15), Qimen (LR14), Fenglong (ST40).

3. **Explanation**

    Tanzhong (CV17) is the Sea of Qi, and when punctured with the reducing method benefits Qi; Wuyi (ST15) and Rugen (ST18) can smooth the Qi of the Large Intestine Meridian of Hand-Yangming and the Stomach Meridian of Foot-Yangming, and regulate local Qi circulation and Blood; Qimen (LR14) is used for dispersing stagnant Liver Qi and regulating the Conception Vessel and the Thoroughfare Vessel; Fenglong (ST40) is the Luo-Connecting point of the Stomach Meridian and can eliminate Damp and Phlegm, open the collaterals and relieve swelling.

4. **Modification**

- *Stagnation of Liver Qi*: + Taichong (LR3) and Jianjing (GB21) to disperse stagnant Qi of both the Liver and the Gallbladder, and relieve stagnation and pain.

- *Obstruction of Phlegm and Damp in the collaterals*: + Neiguan (PC6), Zhongwan (CV12) and Zusanli (ST36) to eliminate Phlegm, open the collaterals, and relieve swelling and pain.

- *Irregularity of the Conception Vessel and the Thoroughfare Vessel*: + Guanyuan (CV4), Sanyinjiao (SP6), Ganshu (BL18) and Shenshu (BL23) to benefit both the Liver and the Kidney, regulate the Conception Vessel and the Thoroughfare Vessel.

5. **Manipulation**

Puncture Tanzhong (CV17) transversely to the affected breast; puncture Rugen (ST18) upwards to the base of the breast, avoiding needling perpendicularly or deeply so as not to hurt the internal organs; puncture Wuyi (ST15) and Qimen (LR14) outwardly along spatia intercostalia or towards the breast, avoiding needling perpendicularly or deeply so as not to hurt the internal organs. Routine acupuncture technique is applied to other acupoints.

Other therapies

1. **Auricular acupuncture**

Points: Endocrine, Sympathetic Nerve, Subcortex, Mammary Gland, Pituitary Gland, Ovary, Liver. Puncture with filiform needle with moderate stimulation, or apply Vaccaria seeds to auricular points.

2. **Intradermal needle**

Intradermal needle is embedded in Wuyi (ST15) by puncturing outward horizontally. It is required to be painless in the chest when patients move both arms. The needle is fixed with plaster and remains for 2–3 days. Press the point 2–3 times a day during retention.

3. **Point injection**

Angelica Sinensis injection or Danshen (丹参 *Angelica Pubescens Maxim*) injection is mixed with vitamin B_{12} injection at the ratio of 1:1 and injected in 2–3 points from the prescription in each treatment, about 0.5ml in each point.

Notes

1. The treatment of acupuncture and moxibustion for this disease has quite a good effect and makes the mass reduce in size or dissolve.

2. Irregular menstruation as well as chronic inflammation of uterus and adnexa should be treated early.

3. Cancer is a possible development for a few patients, in which case surgery should be applied if necessary.

4. The patient should maintain a happy mood and control the amount of fatty food intake.

5. ACUTE APPENDICITIS

Brief introduction

Acute appendicitis is characterized by continuous pain in the right lower abdomen, accompanied by paroxysmal aggravated pain, muscular tension and rebound tenderness. It pertains to the category of 'intestinal abscess' in Chinese medicine. It can attack people at various ages, especially young people, and is frequently seen as one of the acute abdomen diseases in surgery.

Aetiology and pathogenesis

It is caused by an irregular diet and gluttony; or by overeating greasy, raw, cold and unsanitary food, which damages the Stomach and the intestines, leading to internal accumulation of Damp Heat in the intestines; or by walking too fast after a meal, resulting in stagnation of Qi and Blood and impairment of the intestine collaterals; or by attack by Cold or Heat, falling, sprains and emotional factors, which can all lead to stagnation of Qi and Blood, retention of Dampness Heat and rotting of flesh and Blood.

Syndrome differentiation

Acute appendicitis features migratory pain in the right lower abdomen. The abdominal pain typically begins in the upper abdomen, then gradually moves to the umbilical region, finally to the right lower abdomen and stays there after 6–8 hours. The accompanying symptoms are poor appetite, vomiting, nausea, constipation or diarrhoea, fatigue, body temperature rising along with aggravation of the symptoms, McBurney's point tenderness and rebound tenderness in the right lower abdomen.

Chronic appendicitis does not have typical symptoms, with a history of acute appendicitis, pain and discomfort in the right lower abdomen. The disease can be induced due to violent exercise or irregular diet.

1. **Stagnation of Qi and Blood**: Pain in the upper abdomen or around the umbilicus and intermittent dull pain initially, then the pain transfers to the right lower abdomen after several hours, accompanied by aversion to cold, fever, nausea, vomiting, white and sticky tongue coating, wiry and tense pulse.

2. **Heat transformation from stagnation**: Aggravated pain fixed at right lower abdomen, tension in and contraction of abdominal muscles that is worse on pressure, touchable regional mass, obvious tenderness and rebound tenderness; constant high fever, constipation, yellow urine, red tongue with yellow and sticky coating, wiry, rolling and rapid pulse. This falls into the category of a critical syndrome of intestinal abscess, and should be treated by comprehensive therapy.

3. **Purulence due to accumulation of excessive Heat**: Severe pain with fixed region, obvious tenderness and rebound tenderness, touchable regional mass, high fever, nausea, vomiting, constipation or diarrhoea, scanty and yellow tongue coating, dark red and dry tongue, surge and rapid pulse.

Treatment

Body acupuncture

1. **Principles of treatment**

    To dispel Heat to remove stagnation, promote circulation of Fu organ to resolve the mass; apply acupuncture with the reducing method only.

2. **Prescription**

    Select the acupoints in the Stomach Meridian of Foot-Yangming as the principle points. Lanwei (EX-LE7), Shangjuxu (ST37), Tianshu (ST25), Quchi (LI11), Ashi points.

3. **Explanation**

    Lanwei (EX-LE7) is selected as the principal point to treat acute appendicitis; Shangjuxu (ST37) is used for conducting Qi circulation of the Yangming meridians; Quchi (LI11) is the He-Sea point of the Large Intestine Meridian of Hand-Yangming and can remove pathogenic Heat of the Large Intestine; Tianshu (ST25) can regulate Qi of the Large Intestine; Ashi points are combined for conducting Qi to disperse stagnation and resolving mass at affected region directly.

4. **Modification**

- *Qi stagnation and Blood stasis*: + Hegu (LI4) and Zhongwan (CV12) to promote Qi and activate Blood, promote circulation of Fu organ and relieve pain.

- *Heat transformation from stagnation*: + Dachangshu (BL25) and Hegu (LI4) to remove Heat, eliminate stasis, promote Qi and eliminate stagnation.

- *Purulence due to accumulation of excessive Heat*: + Dachangshu (BL25) and Zhigou (TE6) to clear away Heat and toxins, conduct stagnated Qi and resolve mass.

- *Excessive Heat*: + Dazhui (GV14) to remove Heat and Fire.

- *Nausea and vomiting*: + Neiguan (PC6) and Zusanli (ST36) to sooth chest, benefit diaphragm, and keep the adverse Lung Qi or Stomach Qi downwards so as to stop vomiting.

5. **Manipulation**

Routine puncturing by filiform needle with the reducing method is applied. Needles are retained for 60–120 minutes, and the treatment is applied twice a day.

Other therapies

1. **Auricular acupuncture**

   Points: Appendix, Large Intestine, Sympathetic Nerve and Ear-Shenmen are stimulated strongly by filiform needle, once or twice a day.

2. **Point application**

   Select Mangxiao (芒硝 *Natrii Sulfas*) 30g, Shengdahuangfen (生大黄粉 *Rheum Palmatum L.*) 10g, Pingpian (冰片 *Borneolum*) 5g, and one clove of garlic. Mix and mash into a paste and apply on Ashi points. Apply a few times a day.

Notes

1. The treatment of acupuncture and moxibustion has quite a good effect on acute appendicitis occurring without purulency. Surgery should be given if the disease develops to purulency or perforation.

2. Warming moxibustion with moxa stick or indirect moxibustion with ginger is applicable locally in combination for chronic appendicitis.

3. Light and liquid diet is recommended during treatment.

6. CHOLELITHIASIS

Brief introduction

Cholelithiasis refers to a stone in the Gallbladder or the bile duct. It belongs to the categories of 'hypochondriac pain' and 'jaundice' in Chinese medicine.

Aetiology and pathogenesis

The Liver and the Gallbladder are mainly responsible for this disease with which the Spleen, Stomach and Kidney are also involved. The Gallbladder is one of the Fu organs for storing bile; the Liver maintains the free flow of Qi and is characterized as 'flourish'. In the condition of overeating rich fatty food, Qi stagnation in the Liver and the Gallbladder, or obstruction and accumulation of Dampness Heat and parasite toxins, the Liver fails to flourish and maintain the free flow of Qi, the Gallbladder fails to maintain the smooth circulation and descending of Qi; thus, bile is not discharged smoothly. Long-term stagnation and accumulation of bile transforms into Heat. Heat may evaporate the bile together with Damp into stone. The main symptoms are Qi stagnation, Blood stasis and Damp Heat at the initial stage. But, Heat may be transformed and Yin is injured, leading to Yin deficiency of Liver and Kidneys in the long term.

Syndrome differentiation

About 20–40% of the patients of cholelithiasis may have no symptom all their life and the disease only be occasionally found during medical examination. The main manifestations are discomfort or pain in the upper abdomen after eating food, especially greasy food, accompanied by belching, hiccups, nausea and vomiting. Biliary colic lies in the upper abdomen or right upper abdomen, which is paroxysmal and radiates to the right shoulder and back.

Normally, there is no symptom in choledocholithiasis, but typical abdominal pain could appear when the stone blocks the bile duct and causes secondary infection (mostly occurring beneath the xiphoid process as well as in the right upper abdomen, with colic pain which could radiate to the right shoulder and back paroxysmally or continuously), accompanied by nausea, vomiting, chills, high fever and jaundice.

1. **Qi stagnation of the Liver and Gallbladder**: Distending or colic pain in the right hypochondria and beneath the xiphoid process which changes in severity according to emotional changes, accompanied by frequent belching, bitter mouth, oppression in the chest and poor appetite; thin and white tongue coating and wiry pulse.

2. **Damp Heat of the Liver and Gallbladder**: Continuous stabbing pain in the chest and hypochondria, accompanied by aversion to cold, high fever, bitter mouth, irritability, dislike of fatty and greasy food, nausea, vomiting, yellowness in the eyes and body, deep yellow urine, constipation; red tongue with yellow and sticky coating, rolling and rapid pulse.

3. **Yin deficiency of the Liver and Kidney**: Dull and lingering pain in the hypochondria, aggravated after fatigue, dry mouth and throat, dizziness, blurred vision, and lassitude; red tongue with scanty coating and thready pulse.

Treatment

Body acupuncture

1. **Principles of treatment**

   Qi stagnation of the Liver and Gallbladder, Damp Heat in the Liver and Gallbladder: to disperse and regulate stagnated Liver Qi, remove Heat and Damp; acupuncture is applied only with the reducing method. Yin deficiency of the Liver and Kidneys: to tonify and benefit the Liver and Kidneys, benefit the Gallbladder and promote stone discharge; acupuncture is applied as the main therapy with even method.

2. **Prescription**

   The Back-Shu point, Front-Mu point and Lower He-Sea point of the Gallbladder are selected as the principle acupoints. Riyue (GB24) (right side), Qimen (LR14) (right side), Danshu (BL19), Yanglingquan (GB34).

3. **Explanation**

   Riyue (GB24) is the Front-Mu point of the Gallbladder, and Danshu (BL19) is the Back-Shu point of the Gallbladder; both points are used in combination according to the application of the Back-Shu point and the Front-Mu point to disperse and regulate Qi of both the Liver and Gallbladder so as to promote stone discharge. Qimen (LR14) is the Front-Mu point of the Liver and can disperse the Liver and benefit the Gallbladder; Yanglingquan (GB34) is the one Eight Confluent Point concerning the tendons and the

Lower He-Sea point of the Gallbladder. 'The Lower He-Sea point is indicated in the disorders of Fu organs', thus, acupuncture on it can relieve spasm, promote circulation in the collaterals and stop pain.

4. **Modification**

- *Qi stagnation of the Liver and Gallbladder*: Penetrating needling from Neiguan (PC6) to Zhigou (TE6) is used to regulate Qi and relieve pain.

- *Damp Heat in the Liver and Gallbladder*: + Xingjian (LR2) and Xiaxi (GB43) to clear away Heat and eliminate Damp.

- *Liver and Kidney Yin deficiency*: + Taixi (KI3) and Sanyinjiao (SP6) to benefit Yin and open collaterals.

- *Bitter mouth, poor appetite, nausea and vomiting*: + Zhongwan (CV12), Zusanli (ST36) and Neiguan (PC6) are added to regulate and lower the adverse flow of Stomach Qi.

- *Jaundice*: + Zhiyang (GV9), Sanyinjiao (SP6) and Yinlingquan (SP9) to eliminate Damp and benefit jaundice.

5. **Manipulation**

Puncture Riyue (GB24) and Qimen (LR14) outwardly along spatia intercostalia, avoiding needling perpendicularly or deeply so as not to hurt the internal organs; puncture Danshu (BL19), avoiding needling perpendicularly or deeply. Routine acupuncture technique is applied to other acupoints. Acupuncture is given twice a day in the attack stage of the disease and needles are retained for 30–60 minutes; and treatment is given 2 or 3 times a week in the interval stage.

Other therapies

1. **Finger pressure**

Select the tender spots around Ganshu (BL18) and Danshu (BL19) of the Bladder Meridian of Foot-Taiyang in right side of back; press them forcefully by thumb, for 5–10 minutes each time.

2. **Auricular acupuncture**

Points: Liver, Gallbladder, Duodenum, Ear-Shenmen, Sympathetic Nerve. Acupuncture is applied with strong stimulation for excess syndromes and mild stimulation for deficiency syndromes, the needles are retained for 30 minutes. Needle-embedding or seed is applicable to auricular points.

3. **Electroacupuncture**

In the attack stage of biliary colic, electroacupuncture is used after the arrival of Qi with continuous wave, high frequency and strong stimulation, lasting 30 to 60 minutes.

4. **Point injection**

10% Glucose injection 10ml or vitamin B_{12} injection 1ml is injected nearby the nerve roots of the Jiaji points of T9–12. After the apparent arrival of Qi, the injection needle is lifted slightly and the medicine is infused. Danggui (当归 *Radix Angelicae Sinensis*) injection or Honghua (红花 *Safflower*) injection is applicable to 2 or 3 acupoints selected according to the principle of treatment each time.

Notes

1. The treatment of acupuncture for this disease has a satisfactory effect. It is more effective on cholelithiasis when the stone is within the diameter of 1cm. Surgery should be applied for the stone over 2–3cm in diameter.

2. The patient is required to take a light diet and less greasy food.

7. ERYSIPELAS

Brief introduction

Erysipelas is an acute contagious disease, manifested as the sudden appearance of flake-like red spots and burning pain, and accompanied by high fever and aversion to cold. It mainly occurs on the legs and face, or in the whole body. The disease is related to acute lymphangitis, often seen in children and the aged in spring and autumn.

Aetiology and pathogenesis

The main causative factor is Fire toxin. It is frequently caused by pathogenic Heat in Xue-Blood stage and invasion of Fire toxin, or by invasion of toxic pathogens after injury of skin and mucous membranes. Fire, Heat and toxic pathogens attack the skin and muscle, block meridians and collaterals and further obstruct Qi and Blood circulations. Hence, the disease occurs. If the affected area is located in the head and face, pathogenic Wind and Heat are commonly combined; if in the chest and hypochondriac region, Liver Fire is combined; if in the lower limbs, Damp Heat are combined; if in neonates, the disease is commonly induced by retention of foetal toxin in the interior and invasion of pathogenic factors from the exterior.

Syndrome differentiation

It primarily occurs in the lower limbs and secondly in the head and face with a history of damage to the skin and mucous membranes. General symptoms occur initially, such as chills, fever, headache, poor appetite, etc. Local skin lesions are reddish, which is reduced on pressure and restored after pressure is released. In severe cases, petechiae appear in the area swelling which gradually turns dark red or orange yellow. Desquamation happens after 5–6 days, thus, the lesion is recovered gradually. The internal attack of pathogenic toxin involves high fever, irritability, unconsciousness, delirium, nausea, vomiting and convulsions, indicating a critical case.

1. **Wind Heat interrupting the Upper Burner**: Usually in the head and face. Redness, burning sensation, swelling pain, or even blisters in the affected local region, accompanied by aversion to cold, fever, pain in the joints, poor appetite, dark urine, constipation, red tongue with thin and yellow coating, rolling and rapid pulse.

2. **Retention of Damp Heat**: Mostly in the lower limbs. Redness, swelling, Heat and pain in the attacked area, or blisters and purpura, even suppuration, leading to skin necrosis, accompanied by fever, upset, thirst, oppression in the chest, swelling pain in the joints, dark and yellow urine, yellow and sticky tongue coating, rolling and rapid pulse.

3. **Retention of foetal Fire and toxin**: Often seen in neonates, frequently occurring around the umbilicus and between the hips and lower limbs. Wandering redness, swelling, burning sensation in the affected local area, accompanied by high fever, upset, vomiting; red tongue with yellow coating, purple and black fingerprints.

Treatment
Body acupuncture

1. **Principles of treatment**

   To remove Fire and clear away toxin, cool Blood and eliminate stasis. Acupuncture alone is applied with the reducing method.

2. Prescription

Select the acupoints located in the skin lesions and the Large Intestine Meridian of Hand-Taiyang as the principle points. Hegu (LI4), Quchi (LI11), Xuehai (SP10), Weizhong (BL40), Ashi points.

3. Explanation

Hegu (LI4) and Quchi (LI11) disperse Heat and toxin from the Large Intestine Meridian of Hand-Yangming and the Stomach Meridian of Foot-Yangming; Xuehai (SP10) activates Blood and eliminates stasis by the reducing method; use the combination of Weizhong (BL40) and Ashi points and apply scattered Blood-letting puncture to clear away Heat of all the Yang meridians and stagnated Heat of the Xue-Blood stage.

4. Modification

- *Flaming up of Wind Heat*: + Dazhui (GV14) and Fengmen (BL12) to disperse pathogenic Wind.

- *Retention of Damp Heat*: + Yinlingquan (SP9), Neiting (ST44) and Fenglong (ST40) to clear away Heat and eliminate Damp.

- *Toxic Fire of foetus*: + Zhongchong (PC9), Dazhui (GV14) and Shuigou (GV26) to cool Blood and clear toxin.

- *Oppression in chest and irritability*: + Neiguan (PC6) and Tanzhong (CV17) to relax the chest and resolve mass.

- *Nausea and anorexia*: + Neiguan (PC6) and Zhongwan (CV12) to regulate Stomach and stop vomiting.

5. Manipulation

Prick to cause bleeding with three-edged needle on Weizhong (BL40) and Ashi points; and then cup after pricking (not allowed on the face). Routine acupuncture technique is applied to other acupoints with the reducing method. 1 or 2 treatments a day.

Other therapies

1. Auricular acupuncture

Points: Ear-Shenmen, Adrenal, Subcortex, Occiput. Puncture with filiform needle with moderate or strong stimulation, or apply Vaccaria seeds to auricular points.

Notes

1. Treatment with acupuncture and moxibustion has quite a good effect on this disease, especially for erysipelas in the lower limbs. Erysipelas in the head and face as well as in neonates is generally severe and should be treated with comprehensive methods.

2. Strict sterilization should be applied to contaminated needles and cups. The needles and cups should be used individually during the treatment to avoid cross infection.

8. THROMBOANGIITIS OBLITERANS

Brief introduction

Thromboangiitis obliterans is a chronic obliterative vascular anomalies of cumulative vessels which occurs inflammatorily, segmentally or periodically. It is characterized by numbness and coldness of the affected limbs, pain, intermittent claudication, weakness or disappearance of the pulsation of affected arteries. Acroanesthesia, soreness and coldness of the limbs in early stage are part of the range of 'Bi syndrome' of Chinese medicine; necrosis and desquamation of acra in late stage are in range of 'gangrene' of Chinese medicine.

Aetiology and pathogenesis

Constitutional Yang deficiency of the Spleen and Kidneys leads to loss of being warmed and nourished. Attack of pathogenic Cold and Damp obstructs the meridians and collaterals, resulting in disturbance of Qi and Blood circulation, and stagnation of both Cold and Damp leads to Heat stagnation in the long term. Indulgence in smoking, alcohol and spicy and strong flavoured food produces Heat, and accumulation of Heat may block the meridians and collaterals. Excessive Heat makes muscles rotten, leading to disease.

Syndrome differentation

The onset of this disease is slow and cyclical. Before or during occurrence, wandering superficial phlebitis appears, manifested as pain, aversion to cold, decline of temperature, intermittent claudication, weakness or disappearance of pulsation of distant arteries. Acra ulceration or necrosis occurs in severe cases.

There are three stages, divided in light of the ischaemic severity on limbs in clinic:

1. **Local ischaemia stage**: This is equivalent to the obstruction of Damp and Cold in meridians. Symptoms are soreness, numbness, coldness of the affected limbs, preference for warmth and aversion to cold, aggravated by cold, mild intermittent claudication relieved after a short break. The examination shows dry and pale skin with lower temperature, weakness or disappearances of pulsation of dorsalis pedis and posterior tibial artery, wandering red and hard streak on the shank in some of the patients; white and sticky tongue coating, deep and thready pulse.

2. **Disturbance of nutrition stage**: This is equivalent to the obstruction of Qi stagnation and Blood stasis type. All of the above symptoms are aggravated, followed by pain when resting, severe pain which disturbs the sleep, difficulty in walking and fatigue. The skin of the affected limbs turns to dark red from pale, wandering erythema, tubercle or hard streak; slow growth of toenail and nail thickening; disappearance of pulsations of dorsalis pedis and posterior tibial artery, muscular atrophy in chronic case; white and sticky tongue coating, deep and thready pulse.

3. **Necrosis stage**: This is equivalent to the retention of Heat and toxin type. Progressive aggravation of all the symptoms above; severe pain of the affected limbs, purple and swelling skin; grey and wizened fingers and toes with diabrosis; dark surface to the wound; followed by fever, dry mouth, constipation and dark yellow urine; yellow and sticky tongue coating, wiry and rapid pulse.

4. **The late stage** of this disease is equivalent to injury of both Qi and Yin. Dark red skin in affected limbs, muscular atrophy, severe pain which disturbs the sleep, disappearance of palpation on the dorsal artery of feet, followed by sallow complexion, thin body, fatigue, palpitations and shortness of breath; pale tongue; deep, thready and weak pulse.

Treatment
Body acupuncture

1. **Principles of treatment**

   • *Obstruction of meridians by Cold Damp, Qi stagnation and Blood stasis*: Warm and open the meridians, eliminate stasis and promote circulation of Blood; apply both acupuncture and moxibustion with reducing or even method.

- *Retention of both Heat and toxin*: Clear away Heat, remove the toxins, eliminate stasis and mass; application of acupuncture with the reducing method.

- *Injury of both Qi and Blood*: Tonify Qi and nourish Yin, regulate both Qi and Blood; application of both acupuncture and moxibustion, the reinforcing method.

2. **Prescription**

   Guanyuan (CV4), Geshu (BL17), Zusanli (ST36), Sanyinjiao (SP6), Xuehai (SP10), Yanglingquan (GB34).

3. **Explanation**

   Guanyuan (CV4) is the Crossing point of the Conception Vessel and the three Yin meridians of foot, and used for regulating the Spleen, Liver, Kidneys, benefiting Qi and nourishing Blood; Geshu (BL17) is the point of the Eight Influential Points dominating Blood, and is used to nourish and harmonize Blood, and eliminate stasis to relieve pain; Zusanli (ST36) is the He-Sea point of the Stomach Meridian of Foot-Yangming that has abundant Qi and Blood, and it can promote Qi and Blood, eliminate stasis to relieve pain with the combination of Xuehai (SP10) and Sanyinjiao (SP6); Yanglingquan (GB34) is the point of the Eight Influential Points dominating the tendons, and is used to relax the tendons, open collaterals, and eliminate stasis to relieve pain.

4. **Modification**

   - *Obstruction of collaterals by Cold Damp*: + Shangqiu (SP5) and Yinlingquan (SP9) to warm meridian and dispel Cold.

   - *Qi stagnation and Blood stasis*: + Hegu (LI4) and Taichong (LR3) to activate Blood and eliminate stasis.

   - *Retention of Heat and toxin*: + Quchi (LI11), Dazhui (GV14) and Weizhong (BL40) to clear away Heat and remove toxin, or Ashi points (the local region with red, swelling, burning and pain) to clear away Heat and toxin by pricking (to cause bleeding) with cutaneous needle.

   - *Injury of both Qi and Yin*: + Qihai (SP6) and Taixi (KI3) to benefit Qi and nourish Yin.

   - *Hands affected*: + Baxie (EX-UE9) to activate Blood and open collaterals.

   - *Feet affected*: + Bafeng (EX-LE10) to activate Blood and open collaterals.

5. **Manipulation**

Perpendicular and deep puncture is prohibited in Geshu (BL17) so as not to hurt the internal organs. Routine acupuncture technique is applied to other acupoints.

Other therapies

1. **Auricular acupuncture**

   Points: Heart, Liver, Kidneys, Sympathetic Nerve, Adrenal, Subcortex, Triple Burner, corresponding points of limbs. Select 3–5 points in every treatment with strong stimulation by filiform needle; or apply 0.5% Procaine 0.2ml for blocking injection.

2. **Point injection**

   Select 0.5% Danggui (当归 *Radix Angelicae Sinensis*) injection or Danshen (丹参 *Angelica Pubescens Maxim*) injection, 2–3 points in every treatment, 0.5ml for each point, once a day.

3. **Catgut implantation**

   Implant with 2cm long surgical catgut No.0 at Fenglong (ST40) and Chengshan (BL57), once every 2 weeks.

Notes

1. Acupuncture and moxibustion treatment has a remarkable effect on thromboangiitis obliterans without ulceration. The treatment should be combined with surgery when ulceration occurs.

2. The patient to keep the affected limbs warm and avoid invasion of Wind, Cold and Damp.

3. The patient should quit smoking and avoid spicy and stimulant food.

9. HERNIA

Brief introduction

Hernia is characterized by swelling and pain in the lower abdomen, testicles and scrotum, etc. This disease is mostly seen in children and the aged. This chapter can serve as a reference to the treatment of inguinal hernia, femoral hernia, indigitation, intestine incarceration and torsion of spermatic cord in Western medicine.

Aetiology and pathogenesis

The onset is mainly associated with the Conception Vessel and the Liver Meridian of Foot-Jueyin. Due to sitting or lying in the wet and walking through water in the rain, pathogenic Cold and Damp invade the Conception Vessel and the Liver Meridian of Foot-Jueyin, and stagnate in the testicles and scrotum. Stagnation of Qi and Blood results in swelling, leading to hernia of the Cold type. The Heat transformation from Cold and Damp accumulation or the attack on the Lower Burner by Damp Heat in both the Liver and Spleen leads to swelling and pain of testicles, hydrocele of scrotum, or redness, swelling and ache of scrotum, thus, hernia of the Damp Heat type occurs. Heavy loads and overstrain may injure tendons and lead to sinking of Qi in the Middle Burner, thus the Small Intestine is herniated into the scrotum from time to time, and inguinal hernia occurs.

Syndrome differentiation

The main symptoms are distension and pain of the lower abdomen, pain in the testicles, or swelling and pain in the scrotum. It is aggravated or induced by long term standing, fatigue, cough and anger, etc. Sometimes, the hernia is enlarged and fails to return naturally, thus causing paroxysmal abdominal pain, nausea and vomiting. Therefore, it is considered an intestine incarceration and requires surgery immediately.

1. **Hernia of Cold type**: Coldness and pain of scrotum, stiffness and contracture of testicles and lower abdominal, coldness of body and limbs, thin and white tongue coating, deep and thready pulse.

2. **Hernia of Damp Heat type**: Redness, swelling and burning pain of the scrotum, swelling and pain of the testicles, or followed with fever with aversion to cold, scanty and dark urine, constipation, yellow and sticky tongue coating, soft and rapid pulse.

3. **Inguinal hernia**: Bearing-down pain of the lower abdomen and scrotum, or even the testicles are involved, bearing-down sensation induced in standing position; distension of the scrotum, the intestine returns to the abdomen in lying position, so that there is self-extinction of swelling of the scrotum; it returns to the original region if pushed by hand in severe cases; poor appetite, short breath and fatigue, pale tongue with white coating, deep and thready pulse.

Treatment

Body acupuncture

1. **Principles of treatment**

   - *Hernia of Cold type:* Warm meridians and open collaterals, dispel Cold to relieve pain; both acupuncture and moxibustion are applied, the reducing method.

   - *Hernia of Damp Heat type:* Clear away Heat, eliminate Damp, dispel swelling and mass; acupuncture alone is applied with the reducing method.

   - *Inguinal hernia:* Tonify Qi, raise collapse, activate collaterals to relieve pain; both acupuncture and moxibustion are applied, the reducing method.

2. **Prescription**

   Taichong (LR3), Dadun (LR1), Guanyuan (CV4), Guilai (ST29), Sanyinjiao (SP6).

3. **Explanation**

   Hernia is the main disease of the Conception Vessel, and the Liver Meridian of Foot-Jueyin curves around the external genitalia; therefore, Guanyuan (CV4), Dadun (LR1) which is the Jing-Well point of Foot-Jueyin, Taichong (LR3) which is the Yuan-Primary point of Liver Meridian, Guilai (ST29) and Sanyinjiao (SP6) which is the Crossing point of the Spleen, Liver and Kidney Meridians are selected to regulate Liver Qi, eliminate swelling and mass, regulate the Conception Vessel and promote Qi so as to relieve pain.

4. **Modification**

   - *Hernia of Cold type:* + Shenque (CV8) and Qihai (CV6) to warm meridian and dispel Cold.

   - *Hernia of Damp Heat type:* Omit Guanyuan (CV4), and add Zhongji (CV2) and Yinlingquan (SP9), to remove Heat and eliminate Damp.

   - *Inguinal hernia:* + Xiajuxu (ST39) and Sanjiaojiu (Extra point) to raise collapse and relieve pain.

   - *Fever and aversion to cold:* + Hegu (LI4) and Waiguan (TE5) to clear away Heat and dispel Cold.

   - *Poor appetite and fatigue:* + Zusanli (ST36) and Dabao (SP21) to strengthen Stomach and benefit Qi.

5. **Manipulation**

Routine needling technique is applied to all the points. Dadun (LR1) is pricked to cause bleeding.

Other therapies

1. **Auricular acupuncture**

   Points: External Genitals, Ear-Shenmen, Sympathetic Nerve, Small Intestine, Kidney, Liver. 2 to 3 points are selected in every treatment; moderate stimulation is induced by filiform needle.

2. **Point injection**

   Inject into Taichong (LR3) and Guanyuan (CV4) with Compound Chlorpromazine or vitamin B_{12} injection, 0.5ml in each point.

Notes

1. Acupuncture and moxibustion treatment are quite effective in treating this disease. However, the surgery should be applied if inguinal hernia occurs, such as incarceration of the Small Intestine into scrotum and failure of recovery due to hydrocele of scrotum.

2. The patient should avoid fatigue and keep a nutritional balance.

10. HAEMORRHOID

Brief introduction

Haemorrhoid is a chronic disease occurring in the anus and rectum, also known as haemorrhoids nucleus. It refers to a venous mass formed by enlargement and varicosis of the venous plexus below the mucous membrane of the rectal end and below the anal canal. It attacks both males and females, often seen in young people and multipara.

Aetiology and pathogenesis

The disease is usually caused by prolonged sitting or standing, being overloaded, long distance walking, pregnancy; or by improper diet, excessive intake of pungent and greasy foods, leading to internal production of Dryness and Heat, and impairment of the Stomach and intestines; or by prolonged diarrhoea and dysentery, constipation, which results in interior Damp Heat, obstructed in the meridians and accumulated in the anus and intestine.

Syndrome differentiation

It is divided into internal haemorrhoids, external haemorrhoids and mixed haemorrhoids according to the location. Internal haemorrhoids refer to haemorrhoids above the dentate line, external haemorrhoids are below the dentate line and mixed haemorrhoids include symptoms of both internal and external haemorrhoids. Internal haemorrhoids are often seen clinically with the major symptoms of bloody stools, protrusion of the haemorrhoid nucleus, pain and pruritus.

1. **Stagnation of Qi and Blood**: Protrusion of the mass from the anus, contraction of the anal canal, down-bearing pain, or even incarcerating, oedema around the anus, obvious tenderness, bloody stools; dark red tongue with white or yellow tongue coating, wiry, thready and rolling pulse.

2. **Retention of Damp Heat**: Fresh red bleeding, protrusion of the mass from the anus on defecation, which can be recovered naturally, down-bearing or burning sensation in the anus, abdominal distension and poor appetite; red tongue, yellow and sticky tongue coating, rolling and rapid pulse.

3. **Spleen deficiency and Qi collapse**: Protrusion of the mass from the anus on defecation, which is unable to be recovered naturally, light-coloured bleeding, down-bearing anus, reluctance to speak and lack of Qi, pale complexion, poor appetite and loose stools; pale tongue with white coating, thready and weak pulse.

Treatment

Body acupuncture

1. **Principles of treatment**

   - *Qi stagnation and Blood stasis, retention of Damp Heat*: To promote Qi, activate Blood, clear away Heat and benefit Damp; acupuncture alone is used with the reducing method.

   - *Spleen deficiency and Qi collapse*: To strengthen Spleen, benefit Qi, elevate Yang from collapse; both acupuncture and moxibustion are applied, the reinforcing method.

2. **Prescription**

The principles acupoints are from the Governor Vessel and the Bladder Meridian of Foot-Taiyang. Changqiang (GV1), Huiyang (BL35), Baihui (GV20), Chengshan (BL57), Erbai (EX-UE2).

3. **Explanation**

Changqiang (GV1), Huiyang (BL35) and Chengshan (BL57) belong to the Bladder Meridian of Foot-Taiyang, and the Divergent Meridian of the Bladder Meridian of Foot-Taiyang derives from the calf and ends at the popliteal fossa, winding round to the anal region; therefore, the three acupoints are selected to dispel Damp Heat in anus and intestines, promote Qi of the Bladder Meridian of Foot-Taiyang so as to eliminate stasis and stagnation; Baihui (GV20) is the distant point to raise sinking of Qi and it is selected according to the principles of 'choosing points on the lower part of the body to treat disease of the upper part'; Erbai (EX-UE2) is the established point to treat haemorrhoids and effective for internal haemorrhoidal bleeding.

4. **Modification**

- *Qi stagnation and Blood stasis:* + Baihuanshu (BL30) and Geshu (BL17) to open the intestines, eliminate stasis and relieve pain.
- *Stagnation of Damp Heat:* + Sanyinjiao (SP6) and Yinlingquan (SP9) to clear away Heat and benefit Damp.
- *Sinking of Qi and Spleen deficiency:* + Qihai (CV6), Pishu (BL20) and Zusanli (ST36) to tonify and benefit Qi in Middle Burner, elevate Yang and make collapsed Qi consolidated.
- *Swelling of anus:* + Zhibian (BL54) and Feiyang (BL58) to promote Qi and relieve pain.
- *Constipation:* + Dachangshu (BL25) and Shangjuxu (ST37) to open and regulate Fu Qi.
- *Haematochezia:* + Kongzui (LU6) and Geshu (BL17) to remove Heat and stop bleeding.

5. **Manipulation**

Changqiang (GV1) is punctured 1–1.5 cun in depth along inner wall of coccyx; routine puncturing method is applied to Huiyang (BL35) and the sensation is induced to be radiated to the anus; upward oblique insertion is used at Chengshan (BL57) to induce the sensations transmitted upward; warming moxibustion with moxa stick is used at Baihui (GV20) for 10–15 minutes.

Other therapies

1. **Auricular acupuncture**

   Points: Rectum, Anus, Ear-Shenmen, Subcortex, Spleen, Triple Burner. Moderate stimulation is induced by filiform needle on 3 to 5 points each time.

2. **Three-edged needle**

   Pricking Yinjiao (GV28) to cause bleeding.

3. **Pricking therapy**

   Finding haemorrhoid spots (one or several red papules), 1–1.5 cun from T7 to sacral vertebrae, pricking them one by one with thick needle and squeezing Blood or mucus. This therapy is used once a week.

4. **Catgut implantation**

   Catgut implantation is applied at Guanyuanshu (BL26), Dachangshu (BL25) and Chengshan (BL57), once every 20–30 days.

Notes

1. Acupuncture and moxibustion treatment for this disease has quite a good effect on reducing pain and bleeding of haemorrhoids.

2. The patient should cultivate good habits of defecating on time and maintain smooth defecation to reduce incidence of haemorrhoids.

3. The patient should drink more warm water, eat more fresh vegetables and fruits, and avoid pungent and stimulant food.

11. PROLAPSE OF RECTUM

Brief introduction

Prolapse of rectum refers to the partial or complete protrusion of the rectal mucosa from the anus, which is the same disease in Western medicine. It is often seen in children, the aged and multipara.

Aetiology and pathogenesis

Deficiency syndrome of the disease is mainly caused by non-abundance of Qi and Blood and deficiency of Kidney Qi in children; deficiency of Qi, Blood and insufficiency of Qi in the Middle Burner in the aged; consumption of Qi and Blood and deficiency of Kidney Qi in grand multipara. Deficiency of Spleen Qi and sinking of Qi in the Middle Burner can result from chronic diarrhoea, dysentery or coughing. Excessive syndromes are mainly due to retention of Damp Heat in the Large Intestines and obstruction of the meridians. The disease lies in the Large Intestines and is also closely related with the Lungs, Spleen and Kidneys.

Syndrome differentiation

The major clinical manifestation is prolapse of the anus. In a mild case, the anus can return to its original location naturally after defecation. In a severe case, slight fatigue and cough may lead to prolapse of the anus and it can not return back naturally, accompanied by fatigue, poor appetite, failure in defecating completely and down-bearing sensation.

1. **Spleen deficiency and sinking of Qi**: Prolapse of anus after fatigue, with a light red coloured swollen part out of the anus on defecation, accompanied by down-bearing sensation of the anus, fatigue, poor appetite, pale and sallow complexion, dizziness and palpitations, pale tongue with thin and white coating, thready and weak pulse.

2. **Failure of Kidney Qi in consolidation**: Onset or aggravation after overwork, with protrusion of the anus, down-bearing and loosing feelings of the anus, accompanied by soreness and weakness of the lumbus and knees, dizziness, tinnitus, pale tongue with thin and white coating, deep and thready pulse.

3. **Damp Heat attacking the Lower Burner**: It is often seen during an acute period of dysentery or the attack of haemorrhoids; red, swelling, itching and painful anus, burning sensation and down-bearing pain on defecation, with a dark purple or dark red swollen part protruding out of the anus, red tongue with yellow and sticky coating, wiry and rapid pulse.

Treatment
Body acupuncture

1. **Principles of treatment**
   - *Spleen deficiency and Qi sinking, unconsolidation of the Kidney Qi*: Tonifying Middle Burner and benefiting Qi, strengthening anti-pathogenic Qi, cultivating and consolidating the primary; both acupuncture and moxibustion are applied with the reinforcing method.

- *Pathogenic Damp Heat attacking the Lower Burner:* Clearing away and benefiting Damp Heat, treating prolapse and relieve pain; acupuncture alone with the reducing method is applied.

2. **Prescription**

Select the acupoints of the Governor Vessel and the Bladder Meridian of Foot-Taiyang as the principle points. Changqiang (GV1), Baihui (GV20), Chengshan (BL57), Dachangshu (BL25).

3. **Explanation**

Changqiang (GV1) can enhance the control ability of the anus; Baihui (GV20) locates on the vertex and functions to excite Yang Qi, raising Yang and sinking Qi. Chengshan (BL57) removes Damp Heat in the intestine and anus, dispels swelling to relieve pain. Dachangshu (BL25) is the place of transfer of Qi of the Large Intestine Meridian, and also the acupoint of the Bladder Meridian. Therefore, the point can regulate Qi of the Large Intestine.

4. **Modification**

- *Spleen deficiency and Qi sinking:* + Pishu (BL20), Qihai (CV6) and Zusanli (ST36) to tonify and benefit Qi of the Middle Burner, raising Yang from collapse, and cultivating and consolidating the primary.

- *Failure of Kidney Qi in consolidation:* + Qihai (CV6), Guanyuan (CV4) and Shenshu (BL23) to tonify and benefit Kidney Qi, and strengthening anti-pathogenic Qi.

- *Pathogenic Damp Heat attacking the Lower Burner:* + Sanyinjiao (SP6) and Yinlingquan (SP9) to regulate Qi activity of anus so as to consolidate collapse.

5. **Manipulation**

Acupuncture of the reinforcing method is used on Baihui (GV20), combined with warm moxibustion or sparrow-pecking moxibustion; oblique puncturing is used on Changqiang (GV1) upwards for about 1 cun, parallel to the sacrum. It is necessary that the needling sensation should be radiated to the anus, avoiding penetrating the rectum. Routine needling technique is applied to other points.

Other therapies

1. **Cutaneous needle**

   Tap slightly on musculus sphincter around anus for 10–15 minutes in every treatment.

2. **Auricular acupuncture**

   Points: Rectum, Large Intestine, Subcortex, Ear-Shenmen. Moderate stimulation is applied with filiform needle. Embedding needle or Vaccaria seeds are applicable.

3. **Pricking therapy**

   Prick 1–2 reaction spots on the first lateral line of the Bladder Meridian of Foot-Taiyang between T3 and S2, once or twice a week.

4. **Catgut implantation**

   Catgut implantation at Chengshan (BL57) on both sides alternately, Changqiang (GV1) and Tigang (Extra point), once every 20–30 days.

Notes

1. The treatment of acupuncture and moxibustion has quite a good effect on a mild prolapse of rectum and comprehensive treatment should be taken for a severe case.

2. Primary diseases such as chronic diarrhoea, long standing cough and constipation should be treated proactively in order to reduce abdominal pressure, in combination with frequently functional exercise of abdominal and levator muscles.

3. The patient should take a light diet and avoid cigarettes, alcohol and pungent foods.

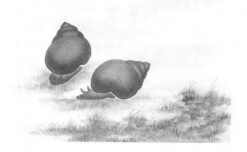

V. ORTHOPAEDIC AND TRAUMATIC DISEASES

1. SPRAIN

Brief introduction

Sprain refers to soft tissue injury of the body or the joints of the limbs, such as muscle, tendon, ligament or blood vessel sprain, without fracture, dislocation of joints and injured skin and muscle. It pertains to the category of 'tendon injury' in Chinese medicine. It mainly occurs in joints.

Aetiology and pathogenesis

Sprain is mostly caused by the injury of soft tissues, local swelling due to Qi obstruction in the meridians, stagnation of Qi and Blood, or even impaired movement of joints resulting from strenuous exercise or overloading, stumbling and falling, traction and oversprain, leading to the joints under external force beyond the limits of their normal activities.

Syndrome differentiation

Swelling and distending pain in the sprained region, with red, blue and purple skin appearance; slightly local swelling and muscular tenderness in a new mild case; red swelling, intense pain and limited movement of joints in a severe case; generally, an old injury does not have obvious swelling and easily relapses due to invasion of pathogenic Wind, Cold and Dampness; sprain often occurs on neck, shoulder, elbow, wrist, waist, hip joint, knee and ankle.

Treatment

Body acupuncture

1. **Principles of treatment**

   To open meridians and activate collaterals, eliminate swelling, relieve pain; acupuncture is applied (moxibustion is applied for old trauma) with the reducing method.

2. **Prescription**

   Select local and nearby points as the principal points.
   - *Neck*: Dazhui (GV14), Tianzhu (BL10), Fengchi (GB20), Houxi (SI3).
   - *Shoulder*: Jianyu (LI15), Jianliao (TE14), Naoshu (SI10), Jianzhen (SI9).

- *Elbow*: Quchi (LI11), Xiaohai (SI8), Tianjing (TE10), Shaohai (HT3).
- *Wrist*: Yangchi (TE4), Yangxi (LI5), Yanggu (SI5), Waiguan (TE5), Daling (PC7).
- *Lumbus*: Shenshu (BL23), Yaoyangguan (GV3), Yaoyan (EX-B7), Weizhong (BL40).
- *Hip*: Huantiao (GB30), Zhibian (BL 54), Juliao (GB29), Chengfu (BL36).
- *Knee*: Xiyan (EX-LE5), Heding (EX-LE2), Liangqiu (ST34), Yanglingquan (GB34), Xiyangguan (GB33).
- *Ankle*: Jiexi (ST41), KunLun (BL60), Shenmai (BL62), Zhaohai (KI6), Qiuxu (GB40).

3. **Explanation**

Local and nearby points are selected as the principal points to open meridians, promote Qi, activate Blood, eliminate swelling and relieve pain effectively, and make injured tissue return to normal.

4. **Modification**

- Add Ashi points at sprain regions.
- Add corresponding Jiaji points for neck and lumbar sprain.

5. **Manipulation**

Apply routine puncturing method at acupoints; ask the patient to move the affected region when manipulating needle on distant points; apply moxibustion for old injury on basis of acupuncture.

Other therapies

1. **Bleeding and cupping**

Select related acupoints or Ashi points at sprain region. Prick with three-edged needle, or tap with cutaneous needle heavily to cause bleeding first, and then apply cupping. It is applicable to fresh trauma with obvious haematoma, old trauma with long-term stasis and invasion of pathogenic Wind and Cold in collaterals, etc.

2. **Auricular acupuncture**

Points: Corresponding sensitive spot, Ear-Shenmen, Subcortex. Puncture with filiform with moderate stimulation; asking the patients to move the injured joints when twirling needles; retain for 30 minutes.

3. Point injection

Select Danggui (当归 *Radix Angelicae Sinensis*) injection, Chuanxiong (川芎 *Rhizoma Chuanxiong*) injection, Honghua (红花 *Safflower*) injection or a solution made of 5%–10% Glucose injection, Hydrocortisone and 0.5%–1% Procaine. Once every other day.

Notes

1. The treatment of acupuncture and moxibustion is quite effective on soft tissue sprain. The patient should be advised to limit movement of the sprained area after injury to avoid it being aggravated.

2. Combine with application of a cold compress to stop bleeding and then apply a hot compress to help relieve swelling during the treatment of sprain.

3. Pay attention to protection of the local affected region in a prolonged case. The patient should do appropriate exercise and keep the whole sprained area warm to avoid getting injured again and invasion of pathogenic Wind, Cold and Dampness.

2. STIFF NECK

Brief introduction

Stiff neck is a disease involving stiffness and pain in the nape and impaired movement of the neck. It is mainly caused by muscular spasm in the neck due to invasion of pathogenic Cold or long-term overtraction of cervical muscles. This disease is mostly seen in adults, usually a sign of cervical damage for patients in middle or old age and easily recurrent. Stiffness, pain and limited movement in the neck in Western medicine, induced by strain, rheumatism, neck sprain, degenerative change in cervical vertebra, synovial interposing of the cervical small joints, subluxation or muscular fascitis can be treated with reference to this disease.

Aetiology and pathogenesis

The condition is usually caused by disharmony of Qi and Blood and contraction of tendons in the neck due to improper sleeping posture and the height of the pillow. It can be caused by neck sprain or invasion of Wind Cold on the neck and back, and also irregular Qi in the meridians.

Syndrome differentiation

Sudden stiffness on one side of the neck and nape after getting up in the morning; inability to bend, lift or turn the head; pain spreads to the shoulder, back and upper extremities of the same side; local muscular spasm and obvious pressing tenderness without swelling when examined.

Pain and obvious tenderness in the neck and back, limited movement of the head in bending and lifting, indicates major pathological changes of the Governor Meridian and Taiyang meridians; pain in the neck and arms, inability of the neck to swing and lean towards both sides, obvious tenderness in one side of the neck, demonstrates major pathological changes of the Shaoyang meridians.

Treatment
Body acupuncture

1. **Principles of treatment**

   Relax the tendons, activate the collaterals, promoting Qi and relieving pain; both acupuncture and moxibustion are applied, the reducing method.

2. **Prescription**

   Dazhui (GV14), Ashi points, Houxi (SI3), Xuanzhong (GB39), Luozhen (EX-28).

3. **Explanation**

   Dazhui (GV14) on the neck and back belongs to the Governor Vessel and promotes local Qi of the meridians to relieve pain in combination with Ashi points. Houxi (SI3) belongs to the Lung Meridian of Hand-Taiyang, and is the one of the Eight Confluent Points which communicates with the Governor Vessel, and can promote Qi in meridians distributed on the neck and back. Xuanzhong (GB39) is the point of the Gallbladder Meridian of Foot-Shaoyang and functions on opening meridians and promoting circulation of Qi and Blood. Luozhen (EX-28) is the established point for treating neck stiffness by activating Blood, opening the collaterals, and relieving spasm and pain.

4. **Modification**
   * *Invasion of the Governor Vessel and Taiyang meridians:* + Fengfu (GV16), Tianzhu (BL10) and Jianwaishu (SI14).
   * *Invasion of the Shaoyang meridians:* + Fengchi (GB20) and Jianjing (GB21).
   * *Radiating pain to scapular region:* + Tianzong (SI11) and Bingfeng (SI12).

5. **Manipulation**

Apply routine puncturing method at acupoints; asking the patients to turn the neck in every direction at the same time; apply moxibustion for local invasion of Wind Cold.

Other therapies

1. **Auricular acupuncture**

Points: Neck, Cervical Vertebrae, Ear-Shenmen. Puncture superficially with twirling manipulation, retain needles for 30 minutes, and ask the patients to move the neck simultaneously.

2. **Finger pressure**

Selecting Chengshan (BL57) at affected region. Nipping the local region heavily with thumbs until sore and distend sensations appear, and applying finger pressing while asking the patients to move the neck. It is applicable to the syndromes at the early stage.

3. **Cutaneous needle**

Tap on the painful region of neck, and tender spots of shoulders and back to cause slight redness in the local skin.

4. **Cupping**

Dazhui (GV14), Jianjing (GB21), Tianzong (SI11) and Ashi points. For mild pain, applying cupping; for severe pain, tap on local region with cutaneous needle to cause bleeding, then apply cupping or moving cupping.

Notes

1. Acupuncture and moxibustion achieve quick and significant therapeutic effect on neck stiffness. The key to treatment is the selection of local points and the emphasis on 'choosing the painful points as acupoints'. It is necessary to give strong stimulation on distant points and to advise the patient to do neck exercises in combination with the treatment.

2. The patient should maintain a correct sleeping posture, with a pillow of suitable height; put the pillow in neck region; also avoid invasion of exogenous pathogens, such as Wind and Cold.

3. CERVICAL SPONDYLOSIS

Brief introduction

Cervical spondylosis, also known as cervical vertebral syndrome, is a series of syndromes induced by stimulation and compression of a nerve root, the spinal cord, vertebral artery or a neck sympathetic nerve in hyperplastic cervical vertebral inflammation, protrusion of intervertebral disc as well as degeneration changes in intervertebral joints and ligaments. Some of the symptoms are seen in stiff neck, pain of the shoulder and neck, headache and dizziness successively in Chinese medicine. The disease is commonly seen in people aged from 40 to 60 years old.

Aetiology and pathogenesis

The disease is caused by weakness in the aged, insufficiency of the Liver and Kidneys, malnutrition of tendons and bones; consumption of Qi due to sitting a long time, impairment of tendons and muscles; invasion of exopathogenic factors to the meridians; or by sprain, stagnation of Qi and Blood and obstruction of the meridians.

Syndrome differentiation

The main symptoms are slow onset, with pain in the occiput, neck, shoulders, back and upper limbs as well as progressive sensory and motor disturbance of the body. In mild cases there is dizziness, headache, nausea, pain in the neck and back, pain, numbness and weakness in the upper extremities; a severe case indicates paralysis or even death.

The disease primarily occurs in the disc of C5–6, and secondarily in the discs of C6–7 and C4–5. Generally, the condition can be classified into nerve root type, spinal cord type, sympathetic nerve type, vertebral artery type and mixed type according to different compressed regions. At the beginning, the main manifestations are nerve root compression and stimulation, and then gradually it develops to functional or structural damage in the vertebral artery, sympathetic nerve, and the spinal cord, with corresponding clinical symptoms.

1. **Obstruction due to Wind Cold**: Stiffness and pain in the neck and spine, soreness in the shoulder and back, limited movement of the neck, or even coldness and numbness in the hands and arms, aggravated on exposure to cold, or accompanied by aversion to cold and general aching, resulting from exposed shoulders at night or long-term lying on wet ground. Thin and white or white and sticky tongue coating, wiry and tense pulse.

2. **Blood stasis due to overstrain and injury**: For people who have a trauma history or a sedentary job with the head bent, pain in the neck, shoulders and arms, or even radiating to the forearms; numb fingers, aggravated after overwork; stiffness, swelling and impaired movement of the neck; dark and purple tongue with petechiae, hesitant pulse.

3. **Deficiency of the Liver and Kidney**: Pain in the neck, shoulders and arms, weakness and numbness in the four limbs, accompanied by dizziness, blurred vision, tinnitus, soreness and weakness of the lumbus and knees, seminal emission or irregular menstruation; red tongue with scanty tongue coating, thready and weak pulse.

Treatment

Body acupuncture

1. **Principles of treatment**

   Expelling Wind Cold, relaxing tendons and activating collaterals; both acupuncture and moxibustion are applied, reducing or even method.

2. **Prescription**

   Select local acupoints of neck as the principal points. Dazhui (GV14), Houxi (SI3), Tianzhu (BL10), Jiaji points of the cervical vertebra.

3. **Explanation**

   Dazhui (GV14) is the acupoint of the Governor Vessel and the meeting point of all the Yang meridians; Qi of the Yang meridians is excited to promote and activate the meridians and collaterals by acupuncture; Houxi (SI3) and Tianzhu (BL10) belong to the Hand and Foot-Taiyang Meridians respectively; Tianzhu (BL10) is the local acupoint. Houxi (SI3) is the one of the Eight Confluent Points communicating with the Governor Vessel; the combination of the two acupoints regulate Qi of the Taiyang meridians and the Governor Vessel and open the collaterals to relieve pain; Jiaji point of the cervical vertebra functions to regulate local Qi and Blood to relieve pain. All the acupoints are applied by distal and nearby combination to dispel Wind Cold, relax tendons, activate collaterals, and regulate Qi to relieve pain.

4. **Modification**

   - *Wind and Cold*: + Fengmen (BL12) and Fengfu (GV16) to dispel Wind and open collaterals.

- *Strain and stasis*: + Geshu (BL17), Hegu (LI4) and Taichong (LR3) to activate Blood, eliminate stasis, open collaterals and relieve pain.

- *Deficiency of Liver and Kidneys*: + Ganshu (BL18), Shenshu (BL23) and Zusanli (ST36) to tonify and benefit the Liver and Kidneys, produce Blood and nourish tendons; Jianjing (GB21) and Tianzong (SI11) according to the location of tender point to promote Qi of the meridians, activate the collaterals and relieve pain.

- *Numbness of the upper limbs and fingers*: + Quchi (LI11), Hegu (LI4) and Waiguan (TE4) to open meridians, regulate Qi and Blood.

- *Vertigo, headache and dizziness*: + Baihui (GV20), Fengchi (GB20) and Taiyang (EX-HN5) to dispel Wind, refresh the Mind, brighten the eyes and relieve pain.

- *Vomiting*: + Tiantu (CV22) and Neiguan (PC6) to regulate the Stomach and intestines.

5. **Manipulation**

Puncture Dazhui (GV14) perpendicularly for 1–1.5 cun to conduct the needling sensation to the shoulders and arms; puncture Jiaji points of cervical vertebra perpendicularly or obliquely to cervical vertebra with even method and inducing the needling sensation to the neck, shoulders and arms; apply routine puncture method to other points.

Other therapies

1. **Auricular acupuncture**

   Points: Cervical vertebrae, Shoulder, Neck, Ear-Shenmen, Sympathetic Nerve, Adrenal, Subcortex, Kidney. Puncture on 3–4 points with filiform with strong stimulation in every treatment; retain for 20–30 minutes; or apply Vaccaria seeds to auricular points.

2. **Electroacupuncture**

   Jiaji points of cervical vertebra, Baihui (GV20), Fengchi (GB20), Jianzhongshu (SI15), Dazhu (BL11) and Tianzong (SI11). Select 2–4 points in every treatment. After Qi has arrived, electroacupuncture is used, lasting 20 minutes.

3. **Cutaneous needle**

   Tap Dazhui (GV14), Dazhu (BL11), Jianzhongshu (SI15) and Jianwaishu (SI14) to make the skin red with a little bleeding, and then apply cupping.

4. **Point injection**

Dazhu (BL11), Jianzhongshu (SI15), Jianwaishu (SI14), Tianzong (SI11). Apply 1% Procaine injection 2ml or vitamin B$_1$ injection 2ml and vitamin B$_{12}$ injection 2ml; 0.5ml for each point.

Notes

1. Acupuncture and moxibustion treatment has a certain curative effect in cervical spondylosis, especially for relieving neck, shoulder and back pain, upper limb pain, vertigo and headache, etc. Acupuncture treatment alone is applicable; a better effect will be achieved in combination with Tuina and external application.

2. Those who work at a desk, with the head held low for a long time should do neck exercises, or self-massage on local region to relax the muscles of the neck once every 1–2 hours while working.

3. Cervical spondylosis is aggravated by neck stiffness; thus, it is necessary to keep the correct sleeping posture with the proper height of pillow placed under the neck; and keep neck warm, avoiding invasion of pathogenic Wind Cold.

4. PERIARTHRITIS OF THE SHOULDER

Brief introduction

Periarthritis of the shoulder refers to the clinical symptoms of a sore, heavy sensation, limitation of shoulder in movement and stiffness of shoulders. It belongs to 'shoulder Bi' in Traditional Chinese Medicine. Women have a higher incidence of the disease than men.

Aetiology and pathogenesis

Pathological changes of this disease distribute in the meridians of the shoulder. People aged about 50 years begin to get deficiency of anti-pathogenic Qi, and insufficient Ying-nutrient Qi and Wei-defensive Qi. Shoulder Bi results from the obstruction of Qi and Blood circulation due to the local attack of Wind Cold, sudden sprain, or long term compression of muscle and meridians due to habitual unilateral position in sleep. Long-term compression of muscles leads to blockage of Qi and Blood, thus shoulder Bi occurs. Long-term shoulder pain results in retarded Qi and Blood circulation in the local area and stagnation. Hence, swelling and adhesion occur in the affected area. Ultimately, joint stiffness and limited movement of the shoulder result.

Syndrome differentiation

This disease is mainly characterized as severe pain with fair motor function in the early stage; and motor disturbance of shoulder is more predominant in the late stage when pain is alleviated rather than acute. In the early stage, it happens unilaterally or bilaterally with soreness and pain of the shoulders radiating to the neck and the whole of the upper limbs, alleviated during the day and aggravated at night, aversion to Wind Cold, numbness and swelling of fingers in the affected limbs, stiffness of the shoulder to different degree, and limitation of superduction, forward extension, external rotation and backward extension of the arm, etc. In a prolonged condition, muscular atrophy is caused by stagnation of Cold Damp, and obstruction of Qi and Blood; however, pain is alleviated rather than aggravated.

The syndrome of the Taiyang meridians is indicated if it is manifested as pain in Zhongfu (LU1) of the scapuloanterior, and the pain is aggravated when the upper limbs extend backwards; the syndrome of Yangming and Shaoyang meridians is predominant if manifested as pain in Jianyu (LI15) and Jianliao (TE14) on the lateral side of shoulder, and there is tenderness of the muscles triangularis and aggravated pain in abduction; the syndrome of Taiyang meridians is determined if manifested as pain in Jianzhen (SI9) and Naoshu (SI10) of scapuloposterior, and pain is aggravated in adduction.

Treatment
Body acupuncture

1. **Treatment principles**

   Relaxing tendons, opening the collaterals, promoting Qi and activating Blood circulation; both acupuncture and moxibustion are applied with the reducing method.

2. **Prescription**

   Select local acupoints in shoulder joints as the principal points. Jianyu (LI15), Jianqian (EX-23), Jianzhen (SI9), Ashi points, Yanglingquan (GB34), Extra Zhongping (1 cun below Zusanli (ST36)).

3. **Explanation**

   Select nearby points, Jianyu (LI15), Jianqian (EX-23), Jianzhen (SI9), which are called 'Three Needles of Shoulder'; add Ashi points in the local region as supplementary points; application of acupuncture with the reducing method in combination with moxibustion to expel Wind Cold and open meridians. Select Yanglingquan (GB34) as the distant point of the meridian to relax and activate the collaterals, and open the meridians to relieve pain; Extra point, Zhongping (1 cun below Zusanli (ST36)) has been discovered in modern times to be the effective experiential point for treating periarthritis of shoulder. The combination of the nearby and distant points is applied to dispel pathogenic factors, relax and open the meridians, and regulate Qi and Blood so as to relieve pain naturally.

4. **Modification**

- *Syndrome of Taiyang meridians*: + Chize (LU5) and Yinlingquan (SP9).

- *Syndrome of Yangming and Shaoyang meridians*: + Zusanli (ST36) and Waiguan (TE5).

- *Syndrome of Taiyang meridians*: + Houxi (SI3), Dazhu (BL16) and Kunlun (BL60).

- *Pain of Yangming and Taiyang meridians*: Penetrating needling from Tiaokou (ST38) to Chengshan (BL57).

5. **Manipulation**

- *Jianqian (EX-23) and Jianzhen (SI9)*: Attention is paid to the angle and depth of insertion, avoiding inward oblique and deep insertion.

- *Yanglingquan (GB34)*: Deep insertion or penetrating needling to Yinlingquan (SP9).

- *penetrating needling from Tiaokou (ST38) to Chengshan (BL57)*: Puncture with strong stimulation.

- *Coldness and aversion to Wind*: Moxibustion; cupping and moving cupping are applicable after acupuncture in shoulder. Routine acupuncture technique is applied to other acupoints. Ask the patient to move the shoulder when manipulating distant points.

Other therapies

1. **Long needle**

Penetrating needling from Jianyu (LI15) to Jiquan (HT1), Jianzhen (SI9) to Jiquan (HT1), Tiaokou (ST38) to Chengshan (BL57), etc. Limited movement of shoulder: penetrating needling to multiple directions locally to improve motor function of the shoulder. Ask the patient to move the affected limb during penetrating needling from Tiaokou (ST38) to Chengshan (BL57).

The movement of the affected limb should be slow and get faster gradually, avoiding forceful movement to avoid pain.

2. **Needling and cupping**

Obvious swelling and pain with superficial Blood stasis: tap affected region by cutaneous needle with moderate force to cause slight bleeding, and apply cupping; severe Blood stagnation: prick with three-edged needle until 2–3 drops appear, to cause slight bleeding, and apply cupping to dispel Blood stasis and pathogenic factors and to open the meridians. Twice a week.

3. **Ear acupuncture**

Points: Shoulder, Shoulder Joint, Clavicle, Ear-Shenmen and corresponding acupoints, etc. Choose 3–4 points in every treatment, connecting with electronic apparatus and stimulating for 10–15 minutes with persistent wave in the early stage and interrupted wave in the late stage.

4. **Electroacupuncture**

JianHai (Extra point), Jianti (Extra point), Jianqian (EX-23), Tianzong (SI11), Quchi (LI11), Waiguan (TE5). Choose 3–4 points in every treatment, connecting with electronic apparatus and stimulating for 10–15 minutes with continuous wave in early stage and intermittent wave in late stage.

5. **Point injection**

Point injection in shoulder with injection solution of Dangui (当归 *Angelica Sinensis*), Chuanxiong (川芎 *Rhizoma Chuanxiong*), Yuanhu (元胡 *Rhizoma Corydalis*), Honghua (红花 *Safflower*), or 10% Glucose injection, vitamin B_1 injection. 0.5ml for each point. Injection is applied to 2–3 of the most obvious tender spots over the larger pain area.

Notes

1. Acupuncture and moxibustion treatment is effective in the treatment of periarthritis of shoulder that makes it preferable to other treatments. Proper diagnosis is required to exclude tuberculosis of shoulder joint, tumour, fracture and dislocation, and distinguish it from the referred pain of cervical spondylosis and visceral disorder.

2. Use acupuncture and moxibustion early in treatment; the shorter the course of the disease is, the more effective this treatment. For the adhesion of tissue and muscular atrophy, the treatment should be combined with Tuina therapy to improve the curative effect.

3. Active and passive exercises are necessary to coordinate acupuncture and moxibustion to recover shoulder functions earlier. 'Climbing wall' exercise must be practised 2–3 times every day.

4. Keep shoulder warm and avoid invasion of Wind Cold.

5. ELBOW STRAIN

Brief introduction

Elbow strain is chronic strain manifested as pain in the lateral epicondyle of the elbow, with dysfunction of the wrist extension and forearm rotation. It is often seen in labourers who engage in work with forearm rotation and joint extension, such as woodworkers, locksmiths, plumbers and tennis players, etc. It is similar to external humeral epicondylitis of Western medicine.

Aetiology and pathogenesis

It is mainly caused by chronic strain. It is formed by damage to Qi and Blood and obstruction of the meridians due to injuries of muscle when the forearm repeats twisting and pushing movements over a prolonged period, or invasion of Wind Cold.

Syndrome differentiation

Slow onset, gradual appearance of pain in the external elbow, and weakness in gripping; aggravation of pain when clenching fist and rotating forearms, such as in twisting a towel, radiating to the forearm or shoulder in severe situation, normal motor function of elbow without obvious swelling in local region; a local and sensitive tender spot found on the lateral side of the wrist, epicondyus, humeroradial joint or anterior of caput radii; pain caused by pressing on the dorsum of hands in the dorsal extension of wrist.

Treatment

Body acupuncture

1. **Principles of treatment**

   To relax the tendons, activate Blood, open the collaterals to relieve pain; both acupuncture and moxibustion are applied, the reducing method.

2. **Prescription**

Select local acupoints of the Large Intestine Meridian of Hand-Yangming on elbow joints as the principal ones. Ashi points, Quchi (LI11), Zhouliao (LI12), Shousanli (LI10), Shouwuli (LI13).

3. **Explanation**

Penetrate tender spots in different directions, or puncture with multi-needles. Quchi (LI11), Zhouliao (LI12): promote Qi and Blood in the local region; Shousanli (LI10), Shouwuli (LI13): promote Qi of the Yangming meridians; the other acupoints: relaxing tendons and open collaterals.

4. **Modification**

- *Limited pronation of forearm:* + Xialian (LI8).
- *Limited supination of forearm:* + Chize (LU5).
- *Pain in inferior of elbow:* + Shaohai (HT3).
- *Pain on elbow tip:* + Tianjing (TE10).

5. **Manipulation**

Puncture the points of the Large Intestine Meridian of Hand-Yangming with routine needling method; penetrate from Ashi points in different directions, or triple puncture with multi-needles, retain for 20–30 minutes; apply moxibustion simultaneously or cup on tender spots with small cups.

Other therapies

1. **Fire needling**

Burning a Fire needle to glowing on an alcohol burner after routine disinfection and prick rapidly on the Ashi points (1–2 tender spots). One more treatment is given after 3–5 days if the pain continues.

2. **Bleeding and cupping**

Tap with cutaneous needles to cause slight bleeding on local region, and then cup and retain with small cups for about 5 minutes so as to cause some bleeding.

3. **Auricular acupuncture**

Points: Corresponding sensitive points, Ear-Shenmen, Subcortex, Adrenal, etc. Puncture and retain the needles for 15–30 minutes; or embed needle for 24 hours; for severe pain, prick on ear apex and corresponding sensitive points to cause bleeding with thick filiform needle or three-edged needle.

4. **Electroacupuncture**

   One to two groups of Fu acupoints are selected with electroacupuncture, with strong stimulation of continuous wave or disperse and dense wave for 10–15 minutes.

5. **Point injection**

   Ashi point is injected with 25mg Prednisone injection with 1% Procaine injection 2ml. One more injection is given in 7 days if pain continues.

Notes

1. This condition is treated with satisfying effects by acupuncture and moxibustion, and in general improve after 2–3 treatments.

2. During treatment, patients should avoid over-exertion of the elbow. Elbow movement is prohibited completely during acute attacks. In the case of long-term sickness and local adhesion of tendon or tissue, Tuina and proper exercises can assist in promoting rehabilitation.

3. Keep shoulder warm and avoid invasion of Wind Cold.

6. GANGLION

Brief introduction

A ganglion is a cystic mass which occurs in joints or myelin sheath, with colourless and transparent or light white, light yellow sticky mucus, and belongs to 'tendon stasis' and 'tendon tumour' in Traditional Chinese Medicine. It often occurs in joints or near myelin sheath and appears more frequently on the dorsum of wrists and feet. Most patients are young or middle-aged people, females in particular.

Aetiology and pathogenesis

Overstrain, external injury of tendons and meridians commonly lead to Phlegm stagnation in the tendons and vessels. Long-term standing and the strain associated results in a disharmony of the tendons and vessels, disorders of Qi and Blood circulation and obstruction in tendons and vessels. Hence, the disease occurs.

Syndrome differentiation

Rounded masses in the wrist joint, dorsum of finger or palm, foot, toe and popliteal fossa, protruding from body surface, and varies in size, roughly ranging from the size of soybean to a walnut; it has a smooth surface and clear edges without adhesion, movable, has a cystic or stiff sensation on touching, and a slightly sore sensation on pressing; slight soreness and fatigue sensation of affected limbs. There are no general symptoms other than the local symptoms, with unlimited or mildly limited function of the joints.

Treatment

Body acupuncture

1. **Principles of treatment**

   Promote Qi and activate the Blood, eliminate stasis and dispel stagnation; acupuncture is mainly applied with the reducing method.

2. **Prescription**

   Local acupoints are selected as the principal ones. Cyst areas (Ashi points).

3. **Explanation**

   Ashi points are selected to promote Qi of the meridians and collaterals, relax the tendons, activate Blood, open the collaterals and resolve the mass.

4. **Modification**

   - *Soreness and weakness of limbs*: The acupoints are selected from meridians according to the affected areas to activate Blood, open collaterals, relax tendons to relieve pain.

5. **Manipulation**

   Routine disinfection is applied locally. Filiform needles are inserted to the base around the cyst at 45° by penetrating the cystic wall, and the needles are retained for 10 minutes. Or a three-edge needle is used to be inserted from the top of cyst perpendicularly to penetrate the cystic wall. Afterwards, the needle is lifted and inserted obliquely around the cyst to penetrate the wall. In removal of needle, the needle is rotated to enlarge the point; then, the cyst is pressed by the finger gently, and the pressure is gradually increased to squeeze out the entire liquid if possible. Finally, the local area is sterilized and dressed. If the cyst recurs, the same needling technique is repeated.

Other therapies

1. **Fire needling**

   Making 2–3 marks on cyst; prick quickly with Fire needle. After withdrawing the needle, squeeze the mucus by finger gently and gradually increasing the pressure. Then the local area is sterilized and dressed.

2. **Warming needle**

   Warm needling is used after perpendicular insertion in the centre of the cyst. After the needle is withdrawn, the cyst is pressed to squeeze mucus and the local area is bandaged.

Notes

1. Acupuncture and moxibustion treatment achieves quite a good effect on the condition.

2. Keep the affected region warm and avoid invasion of Damp Cold.

7. HEEL PAIN

Brief introduction

Heel pain is induced by acute or chronic injury. Although the symptoms are simple, the etiological factors are complex and the condition can linger. Generally, the disease is induced by jumping from high place, drastic and sudden hitting of heel, or walking on an uneven road and injury by a small stone. The heel pain is also related to occupation, flat feet, excessive running and jumping by athletes, tension of plantar fascia of the sole, muscle and tendon over a long period, and repeated traction in the attachment of calcaneus. Repeated traction of aponeurosis plantaris, flexor digitorum brevis, quadratus plantae and ligamentum plantare longum may also induce the disease.

Aetiology and pathogenesis

Deficiency of the Liver and Kidney, disharmony of Qi and Blood, malnourishment of the tendons and vessels are the preconditions of the disease. The disease is induced by obstruction of Qi and Blood due to pathogenic Wind, Cold and Damp invasion, external injury and strain, etc.

Syndrome differentiation

Most patients are over middle age and have a history of acute or chronic heel injury. Severe pain of the heel and sole occurs in standing or walking. The pain radiates to the anterior sole, and is aggravated after exercising and walking, and alleviated after resting.

Treatment

Body acupuncture

1. **Principles of treatment**

   Relax the tendons, open the collaterals, eliminate stasis to relieve pain; both acupuncture and moxibustion are applied, reducing or even methods.

2. **Prescription**

   Select acupoints of the Kidney Meridian of Foot-Shaoyin and the Bladder Meridian of Foot-Taiyang as the principal ones. Taixi (KI3), Zhaohai (KI6), Kunlun (BL60), Shenmai (BL62), Xuanzhong (GB39), Ashi.

3. **Explanation**

   Taixi (KI3) is the Yuan-Primary point of the Kidney Meridian of Foot-Shaoyin; the Kidney Meridian of Foot-Shaoyin enters into heel; Zhaohai (KI6) is applied as a supplementary point to strengthen tendons and bones, disperse Bi and relieve pain; Kunlun (BL60) and Shenmai (BL62), located in the heel, belong to the Bladder Meridian of Foot-Taiyang, are externally–internally related with the Kidneys, and function to relax the tendons and vessels, promote Qi and Blood, and open collaterals to relieve pain; Xuanzhong (GB39) is the marrow Influential point of the Eight Influential Points which can not only tonify the marrow and strengthen bones, but also open the meridians and activate circulation of the collaterals; the Ashi points function to arrive at the affected region to promote the Qi of the meridians in the local region.

4. Modification

   - *Pain in shank*: + Chengshan (BL57) and Yanglingquan (GB34) to soften the tendons and relieve pain.

   - *Qi deficiency*: + Pishu (BL20) and Zusanli (ST36) to strengthen the Spleen and benefit Qi.

   - *Blood stasis*: + Geshu (BL17) and Taichong (GB9) to activate Blood and disperse stasis.

- *Deficiency of both the Liver and Kidney:* + Ganshu (BL18), Shenshu (BL23) and Fuliu (KI7) to benefit the Liver and Kidneys.

5. **Manipulation**

   Taixi (KI3) and Kunlun (BL60): apply mutual penetration method; Shenmai (BL62) and Zhaohai (KI6): puncture towards heel and sole; routine acupuncture technique is applied to other acupoints. The curative effect can be increased by both acupuncture and moxibustion treatments.

Other therapies

1. **Auricular acupuncture**

   Points: Heel, Kidney, Ear-Shenmen, Subcortex. Twirl the needles quickly after inserting, and retain for 0.5–1 hours; needle-embedding is applied if necessary; for mild cases, Vaccaria seeds is applicable.

2. **Electroacupuncture**

   After Qi arrival, electroacupunture is used on Taixi (KI3) and Pushen (BL61), for 15–20 minutes with persistent wave.

3. **Scalp acupuncture**

   Upper one fifth of Posterior Oblique Line of Vertex-Temporal, Lateral Line 1 of Vertex. After inserting, swift rotation or electroacupuncture is used for 30 minutes with continuous wave.

4. **Point injection**

   Inject Ashi points with 15mg Prednisolone and 1% Procaine solution. Once a week.

Notes

1. Acupuncture and moxibustion treatment achieves reliable efficacy on the disease. But, for some cases, it requires a long treatment. Thus, the patient must continue the treatment or combine it with other comprehensive therapies.

2. In the acute stage, patient should have sufficient rest; reduce standing and walking time when the syndromes are relieved; wear soft shoes or put a spongy cushion in the shoes of affected foot.

3. Keep good coordination of physical exercise and rest and avoid Wind Cold and Damp.

8. TEMPOROMANDIBULAR JOINT DISTURBANCE

Brief introduction

Temporomandibular joint disturbance syndrome refers to a series of symptoms, such as pain in the temporomandibular joint areas, clicking, muscular ache, fatigue, limitation of gape, dysfunction of temporomandibular joint, etc. It belongs to 'jaw pain', 'cheek pain', 'lockjaw', and 'jaw dislocation' in Chinese medicine. It happens both unilaterally and bilaterally.

Aetiology and pathogenesis

Wind Cold invades the cheek and causes contracture of the local tendons and muscles because pathogenic Cold is characterized as contraction. Traumatic injury of the cheek or over opening of the mouth leads to injury of the temporomandibular joints. Deficiency of congenital Essence, insufficient of Kidney Qi and maldevelopment of the mandibular joint may result in a clenched jaw, clicking and soreness.

Syndrome differentiation

Ache in the temporomandibular joint, stiffness, clicking, weak chewing, and limited opening of the mouth, abnormality of jaw movement when opening or closing the mouth. Some cases are complicated by dizziness, tinnitus and dysaudia, etc.

1. **Stagnation of Cold Damp**: Dysfunction in opening the mouth, disturbance of the jaw, clicking in the joint, pain in the joint when chewing, soreness, distension and numbness at ordinary times; aggravation by attack of Cold, Damp and Wind; pale tongue with thin and white tongue coating, wiry and slight tense pulse.

2. **Deficiency of Liver and Kidney**: Dysfunction in opening the mouth, disturbance of jaw, clicking in joint areas, sometimes ache in joint areas, dizziness, tinnitus, soreness and weakness of the lumbar region and knees; red tongue, thready and weak pulse.

Treatment

Body acupuncture

1. **Principles of treatment**

   To disperse Wind and Cold, relax the tendons and activate the collaterals; both acupuncture and moxibustion are applied, reducing or even methods.

2. **Prescription**

Local acupoints are selected as the principal ones. Xiaguan (ST7), Jiache (ST6), Tinggong (ST19), Hegu (LI4).

3. **Explanation**

Xiaguan (ST7), Jiache (ST6) and Tinggong (ST19) are nearby points in the local region to promote the Qi of the meridians of the face, and they are the principal ones for treating pathologic changes of the temporomandibular joint; Hegu (LI4) is good for diseases of the face and head. A combination of the local and the distant points is applied to open the meridians, activate the collaterals, disperse pathogenic Wind, open the jaw and relieve pain.

4. **Modification**

- *Deficiency of the Liver and Kidneys*: + Ganshu (BL18) and ShenShu (BL23) to tonify and benefit Liver and Kidney.

- *Dizziness*: + Fengchi (GB20) and Taiyang (EX-HN5) to disperse Wind and activate brain.

- *Tinnitus*: + Ermen (TE21) and Yifeng (TE17) to relieve tinnitus and promote hearing.

5. **Manipulation**

The routine acupuncture technique is applied to all the acupoints with the reducing method, and the needling sensation is conducted to the cheek and temporomandibular joint. Moxibustion is applicable for stagnation of both coldness and Dampness.

Other therapies

1. **Finger pressure**

Bilateral Xiaguan (ST7), Jiache (ST6), Tinggong (ST19) and Quanliao (SI18) are selected. Press the points continuously with the finger tip, more forcefully on affected side, 1–2 minutes on each acupoint; once more press the points in order after a 3–5 minutes break; 3–5 times on each point; 2–3 times a week.

2. **Warming needle**

Tinghui (GB2), Tinggong (ST19), Xiaguan (ST7). After the needle is inserted, a moxa stick 1.5–2cm in length is put on the handle of the needle and ignited. Warming needle is given once every day in a new condition, and once every other day in chronic cases.

3. **Auricular acupuncture**

   Points: Jaw, Cheek, Adrenal. *Tinnitus*: add Internal Ear and Temple; *pain of head and face*: add Temple and Forehead. The points are punctured with filiform needle superficially, twirl and retain for 20–30 minutes; or use Vaccaria seeds.

4. **Electroacupuncture**

   Jiache (ST6), Xiaguan (ST7). After Qi arrival, twirl the needles with the reducing method, and then connect with the electronic apparatus, positive electrode on Jiache (ST6) and negative one on Xiaguan (ST7). Stimulate for 20–30 minutes with continuous wave; 2–3 times a week.

5. **Point injection**

   For intractable cases, inject 0.5%–1% Procaine solution 1ml into Xiaguan (ST7); twice a week.

Notes

1. Acupuncture and moxibustion treatment has a good curative effect in the treatment of temporomandibular joint disturbance syndrome. The patient should avoid overexercise of the mandible when subluxation of joint occurs due to loose tendons. In the case of complete dislocation, repositioning should first be applied; otherwise, it is hard for acupuncture and moxibustion to be effective.

2. Patients who suffer from congenital temporomandibular joint dysplasia should avoid overexercise of articulus mandibularis.

3. The patient should pay more attention to diet, and keep away from dry and hard food to protect the articulus mandibularis from further injury. Avoid invasion of Wind Cold. Suggest self-massage to the patient to enhance resistance of the temporomandibular joint to exopathogenic factors.

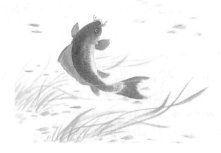

VI. DERMATOPATHY

1. NEURODERMATITIS

Brief introduction

Neurodermatitis is a kind of neurodermal dysfunction, which is relevant to 'psoriasis' and characterized by thickening of the skin, deepening of the dermotoglyph, lichenoid changes and paroxysmal severe itching. According to the size of the skin lesion area, it can be divided into two types, localized neurodermatitis and disseminated neurodermatitis. In Western medicine, this disease is related to the imbalance of excitation and inhibition of the cerebral cortex. Emotional factors are considered to be the main inducing factors causing neurodermatitis; stress, neurasthenia and anxiety can also lead to the occurrence and recurrence of this disease.

Aetiology and pathogenesis

This disease is mainly due to abnormal emotional changes, Liver Qi stagnation transforming into the Fire, prolonged Fire consuming Blood and damaging Yin, Blood deficiency transforming into Dryness and producing Wind, and the poor nourishment of the skin; it can be also due to external pathogenic Wind and Heat attacking the body and blocking the skin.

Syndrome differentiation

This disease has a high incidence in adults. It appears on both sides of the posteriors of the neck, elbow and knee joints, and can also be seen around the eyes and sacral region. In the early stages, the affected area of the skin has normal colour or has slightly red flat papular eruptions. The eruptions are either round or polygonal, are integrated and become a larger area with clear margins. After a long time, the local skin becomes thicker, dry and rough, the dermatoglyph deepens, and starts to have lichenoid changes, with little scales on the surface. Patients experience paroxysmal severe itching, especially at night and in periods of quietness.

This disease has a long course, and sometimes cannot be cured over many years. It will remain the same to a certain degree; some patients, however, can recover naturally within a few weeks without any marks left on the skin. But it recurs easily.

1. **Wind and Dryness due to Blood deficiency**: Papular eruptions are integrated and the surfaces become dry, the colour is light or grey and white, the dermatoglyphs deepen, scales appear on the surface, the patient feels terrible itching especially at night. Female patients may have irregular menstruation; pale tongue with thin coating, soft and thin pulse.

2. **Blood Dryness due to Yin deficiency**: Skin lesions do not heal over a long period; the colour is slightly red or grey and white. The local area is dry and thick; the skin lesions can spread to the whole body. The patient feels severe itching especially at night. Tongue is red with a little coating, and the pulse, wiry and rapid.

3. **Liver Qi stagnation transforming into Fire**: Skin lesions are red in colour, the patient is easily irritated or depressed, insomnia or dream-disturbed sleep, dizzy, bitter taste in mouth and dry throat, red tongue, wiry and rapid pulse.

4. **Accumulation of Wind and Heat**: Eruptions are slightly brown in colour, skin lesions join together and become rough and thick, paroxysmal severe itching which is worse at night, yellow and thin tongue coating, superficial and rapid pulse.

Treatment

Body acupuncture

1. **Principles of treatment**

   To nourish Blood and dispel Wind, replenish Yin to moisten the Dryness for the syndromes of Wind and Dryness due to Blood deficiency, and Blood Dryness due to Yin deficiency, apply acupuncture as the main therapy with even technique; to dispel Wind and clear away Heat, cool the Blood and remove stasis for the syndromes of Liver Qi stagnation transforming into Fire and accumulation of Wind Heat, only apply acupuncture therapy without moxibustion, with reducing technique. Bleeding therapy can be applied as well.

2. **Prescription**

   Fengchi (GB20), Dazhui (GV14), Quchi (LI20), Weizhong (BL40), Geshu (BL17), apply to the area of skin lesions.

3. **Explanation**

   Fengchi (GB20) is located on the back of the neck, where neurodermatitis easily occurs and can dispel Wind, relieve exterior syndrome, promote Qi and Blood circulation; Dazhui (GV14) is the meeting point of Governor Vessel and all the Yang meridians and can reduce Heat and remove the toxic material; Quchi (LI20) can clear away Wind and Heat, and reduce the accumulation of Heat in Blood; bleeding Weizhong (BL40) can clear away Wind and Heat, cool the Blood and remove toxic material; Geshu (BL17) is the Blood Influential point, which can dispel Wind, clear away Heat, activate Blood circulation and stop itching; surrounding techniques can be applied in the affected skin area to promote the Qi and Blood circulation, dispel Wind, remove the toxic material and the stasis.

4. **Modification**

- *Wind and Dryness due to the Blood deficiency:* + Pishu (BL20).

- *To nourish Blood and dispel Wind:* + Xuehai (SP10).

- *To nourish Yin and moisten the Dryness:* + Taixi (KI3) and Xuehai (SP10), if there is Blood Dryness due to Yin deficiency.

- *To soothe Liver Qi and reduce Heat:* + Xingjian (LR2) and Xiaxi (GB43) if the Liver Qi stagnation transforms into the Fire.

- *To dispel Wind and clear away Heat:* + Hegu (LI4) and Waiguan (TE5) for the accumulation of Wind and Heat syndrome.

5. **Application**

Puncture 4–6 points with filiform needles surrounding the affected skin area, puncture horizontally along the base of the skin lesion area; the tip of the needle should point towards the centre of this area; retain the needles for 30 minutes. Several moxa cones can be also applied directly on the skin: make the moxa wool into the size of the head of a match, put the small moxa cone on the point after applying garlic juice to the lesion, and leave 1.5cm space between each moxa cone; remove the moxa ashes after burning off, then cover the area with sterilized material.

Other therapies

1. **Cutaneous needle**

Select the skin lesion area, combined with Back-Shu points, Ciliao (BL32), Huatojiaji (EX-B2) points. Tap the selected areas from outside to inside spirally. Tap gently for mild cases until the skin bleeds slightly and for severe cases create more bleeding by using the heavily tapping method. Tap lightly on the assistant points until the local area becomes red. One treatment every 3 days.

2. **Auricular acupuncture**

Points: Lung, Ear-Shenmen, Adrenal Gland, Subcortex, Endocrine, Liver. Puncture the points shallowly with filiform needles. The embedded-needling technique can be applied or the use of Vaccaria seeds.

3. **Point injection**

    Select Quchi (LI11), Zusanli (ST36), Dazhui (GV14), Feishu (BL13), Baihui (GV20). Choose 2–3 points each time, inject the mixture of 500µg of vitamin B_{12} and 25mg of Promethazine Hydrochloride injection. Inject 0.5ml in each point.

Notes

1. Acupuncture has a good effect in the treatment of neurodermatitis in the short term; it can adjust the excitation and inhibition of the nerve system, and has the obvious functions of calming down the Mind and stopping itching.

2. Patients should relax mentally, avoid scratching the skin lesions, and should not wash the area with hot water or apply any irritating medicine.

3. More fresh vegetables and fruits are recommended, spicy food and seafood are forbidden, no smoking and no alcohol.

2. CUTANEOUS PRURITUS

Brief introduction

Cutaneous pruritus is a type of skin nerve dysfunction without primary skin damage and is characterized by itching of the skin. It belongs to 'Wind itching', 'Wind pruritus' in Traditional Chinese Medicine. It can be divided into general pruritus and localized pruritus. Localized pruritus is related to the friction between the material and the skin, bacteria, parasite or neurosis. General pruritus is related to chronic diseases such as diabetes, Liver and Gallbladder diseases, uraemia and malignant tumour. This disease usually occurs in the lower extremities and has a long course. It has a higher incidence in winter than in spring.

Aetiology and pathogenesis

The main causes of this disease are Liver and Kidney Yin deficiency, Wind and Dryness due to Blood deficiency, poor nourishment of the skin or accumulation of Wind and Dampness in the skin.

Syndrome differentiation

There is no skin damage in the early stage of the disease; paroxysmal severe itching is the main symptom. The itching feeling can be aroused or worsened by drinking alcohol, abnormal emotional changes, being too warm under the covers in bed, and even with psychological suggestion. Often scratching can leave marks and blood scabs on the skin lesion area. Prolonged illness can make the skin thicker and the dermatoglyph deeper; the pigmentation and lichenoid changes are the secondary damage to the skin. Sleeping quality is poor because of the severe itching at night; neurasthenic symptoms such as dizziness, depression, irritability can be seen.

1. **Spleen deficiency and weak Defensive Qi**: Paroxysmal itching, itching is aggravated by coldness and Wind, poor appetite, shortness of breath, lassitude, pale tongue with white coating, thin and weak pulse.

2. **Deficiency of Liver and Kidney**: Itching at night, Dryness and desquamation, skin becomes thick like a straw sheet, soreness and weakness in lumbar and knee joints, poor sleep, pale tongue with yellow coating, deep and thin pulse.

3. **Fire in Qi and Blood**: Diffused redness of the skin, severe itching, bleeding marks due to the scratching, restlessness and thirst, scanty and deep yellow urine, red tongue with yellow coating, rapid pulse.

Treatment

Body acupuncture

1. **Principles of treatment**

   To strengthen the Spleen and resolve the Dampness, tonify Liver and Kidney, nourish Blood and moisten the skin for the syndromes of weak Wei-defence Qi and Spleen deficiency, acupuncture and moxibustion should be combined together with reinforcing technique; to clear away Heat and cool the Blood, dispel Wind and stop itching for Heat in Qi and Blood syndrome, apply acupuncture as the main therapy with reducing technique.

2. **Prescription**

   Quchi (LI11), Xuehai (SP10), Fengshi (GB31), Geshu (BL17).

3. **Explanation**

   Quchi (LI11) is the He-Sea point from the Large Intestine Meridian; it can not only clear away the Heat from the skin, but also remove the Damp Heat from the Stomach and intestine, as well as dispel Wind and stop itching; Xuehai (SP10) can nourish Blood and moisten the Dryness, dispel Wind and relieve itching; Fengshi (GB31) is the key point to dispel Wind; Geshu (BL17) is the Blood Influential point and good for activating the Blood circulation and stopping itching; when it is combined with Xuehai (SP10), it fulfils the direction 'To treat Blood before treating the Wind, Wind can be naturally dispelled when the Blood circulation is promoted.'

4. **Modification**

- *Spleen deficiency and weak Wei-defence Qi*: + Pishu (BL20) and Feishu (BL13) to strengthen the Spleen and Wei-defence Qi.

- *Syndrome of Liver and Kidney deficiency*: + Ganshu (BL18), Shenshu (BL23) and Taixi (KI3) to tonify Liver and Kidney.

- *Syndrome of Fire in Qi and Blood*: + Dazhui (GV14), Waiguan (TE5) and Hegu (LI4) to cool the Ying-nutrient and Blood.

5. **Manipulation**

Apply the routine needling technique for all the above-mentioned points; Geshu (BL17) should be punctured downward or about 1 cun obliquely to the direction of the spinal column.

Other therapies

1. **Auricular acupuncture**

Points: Ear-Shenmen, Sympathetic Nerve, Adrenal Gland, Endocrine, Lung and Itching point. Apply the routine needling technique; retain the needles for 30 minutes.

2. **Point injection**

Select Jianliao (TE14), Xuehai (SP10), Fengmen (BL12), Quchi (LI11), Zusanli (ST36). Choose 2–3 points each time; inject 5–10ml of 0.1%–0.25% Procaine Hydrochloride slowly in the points, 2ml in each point. One treatment every other day.

Notes

1. This disease should be differentiated from other diseases such as eczema, dermatitis, urticaria, scabies and seborrheic dermatitis.

2. The patient should avoid scratching so as to prevent skin damage and causing secondary infection.

3. The patient should avoid using strong alkaline soap and hot water to wash the skin lesion area.

3. URTICARIA

Brief introduction

Urticaria is characterized by general itching of the body, flat-topped wheals which look like measles or are as large as broad beans. It wanders around, comes and goes, no marks remaining after the rashes have disappeared. It is also called Wind rash or Wind wheal. The main symptoms are sudden onset of the rashes with a severe itching feeling. The highest incidence of urticaria is in spring. Acute urticaria occurs suddenly and will not last longer than 3 months, while the chronic type is recurrent and will last more than 3 months.

Aetiology and pathogenesis

Urticaria is mainly caused by congenital weakness and external pathogenic Wind. The acute type is due to weak Wei-defence Qi of the body, the attack of Wind Cold or Wind Heat to the skin leading to the disharmony between Ying-nutrient and Wei defence; or is due to improper food intake causing the accumulation of Damp Heat in the intestines and Stomach. Chronic urticaria is mainly due to Liver Qi stagnation transforming into Fire and consuming the Yin Blood; or due to Spleen Qi deficiency, Damp Heat and parasites; or due to the disharmony between the Thoroughfare Vessel and the Conception Vessel, profuse menstruation; or due to prolonged illness consuming a large amount of Qi and Blood, deficiency of Ying-nutrient and Blood, Wind and Dryness in Blood, and poor nourishment of the skin.

Syndrome differentiation

Acute urticaria has a sudden onset. Wheals appear on the skin suddenly in different shapes and different sizes, and are fused together or appear individually; the colour is slightly red or white with a clear margin. It is red in the surrounding area of the lesion and with a constant severe itching feeling. The oedema can get better and the erythema disappears within a few hours. New wheals will appear again as a result of scratching and attack several times a day. Normally the attacks will stop within 2 weeks.

Chronic urticaria usually has no obvious symptom; the wheals get worse in the morning or at night with or without a regular pattern. It is recurrent and may not be healed over many years.

Urticaria occurs in a localized area of the body or all over the body. If it occurs in the Stomach and intestine, symptoms such as nausea, vomiting, abdominal pain and diarrhoea can be seen. If the hericium mucosa is attacked, the patient may suffer from fullness of the chest, asthma, dyspnoea; asphyxia and other dangerous conditions can result in severe cases.

1. **Wind Heat attacking the exterior**: Wheals are a fresh red colour, itching with burning sensation and aggravated by Heat; combined symptoms are aversion to coldness, swelling and sore throat, thin and yellow tongue coating, superficial and rapid pulse.

2. **Wind Cold blocking the exterior**: Rashes are pale and can be aggravated by Wind and Cold, and alleviated by warmth. Aversion to cold, no thirst, pale tongue with thin and white coating, superficial and tense pulse.

3. **Wind and Dryness due to Blood deficiency**: Rashes are recurrent, linger for a long time, and get worse in the afternoon and at night, combined with symptoms such as restlessness and poor sleep, dry mouth, feverish sensation in palms and soles, red tongue with a little coating, thin, rapid and weak pulse.

Treatment
Body acupuncture

1. **Principles of treatment**

   - *To dispel Wind and clear away Heat for the syndrome of Wind and Heat attacking the exterior*: Only apply acupuncture therapy without moxibustion, with reducing technique.

   - *To remove coldness and relieve exterior syndromes for the Wind Cold blocking the exterior*: Acupuncture and moxibustion are combined together, with reducing technique.

   - *To nourish Blood and moisten the Dryness, dispel Wind and stop itching for the Blood deficiency and Wind Dryness syndrome*: Apply acupuncture as the main therapy, with even needling technique.

   - *To clear away Heat and Fire, promote Qi in Fu organs for the excessive Heat in the intestine and Stomach*: Only apply acupuncture without moxibustion, with reducing technique.

2. **Prescription**

   The points are mainly selected from the Large Intestine Meridian of Hand-Yangming and the Spleen Meridian of Foot-Taiyin. Quchi (LI11), Hegu (LI4), Xuehai (SP10), Sanyinjiao (SP6), Geshu (BL17).

3. **Explanation**

   Qichi (LI11) and Hegu (LI4) are the points from the Large Intestine Meridian of Hand-Yangming and can promote the Qi and Blood circulation, dispel

Wind and clear away Heat; Xuehai (SP10) belongs to the Spleen Meridian of Foot-Taiyin, and can nourish and cool the Blood; Geshu (BL17) is the Blood Influential point, and has the function of activating Blood circulation and stopping itching, combined with Xuehai (SP10) it acts 'To treat Blood before treating the Wind, Wind will be naturally dispelled if the Blood circulation is promoted'; Sanyinjiao (SP6) is the point of the Spleen Meridian of Foot-Taiyin as well as the meeting point of the three foot Yin meridians, and it can nourish Blood and activate Blood circulation, moisten Dryness and stop itching.

4. **Modification**

- *Wind Heat syndrome:* + Dazhui (GV14) and Fengmen (BL12) to dispel Wind and clear away Heat, harmonize Ying-nutrient and Wei defence.

- *Syndrome of Wind and Cold blocking the exterior:* + Fengmen (BL12) and Feishu (BL13) to dispel Wind and remove coldness, harmonize Lung and Wei defence.

- *Blood deficiency and Wind Dryness:* + Fengmen (BL12) and Pishu (BL20) and Zusanli (ST36) to nourish Qi and Blood, moisten Dryness and dispel Wind.

- *Syndrome of excessive Heat in the intestine and Stomach:* + Neiguan (PC6), Zhigou (TE6) and Zusanli (ST36) to clear the Stomach and intestine, promote the Qi in Fu organs.

- *To clear throat for difficulties in breathing:* + Tiantu (CV22), Tianrong (SI17), Lieque (LU7) and Zhaohai (KI6).

- *Irregular menstruation for females:* + Guanyuan (CV4), Ganshu (BL18) and Shenshu (BL23) to regulate Thoroughfare Vessel and Conception Vessel.

5. **Manipulation**

Apply the routine needling technique for all the points; add moxibustion on Fengmen (BL12) and Dazhui (GV14) for the syndrome of Wind and Cold blocking the exterior. One treatment every day for the acute type; one treatment every other day for the chronic type; if the attack of urticaria is related to the menstruation period, the treatment should be started 3–5 days before the menstrual flow comes.

Other therapies

1. **Three-edged needles**

   Select Fengchi (GB20), Quchi (LI20), Xuehai (SP10), Jiaji (EX-B2). Select one point from the four extremities and one point from the body trunk each time. Prick Quze (PC3) or Weizhong (BL40) about 1 cun deep quickly with a three-edged needle and let the dark red Blood come out slowly, until the colour of the Blood becomes slightly red, then apply the cupping method for about 10–15 minutes; pricking Dazhui (GV14) or Fengmen (BL12) about 0.5–1cm deep with a three-edged needle and follow by the cupping method for 10–15 minutes.

2. **Cupping**

   Select Shenque (CV8), applying cupping method with a big cup, retain the cup for 5 minutes, then cup again after removing it, repeat this method 3 times; or apply the flashing cupping method on this point until the Blood vessels become congested on the local area.

3. **Cutaneous needle**

   Select Fengchi (GB20), Quchi (LI20), Xuehai (SP10), Jiaji (EX-B2). Tap the points with moderate strength until the skin becomes red or bleeds slightly. 1 to 2 treatments every day for the acute type, 1 treatment every other day for the chronic type.

4. **Auricular acupuncture**

   Points: Lung, Stomach, Intestine, Liver, Kidneys, Adrenal Gland, Ear-Shenmen, Fengxi. Puncture the auricular points with filiform needles shallowly, with moderate stimulation, or bleed a few drops of Blood from the veins on back of the ear.

5. **Point injection**

   Select Hegu (LI4), Quchi (LI11), Tianzhu (BL10), Sanyinjiao (SP6), Dazhui (GV14), Geshu (BL17). Choose 1–2 points each time, inject complex Danshen (丹参 *Radix Salviae Miltiorrhizae*) injection, or inject auto-Blood from the vein with anticoagulant, 2–3ml in each point.

Notes

1. Acupuncture is very effective in treating urticaria; after 1–4 treatments, the eruptions will disappear and the itching will be relieved.

2. The root cause of chronic urticaria should be clarified, and the proper treatment should be given indicating the root cause, such as parasites in the intestines, endocrine disorders. The combined therapies should be applied if the patient has fullness of the chest and dyspnoea.

3. During treatment, the patient should try to avoid contacting items and medicine that may cause irritation. Irritating and spicy foods such as fish, shrimps and crabs, alcohol, coffee, spring onion and garlic should be forbidden. The patient should maintain a regular bowel movement.

4. ECZEMA

Brief introduction

Eczema is characterized by unfixed skin eruptions in different shapes, with erosion and exudation with itching. Eczema occurs symmetrically on the body. It is recurrent and very easily becomes chronic. It occurs in different types of people, especially those with a sensitive constitution. Acute eczema appears all over the body; the chronic type normally occurs on certain fixed areas.

Aetiology and pathogenesis

It is due to the combination of congenital deficiency and Wind, Damp and Heat attacking the skin. Pathogenic Dampness is the main causative factor and the Spleen is the main Zang organ involved.

Syndrome differentiation

The eruptions cause different types of damage to the skin, such as papules, herpes, erosion, exudation, scab, scale, hypertrophy, lichenoid changes and pigmentation of the skin. According to the symptoms, eczema can be divided into three types: acute, subacute and chronic. Acute eczema has a sudden onset, and initially there are intensive erythema spots and miliary-sized papules and herpes; soon these turn into small blisters, then erosion spots can be seen after the blisters get broken, in the meantime, there is also a severe itching sensation; pustules and pus exudation can be seen when there is infection. Subacute eczema develops from acute eczema; the symptoms are small papules, herpes and blisters with mild erosion, severe itching. Acute and subacute eczema are recurrent and do not heal easily, and easily change into the chronic type; but patient may also have chronic eczema from the beginning, which is manifested as paroxysmal pruritus, with the itching getting worse with Heat or during sleep, rough, hard and thickened skin, lichenoid changes, pigmentation, scratch marks, erosion, exudation, blood scabs and scales. In long-term cases, the disease may last a few months or years.

1. **Invasion of Damp Heat**: It has an acute onset, can be generalized on the whole body. At the beginning, the affected skin is slightly red with burning sensation and swelling, followed by intensive miliaria or blisters, exudation with persistent itching, combined symptoms such as fever, irritability and thirst, dry stools, scanty and dark yellow urine, red tongue with yellow and sticky coating, rolling and rapid pulse.

2. **Spleen deficiency and retention of Dampness**: This has a moderate onset, there is a flushing of the skin lesion, itching, exudation after scratching, with other symptoms such as scaling of the skin, poor appetite, lassitude, abdominal distension, loose stools, pale and tender tongue with teeth marks, white tongue coating; soft, weak, superficial and slow pulse.

3. **Wind Dryness due to Blood deficiency**: This is recurrent in onset, and there is a long course of the disease; skin lesions are dark in colour or with pigmentation, roughness and hypertrophy, lichenoid changes, severe itching, scratch marks on the surface of the skin lesions, blood scab and scales, also combined with symptoms such as dizziness, lassitude, soreness and weakness of the lumbar region and limbs, dry mouth with no desire to drink, pale tongue with white coating, wiry and thin pulse.

Treatment
Body acupuncture

1. **Principles of treatment**

   - *Invasion of Damp Heat syndrome*: To clear away Heat and resolve Dampness, only apply acupuncture without moxibustion with reducing technique.

   - *Syndrome of Spleen deficiency and retention of Dampness*: Acupuncture and moxibustion are combined with reinforcing technique to strengthen Spleen and drain the Dampness.

   - *Blood deficiency and Wind Dryness syndrome*: Acupuncture is the main therapy with even-needling technique to nourish the Blood and moisten Dryness.

2. **Prescription**

   Select the points mainly from the skin lesion area and the Spleen Meridian of Foot-Taiyin. Quchi (LI11), Zusanli (ST36), Sanyinjiao (SP6), Yinlingquan (SP9), skin lesion area.

3. **Explanation**

   Quchi (LI11) is the He-Sea point of the Large Intestine Meridian of Hand-Yangming, it can remove Dampness from the skin as well as Damp Heat from the intestine and Stomach; Zusanli (ST36) can strengthen the Spleen and remove Dampness, tonify the Qi and Blood, as well as treat both the secondary symptoms and the root cause; Sanyinjiao (SP6) and Yinlingquan (SP9) can help the Spleen to resolve Dampness and remove Damp Heat from the skin; the points on the skin lesion area can promote the Qi movement in the local meridians and collaterals as well as dispel Wind and stop itching.

4. **Modification**

   - *Invasion of Damp Heat syndrome:* + Pishu (BL20), Shuidao (ST28) and Feishu (BL13) can be added to clear away Heat and resolve the Dampness.

   - *Spleen deficiency and retention of Dampness:* + Taibai (SP3), Pishu (BL20), Weishu (BL21) to strengthen the Spleen and remove the Dampness.

   - *Wind Dryness due to the Blood deficiency:* + Geshu (BL17), Ganshu (BL18) and Xuehai (SP10) can be added to nourish Blood and moisten the Dryness.

   - *For the patient who suffers from severe itching and insomnia:* + Fengchi (GB20), Anmian (EX point), Baihui (GV20) and Sishencong (EX-HN1).

5. **Manipulation**

   Apply the routine acupuncture technique, retain the needles for 15 minutes; tap the affected skin area heavily with a cutaneous needle until it bleeds, then followed by cupping therapy. One treatment every day in the acute stage, and one treatment every other day in the chronic stage.

Other therapies

1. **Auricular acupuncture**

   Points: For acute eczema, select Lung, Ear-Shenmen, Adrenal Gland, tiny vein on the back of the ear; for the chronic eczema, add Liver and Subcortex. Bleed the vein on the back of the ear; the rest of the points should be punctured with filiform needles with a rapid rotation technique; retain the needles for 1–2 hours.

2. **Cutaneous needle**

Slightly tap the Jiaji (EX-B2) and the first line of the Bladder Meridian of Foot-Taiyang on the back, until the skin gets slightly red, once a day.

3. **Point injection**

Select Quchi (LI11), Zusanli (ST36), Xuehai (SP10), Dazhui (GV14), etc. Choose 2 points each time, inject vitamin B_1, vitamin B_{12} and Banlangen (板蓝根 *Radix Isatidis*) injection, or add 2.5% Sodium Citrate injection, inject 1–2ml in each point, once every other day.

Notes

1. Acupuncture therapy has a very obvious effect in the treatment of eczema; it can enhance the immune response ability of the human body. In particular, it can alleviate the symptoms quickly, although it is very difficult to cure it.

2. The patient should avoid scratching the affected areas, washing the areas with hot water and soap or irritants, and improper external applications.

3. The patient should avoid external stimuli and allergic factors. They should not wear underwear and socks made of nylon or synthetic fibres. Food such as fish, shrimp, and drinks such as strong tea, coffee, alcohol are forbidden.

4. Patients should regulate their emotions and avoid mental stress and over exertion.

5. ACNE

Brief introduction

Acne is a common inflammation of the sebaceous follicles that is usually seen in young people. It particularly occurs in areas such as the face, chest and back, and most cases have a natural recovery after adolescence; in a small number of severe cases, life-long scars are left.

Aetiology and pathogenesis

Acne is mainly due to Wind Heat in the Lung Meridian steaming the skin; or due to overeating spicy, hot, greasy and oily food, the accumulation of Damp Heat in the Spleen and Stomach affecting the skin; or due to the disharmony between the Thoroughfare and Conception Vessels, and dysfunction of the skin in maintaining dispersion.

Syndrome differentiation

Lesions mainly occur in the places with rich sebaceous glands, such as the face, chest and back. In the early stage, it shows as acne (acne with a black spot on the top is most commonly seen) which appears as a pore with a little black spot, out of which some yellow and white fat deposit can be squeezed; acne with a white spot is a gray papule, without a black spot on the top and the fatty deposit is not easily squeezed out. This disease can evolve into inflammatory papules, pustules, nodules, cysts or scars. If the inflammation is obvious, it can cause pain and tenderness as well.

1. **Wind Heat in the Lung Meridian**: Mainly shown as papule damage, may have pustules, nodules, cysts, etc., thin and yellow tongue coating, rapid pulse.

2. **Accumulation of Damp Heat**: The symptoms are discomfort of the face with oily irritation, rashes with impetigo, nodules, cysts, etc., constipation, yellow sticky tongue coating, soft, weak, superficial and rapid pulse.

3. **Stagnation of Phlegm and Dampness**: Papules with pustules, nodules, cysts, scarring and other damages, combined with other symptoms such as poor appetite, loose stools. Pale tongue with sticky coating, rolling pulse.

4. **Disharmony between the Thoroughfare Vessel and the Conception Vessel**: Symptoms are related to the menstrual cycle, and may be associated with irregular menstruation, dysmenorrhoea, dark red tongue, thin yellow coating, wiry and rapid pulse.

Treatment

Body acupuncture

1. **Principles of treatment**

    To clear away Heat, remove Dampness, cool the Blood and remove the toxic material for the syndromes of Wind and Heat in the Lung Meridian, accumulation of Damp Heat, stagnation of Phlegm and Dampness; to activate Qi and Blood, regulate the Thoroughfare Vessel and Conception Vessel for the syndrome of disharmony between Thoroughfare Vessel and Conception Vessel; only apply acupuncture therapy without moxibustion, with reducing technique.

2. **Prescription**

Select points mainly from the local area and the Large Intestine Meridian of Hand-Yangming. Yangbai (GB14), Quanliao (SI18), Dazhui (GV14), Hegu (LI4), Quchi (LI11), Neiting (ST44).

3. **Explanation**

Yangbai (GB14) and Quanliao (SI18) can activate the Qi and Blood movement in the local area in order to promote the dispersing function of the skin. Dazhui (GV14) can clear away Heat and reduce the Fire, cool the Blood and remove toxic materials; Hegu (LI4), Quchi (LI11) can reduce the Heat from the Yangming meridians; the Yangming meridians are the meridians full of Qi and Blood which also run to the facial region, therefore Neiting (ST44) can reduce Heat from the Yangming meridians.

4. **Modification**

- *Syndrome of Wind Heat in the Lung Meridian:* + Shaoshang (LU11), Chize (LU5), Fengmen (BL12) to clear away Lung Heat.

- *Accomulation of Damp Heat Syndrome:* + Zusanli (ST36), Sanyinjiao (SP6), Yinlingquan (SP9) to clear away the Heat and resolve the Dampness.

- *Stagnation of Phlegm and Dampness:* + Pishu (BL20), Fenglong (ST40), Sanyinjiao (SP6) to drain the Dampness and resolve the Phlegm.

- *Disharmony between the Thoroughfare Vessel and the Conception Vessel:* + Xuehai (SP10), Geshu (BL17) and Sanyinjiao (SP6) to harmonize the Thoroughfare Vessel and Conception Vessel.

5. **Manipulation**

Apply the routine needling technique with the reducing method. Prick and bleed Dazhui (GV14). Once every other day.

Other therapies

1. **Auricular acupuncture**

Points: Lung, Spleen, Large Intestine, Endocrine, Adrenal Gland, Ear Apex. Moderate stimulation with filiform needles, retain the needles for 15–20 minutes; Vaccaria seeds can be also used.

2. **Pricking therapy**

Look for the positive reaction papule points 0.5–3 cun lateral to T1–T12 on the back. Prick those points with a three-edged needle, and break some of the subcutaneous fibro tissues and bleed them slightly, once or twice a week.

3. **Bleeding and cupping**

Select Dazhui (GV14), Feishu (BL13), Geshu (BL17), Taiyang (EX-HN5), Chize (LU5), Weizhong (BL40). Choose 2 points each time, use a three-edged needle to bleed the stagnant veins on the points, the flashing cupping method should be applied after the Blood colour becomes light. Once every 2–3 days.

Notes

1. Acupuncture has a certain amount of success in treating acne. Some patients can be healed completely. No treatment is needed if facial hygiene is well maintained for mild cases.

2. Seborrheic acne is the main type of this disease. The patient should not use cosmetics and facial cream during the treatment. Sulphur soapy water is recommended to wash the face so as to reduce the fat which block the pores in the face.

3. The patient should not squeeze the pimples by hand, so as to avoid secondary infection and scarring.

4. The patient should eat no spicy, fatty and sweet food. Patients should eat more fresh vegetables and fruit and maintain regular bowel movement.

6. FLAT WART

Brief introduction

Flat wart is a kind of small vegetation that occurs on the superficial part of the skin. It usually occurs in young people, mainly on the dorsum of the hand or face.

Aetiology and pathogenesis

They are usually due to the combination of pathogenic Wind and Heat attacking the skin, or due to Liver Qi stagnation, or Qi and Blood stagnation. In Western medicine, they are considered a virus infection.

Syndrome differentiation

Occurring mainly on the face, dorsum of the hand and forearm, flat warts are flat bulging papules the size of a grain of rice or a soybean, and the shapes are round, oval or an irregular polygon. The surface of the papules is smooth but hard, the colour is light brown or normal skin colour. They are scattered or distributed in density, and mixed together. Generally, the patient has no subjective symptoms, but may experience itching after the disappearance of the warts.

1. **Accumulation of Heat in the Lungs and Stomach**: Brown flat warts, scattered distribution, strip-like or bead-like shape after scratching. Associated symptoms are seborrheic secretion and acne, thirsty with dry lips. Red tongue with yellow coating, superficial and rapid pulse.

2. **Spleen Dampness and Phlegm retention**: This happens mainly on the face, fewer flat warts in numbers, prominent and mostly of skin colour, sometimes with itching. Other symptoms are poor appetite and epigastric distension. Pale tongue with sticky coating, deep and rapid pulse.

Treatment
Body acupuncture

1. **Principles of treatment**

   To dispel Wind and clear away Heat, reduce the Fire from the Lungs and Stomach for the syndrome of accumulation of Heat in the Lungs and Stomach, apply acupuncture alone therapy without moxibustion, with reducing technique; to remove Dampness and resolve Phlegm, promote the Qi and Blood in the meridians and collaterals for the syndrome of Spleen Dampness and Phlegm retention, use both acupuncture and moxibustion, with reducing technique.

2. **Prescription**

   Hegu (LI4), Quchi (LI11), Taichong (LR3), Sanyinjiao (SP6), local wart area.

3. **Explanation**

   Flat wart occurs mainly on the face and back of the hands, which are the areas of the Large Intestine Meridian of Hand-Yangming, therefore, Hegu (LI4), Quchi (LI11), Sanyinjiao (SP6) should be selected to reduce the Wind and Heat from the Large Intestine Meridian of Hand-Yangming and the Spleen Meridian of Foot-Taiyin; Hegu (LI4) and Taichong (LR3) are considered as 'the Four Gates' points, they can harmonize the Qi and Blood, and soothe Liver Qi; Sanyinjiao (SP6) can nourish the Liver and Kidneys, regulate the Qi and Blood of the skin; treatment in the local warts area can help the circulation of Qi and Blood in order to remove the warts.

4. **Modification**

   - *Syndrome of excessive Heat in the Lung and Stomach:* + Chize (LU5), Neiting (ST44) to clear away Heat, cool the Blood and harmonize Ying-nutrient and Blood in order to remove warts.

   - *Syndrome of Spleen Dampness and Phlegm retention:* + Shangqiu (SP5) and Yinlingquan (SP9) to strengthen the Spleen and remove the Dampness, resolve the Phlegm and promote the collaterals.

5. **Manipulation**

   Apply the routine acupuncture technique; use a short and thick filiform needle to puncture the base of the wart horizontally after strict disinfection procedure, and puncture the centre with another needle, retain the needles for 20 minutes, squeeze a little Blood out when the needles are removed. Once every day.

Other therapies

1. **Fire needle**

   Select the wart areas, use a heated Fire needle to puncture into the wart body rapidly about 2–3mm deep, then remove the needle after a few seconds, repeat this method 2–3 times. One treatment every day. The area must not touch water within one day of the therapy, so as to avoid infection.

2. **Auricular acupuncture**

   Points: Lung, Ear-Shenmen, Adrenal Gland, Subcortex, Endocrine and the corresponding areas of the warts on the ear. Select 3–4 points each time, with moderate stimulation, retain the needles for 15 minutes. Once every day.

3. **Cutaneous needle**

   Select the first line of the Bladder Meridian of Foot-Taiyang on the back, tap it from up to down with moderate force, until the skin becomes slightly red. One treatment every day.

4. **Point injection**

   Select Quchi (LI11), Zusanli (ST36) on the same side as the wart area. Inject 1ml Banlangen (板蓝根 *Radix Isatidis*) injection in each point.

Notes

1. Acupuncture is a simple and effective method for treating flat wart. After the treatment, the flat warts of some patients may change, for example, the wart turns red or itching becomes severe, this is considered a normal reaction because of the Qi and Blood being strongly promoted by acupuncture stimulation, and the same treatment should be continued.

2. During the treatment, no spicy and seafood is allowed, and the patient must not scratch the skin so as to avoid autoinfection.

7. HERPES ZOSTER

Brief introduction

Herpes zoster is clustered along one side of the body, distributed in a belt shape like a snake and characterized by severe pain. The eruptions and blisters appear like beads, and occur around the waist, so it is also known as 'Red Fire around the waist'. It also appears on the chest and face, and is particularly prevalent in spring and autumn, but rarely relapses after the recovery. This disease is aroused by the herpes zoster virus.

Aetiology and pathogenesis

The causative factors are pathogenic Wind Fire or toxic Dampness. It is due to the internal retention of Damp Heat in the Liver and Spleen, combined with external pathogens.

Syndrome differentiation

Before the onset of the disease, the patient may have mild fever, fatigue and weakness, loss of appetite, general malaise, and burning pain of the skin. It can start without premonitory symptoms; the papuloid herpes just appear directly.

Neuralgia of the skin lesion is the main symptom; the pain occurs in varying degrees, and is not directly related to the severity of the skin lesion.

Herpes appears normally between the lower back and the abdomen, then the neck and face region; it is distributed in a belt shape with severe stabbing pain. After the herpes disappears, some patients still have the neuralgia left over.

1. **Accumulation of Heat in the Liver Meridian**: Bright red skin lesions, the blisters have a tense wall, burning stabbing pain, also combined with symptoms such as sore throat, irritability, hot temper, dry stools or yellow urine, red tongue with yellow thick coating, rolling, wiry and rapid pulse.

2. **Damp Heat in the Spleen Meridian**: Light colour of the skin lesions, loose blisters walls, combined with the symptoms such as thirst with no desire to drink, poor appetite, chest and epigastric fullness, loose stools, red tongue with yellow and sticky coating, soft, superficial, weak and rapid pulse.

3. **Blood stagnation in the collaterals**: Constant pain after the herpes disappear combined with symptoms such as irritability, insomnia, purple tongue body with thin and white coating, wiry and thin pulse.

Treatment

Body acupuncture

1. **Principles of treatment**

   Clear away Heat and remove the Dampness, reduce the Fire and remove the toxic materials, activate Blood circulation and promote the collaterals, remove the Blood stagnation and stop the pain; acupuncture and moxibustion are combined, with reducing technique.

2. **Prescription**

   Zhigou (TE6), Yinlinquan (SP9), Xingjian (LR2), Jiaji (EX-B2), on the affected skin area.

3. **Explanation**

   Zhigou (TE6) is the point from the Triple Burner Meridian of Hand-Shaoyang, Yinlingquan (SP9) is the He-Sea point of the Spleen Meridian of Foot-Taiyin; the combination of these 2 points can reduce the pathogenic Heat from the Triple Burner Meridian, strengthen the Spleen and resolve the Dampness; Xingjian (LR2) is the Ying-Spring point from the Liver Meridian of Foot-Jueyin, which has the function of soothing Liver Qi and reducing the Heat; after needling the affected skin area, add the moxibustion and cupping so as to activate the Blood circulation and promote the collaterals, remove the stagnation and toxic materials; the corresponding Jiaji (EX-B2) points can promote the Qi and Blood circulation of the skin lesion area.

4. **Modification**

   - *Syndrome of accumulation of Heat in the Liver Meridian*: + Taichong (LR3), Xiaxi (GB43) and Yanlingquan (GB34) to clear away the Damp Heat from the Liver and Gallbladder.

- *Syndrome of Damp Heat from the Spleen Meridian:* + Dadu (LR1), Sanyinjiao (SP6) and Xuehai (SP10) to strengthen the Spleen and remove the Dampness, resolve the stagnation and relieve pain.

- *Blood stagnation in collaterals:* Add the necessary corresponding points according to the different affected skin area.

- *Herpes appear on the face:* + Yangbai (GB14), Taiyang (EX-HN5) and Quanliao (SI18).

- *Herpes appear on the chest and hypochondriac region:* + Qimen (LR14) and Dabao (SP21).

- *Herpes appear on the waist and abdomen region:* + Zhangmen (LR13) and Daimai (GB26).

5. **Manipulation**

   Apply routine acupuncture technique on all the above-mentioned points; apply surrounding needling technique combined with moxibustion and cupping on the local skin lesion area; once every day.

Other therapies

1. **Auricular needle**

   Points: Liver, Lung and the corresponding skin lesion areas on the ear. Acupuncture, embedded needling therapy or the Vaccaria seeds can be applied.

2. **Cutaneous needle**

   Tap the herpes region and the surrounding skin areas, prick the herpes and let the exudation come out, when the skin gets red and slightly bleed, the cupping method can be followed. Once or twice a day.

Notes

1. Acupuncture has a very obvious analgesic effect for treating this disease and can reduce the post neuralgia as well. If acupuncture treatment is applied in the early stage, most patients can recover within one week.

2. If the herpes lesion area is seriously affected, 2% of gentian violet can be used on the affected area so as to prevent secondary infection. If a disease of the tissues or malignant tumour is combined with the herpes, Traditional Chinese Medicine and Western medicine should be integrated.

3. This disease should be distinguished from eczema, herpes simplex, contact dermatitis and the dermatitis due to insects bite.

8. ALOPECIA AREATA

Brief introduction

Alopecia areata is characterized by the sudden falling out of patches of the hair on the scalp. It usually occurs due to strong mental stress, and may be related to the dysfunction of the central nervous system or endocrine disorders in addition. Infection is the inducing reason, and it is related to the autoimmune system, according to the research.

Aetiology and pathogenesis

The hair needs to be nourished by Blood. The loss of hair can be caused by excessive sexual activity and the deficiency of Kidney Essence; or due to over-thinking which impairs the Spleen function, and the lack of Qi and Blood production; or due to Lung Qi deficiency and both Qi and Blood deficiency; or due to both Liver and Kidney Yin deficiency, deficiency of Essence and Blood producing internal Wind; or due to the impeded emotions, Liver Qi stagnation and Blood stasis; or the poor formation of Blood failing in nourishing the hair; or due to mental stimulation, hyperactivity of Heart Fire and the Wind produced by Heat in Blood.

Syndrome differentiation

It is particularly prevalent in young people with the sudden appearance of round or oval spot baldness in different size and severity. There is no inflammation in the local skin, and the skin looks smooth and shining without any auto-symptoms. Erythema and oedema can be seen on the alopecia area in the early stage in a small number of patients. The hair on the border of the alopecia area is loose and very easily falls out or can be pulled out, and the hair gets very weak at the proximal part of the hair trunk. The lesions on individual patients can be expanded until all the hair falls out.

1. **Qi and Blood deficiency**: It occurs after the illness, the delivery of a baby, or sores, which range from small to big, and from few to many in number. It progressively get worse. The scattered remaining hair can be seen on the alopecia region, but will fall out easily at just a gentle touch. The combined symptoms include pale lips, Heart palpitations, shortness of breath, dizziness, hypnopathia, fatigue. Pale tongue with thin and white coating, thin and weak pulse.

2. **Liver and Kidney deficiency**: Usually seen in persons over the age of 40 with burned-yellow or grey hair. During the disease, the hair is evenly detached in a large area; there will be also eyebrow, armpit hair and pubic hair loss in severe cases. Other symptoms include a pale complexion, chills, dizziness, tinnitus, soreness and weakness in lumbar and knee joints. Pale tongue with cracks, little coating or no coating, deep, thin and weak pulse.

3. **Blood Heat producing Wind**: A sudden hair loss, progressing rapidly, the hair detached in a large area. Accompanied by flushes, irritability, hot temper, anxiety, and individual patient's eyebrows and beard may fall off. Occasionally the patient feels itching on the scalp. Red tongue with less coating, thin and hesitant pulse.

4. **Blood stagnation in collaterals**: Patient has auto-symptoms such as headache or scalp irritation before the hair loss. Hair loss happens first in a small area, then the hair on the whole head falls out. Other symptoms such as nightmares, feverish sensation, insomnia, dark complexion, purple spots on the side of the tongue, thin and hesitant pulse.

Treatment
Body acupuncture

1. **Principles of treatment**

   To tonify the Liver and Kidney in order to nourish the Blood and grow the hair in the syndromes of both Qi and Blood deficiency, and Liver and Kidney deficiency, acupuncture and moxibustion are combined, apply reinforcing or even technique; to activate Qi and Blood circulation, remove stagnation and promote the orifices for the syndromes of Blood Heat producing Wind, and Blood stagnation in the collaterals, only apply the acupuncture therapy without moxibustion, with reducing technique.

2. **Prescription**

   Alopecia area, Baihui (GV20), Tongtian (BL7), Dazhui (GV14), Ganshu (BL18), Shenshu (BL23).

3. **Explanation**

   Alopecia area, Baihui (GV20), Tongtian (BL7) are the local points on the scalp, and they can promote the Qi and Blood in the meridians and collaterals in the local area; Dazhui (GV14) is the appropriate point from the Governor Vessel as well as the meeting point of all the Yang meridians, it can stimulate the Yang Qi of all the Yang meridians and tonify Qi and Blood;

Ganshu (BL18) and Shenshu (BL23) can nourish the Liver and Kidneys, reinforce the Blood and grow the hair.

4. **Modification**

- *Both Qi and Blood deficiency*: + Qihai (CV6), Xuehai (SP10), Zusanli (ST36) to tonify the Qi and nourish the Blood.

- *Deficiency of Liver and Kidneys syndrome*: + Mingmen (GV4), Taixi (KI3) to tonify the Liver and Kidneys.

- *Syndrome of the Blood Heat producing Wind*: + Fengchi (GB20), Quchi (LI11) to reduce the Heat.

- *Syndrome of the Blood stagnation in collaterals*: + Geshu (BL17), Taichong (LR3) to activate the Blood circulation and remove Blood stasis.

- *Alopecia area is on the front part of the head*: + Shangxing (GV23), Hegu (LI4), Neiting (ST44).

- *Alopecia area is on the side of the head*: + Shuaigu (GB8), Waiguan (TE5), Zulinqi (GB41).

- *Alopecia area is on the top of the head*: + Sishencong (EX-HN1), Taichong (LR3), Zhongfeng (LR4).

- *Alopecia area on the back of the head*: + Tianzhu (BL10), Houxi (SI3) and Shenmai (BL62).

5. **Manipulation**

Puncture subcutaneously towards the centre of the alopecia area; do not puncture Ganshu (BL18) perpendicularly and deeply; apply the routine acupuncture technique on the rest of the points.

Other therapies

1. **Cutaneous needles**

Select the hair loss areas, Jiaji (EX-B2) points or related Back-Shu points. Tap the hair loss areas from the edges to the centre spirally, then tap the Jiaji (EX-B2) points or Back-Shu points with the range of 0.5–1cm until the local skin slightly bleeds. One treatment every other day. After tapping the alopecia area, use ginger slices to rub the local area, or apply Banmao (斑蝥 *Mylabris*) tincture, Hanliancao (旱莲草 *Herba Ecliptae*) tincture, or Cebaiye (侧柏叶 *Cacumen Platycladi*) tincture to enhance the effect of hair regeneration.

2. **Point injection**

Select Ashi points, Touwei (ST8), Baihui (GV20), Fengchi (GB20). Inject 4ml of vitamin B$_{12}$ or 5–10mg of Adenosine Triphosphate in the points, 0.5ml in each point. Once every other day.

Notes

Acupuncture is a good therapy for treating this disease except for the completely bald condition. It can adjust the nervous system function, improve the blood circulation and hair nutrition, and enhance the activity of hair follicles to grow new hair.

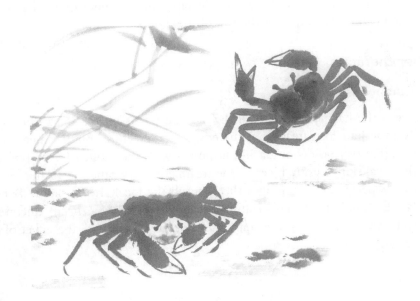

VII. DISEASES OF FIVE SENSE ORGANS

1. CONGESTION, SWELLING AND PAIN OF THE EYE

Brief introduction

Congestion, pain and swelling of the eye is an acute ophthalmic disease, which is characterized by congestion and pain of the eye, photophobia and lacrimation. It is prevalent in spring and summer, contagious and epidemic. In Western medicine, it is referred to as acute conjunctivitis, pseudome conjunctivitis and epidemic kerato-conjunctivitis, etc.

Aetiology and pathogenesis

It is mainly due to the exogenous pathogenic Wind Heat or seasonal epidemic factors that block the meridians, and Qi and Blood stagnation in the eye; or it is due to excessive Fire of the Liver and Gallbladder flaring up along the meridians, together with Qi and Blood stagnation attacking the eye causing the congestion and pain of the eye. In Western medicine, the causes are considered to be bacteria, virus infection or allergy.

Syndrome differentiation

1. **Attacking by exogenous Wind Heat**: Congestion of the eye, burning pain, photophobia, lacrimation, increased clear secretion of the eye, distension and pain of the forehead and head. Red tongue with thin and white coating or thin yellow coating, superficial and rapid pulse.

2. **Excessive toxic Heat**: Congestion of the eye, oedema of the eyelid, photophobia and stabbing pain, increased tears with hot sensation, sticky secretion of the eye. For severe cases, bleeding spots or bleeding patch can be seen on the white part of the eye, the nebula can be seen in the black part of the eye, headache and irritability, thirsty with desire to drink, constipation, red tongue with yellow coating, rapid pulse.

Treatment

Body acupuncture

1. **Principles of treatment**

   To dispel Wind and clear away Heat, reduce the Fire and remove the toxic materials, only apply acupuncture therapy without moxibustion, with reducing technique.

2. **Prescription**

   Select the local points around the eye region. Zanzhu (BL2), Tongziliao (GB1), Hegu (LI4), Taiyang (EX-HN5), Taichong (LR3).

3. **Explanation**

   Zanzhu (BL2) can clear away the Heat from the eye, promote the collaterals and brighten the eyes; Tongziliao (GB1) can reduce the Fire from the Liver and Gallbladder; the Liver opens to the eyes, the Yangming, Shaoyang, Taiyang meridians run through the eye region, Hegu (LI4) can adjust the Qi in the Large Intestine Meridian of Hand-Yangming, and dispel Wind Heat, Taichong (LR3) can promote the Qi from the Liver Meridian of Foot-Jueyin, reduce the Fire and soothe the Liver. These 4 points used together act to 'open the Four Gates' to remove the pathogenic Heat; prick and bleed Taiyang (EX-HN5) in order to reduce the Heat and congestion and relieve the pain.

4. **Modification**

   - *External pathogenic Wind Heat syndrome:* + Fengchi (GB20) and Quchi (LI20) to strengthen the function of dispelling pathogenic Wind.

   - *Syndrome of excessive toxic Heat:* + Dazhui (GV14), Xiaxi (GB43) and Xingjian (LR2) to reduce toxic Heat.

5. **Manipulation**

   Zanzhu (BL2) should be punctured shallowly downward in the direction of Jingming (BL1) or to the lateral side of Sizhukong (TE23). Apply the routine acupuncture method on other points; the bleeding method can be applied for all the points, 1–2 times every day.

Other therapies

1. **Bleeding and cupping**

   Prick Taiyang (EX-HN5) to cause bleeding and follow by cupping method to increase the bleeding. Once every day.

2. **Pricking therapy**

   Prick the reflecting papules between the two scapulars region, or prick Dazhui (GV14) and the point that 0.5 cun lateral to Dazhui (GV14), Taiyang (EX-HN5), Yintang (EX-HN3), or upper eyelid.

3. **Auricular acupuncture**

   Points: Eye, Eye 1, Eye 2, Liver. Use a filiform needle to stimulate the points strongly, retain the needles for 30 minutes; or prick and bleed the tiny veins on the back of the ear.

Notes

1. Acupuncture is a very effective therapy for treating the congestion, swelling and pain of the eye. It can relieve the symptoms immediately and shorten the course of the disease.

2. This disease is a type of commonly seen acute contagious ophthalmic disease and can be epidemic; eye hygiene should be carefully maintained.

3. During the disease, the patient should have plenty of rest and sleep, try to protect the vision, be free from anger and avoid sexual activity. No spicy food.

2. STYE

Brief introduction

Stye refers to the little red scleroma on the edge of the eyelid in the shape of grain, with redness, swelling and pain sensation. It is a common problem of acute suppurative inflammation of the eyelid gland tissue, also known as the hordeolum. It occurs mainly in young people.

Aetiology and pathogenesis

An attack of external pathogenic Wind can produce Heat, then Wind and Heat consume the Body Fluid and result in the stye; or the accumulation of Damp Heat due to over eating spicy food can lead to Qi and Blood stagnation in the skin, meridians and collaterals of the eyelid. Recurrence of this disease is mainly due to retained pathogenic Heat, or a weak constitution and ametropia.

Syndrome differentiation

1. **Attack by external Wind and Heat**: In the early stage, slight itching and pain, slight redness and swelling of the local induration, obvious tenderness. Other symptoms are headache with fever, general malaise; thin yellow tongue coating, superficial and rapid pulse.

2. **Excessive toxic Heat**: Redness and swelling of the eyelid, the induration is large, with burning pain and yellow-white pus spots, congestion of the eye, thirsty with desire to drink, constipation and dark yellow urine, red tongue with yellow or sticky coating, rapid pulse.

3. **Damp Heat due to the Spleen deficiency**: Recurrent stye, but the symptoms are not severe, pale complexion without lustre, with special food preferences, abdominal distension and constipation, red tongue with thin yellow coating, thin and rapid pulse. It is more commonly seen in children.

Treatment
Body acupuncture

1. **Principles of treatment**

   Dispel Wind and clear away Heat, remove the toxic material and the stagnation, only apply acupuncture therapy without moxibustion, with reducing technique.

2. **Prescription**

   Select the local points from the eye region as the main points. Zanzhu (BL2), Taiyang (EX-HN5), Erjian (LR2), Neiting (ST44).

3. **Explanation**

   Zanzhu (BL2) and Taiyang (EX-HN5) are located on the eye area, and they are very good points for clearing away Heat from the eye; Erjian (LI2) and Neiting (ST44) are the Ying-Spring points of the Large Intestine Meridian of Hand-Yangming and the Stomach Meridian of Foot-Yangming. They can strengthen the function of clearing away the Heat and removing the stagnation.

4. **Modification**

- *External Wind Heat syndrome:* + Fengchi (GB20), Hegu (LI4) to dispel the Wind and clear away the Heat.

- *Excessive toxic Heat syndrome:* + Dazhui (GV14), Quchi (LI11) and Xingjian (LR2) to reduce the Heat and remove the toxic material.

- *Syndrome of Damp Heat due to Spleen deficiency:* + Sanyinjiao (SP6), Yinlingquan (SP9) to strengthen the Spleen and drain the Dampness.

- *Stye is on the inner canthus of the upper eyelid:* + Jingming (BL1).

- *Stye is on the lateral canthus:* + Tongziliao (GB1) and Sizhukong (TE23).

- *Stye is between the inner and lateral canthus:* + Yuyao (EX-HN4).

- *Stye is on the lower eyelid:* + Chengqi (ST1) and Sibai (ST2).

5. **Manipulation**

Puncture Zanzhu (BL2) in the direction of Yuyao (EX-HN4) and Sizhukong (TE23), or apply pricking and bleeding methods on these points plus Taiyang (EX-HN5); apply the strong reducing technique or bleeding method on Erjian (LI2) and Neiting (ST44).

Other therapies

1. **Auricular acupuncture**

   Points: Eye, Liver, Spleen and Ear Apex. Stimulate the points strongly with filiform needles, retain the needles for 20 minutes; or bleed the tiny veins on the ear apex or back of the ear.

2. **Bleeding and cupping**

   Prick Dazhui (GV14) with a three-edged needle to cause bleeding, and follow by cupping method.

3. **Pricking therapy**

   Look for the slightly red papules and the sensitive points on both sides of the scapula areas between T1 and T7, prick these points with the three-edged needle, squeeze the liquid or Blood (squeeze 3–5 times); or prick and break the subcutaneous fibre tissues under the papule.

Notes

1. Acupuncture is effective in the treatment of this disease in the early stage, but the patient is advised to drain the pus for the pyopoiesis condition.

2. It is forbidden to squeeze the lesion in the early stage of the pyopoiesis stage of the stye so as to avoid the spread of sepsis.

3. The patient should pay attention to eye hygiene. A light diet is recommended.

3. PTOSIS

Brief introduction

Ptosis is a kind of eye disease in which the eyelid is too weak to lift up, and the narrowed palpebral fissure covers the eyeball partially or completely. This disease can affect the vision. There are two types, congenital and acquired; it may happen to one eye or two eyes. In Western medicine terms, myasthenia gravis, ocular trauma, and oculomotor nerve palsy caused by ptosis may use the similar treatment as a reference.

Aetiology and pathogenesis

Qi is too deficient to lift up the eyelid, Blood is too deficient to nourish the muscles and tendons are the main aetiology and pathogenesis. It may be also due to the congenital weakness, Liver and Kidney deficiency; or due to pathogenic Wind attacking the eyelid and blocking the meridians and collaterals, disharmony between Qi and Blood, the weakness of the muscles and skin; or due to Spleen Qi deficiency in the Middle Burner, or weak and flaccid muscles and tendons because of poor nourishment.

Syndrome differentiation

1. **Pathogenic Wind attacking the collaterals**: Sudden onset of the disease, normally unilateral ptosis of the upper eyelid, in severe cases, the patient is unable to move the eyeball and this will result in external strabismus and double vision. It is often accompanied by the soreness and distension of the eyebrow and forehead, or combined with other muscle paralysis symptoms. Red tongue with thin coating, wiry pulse.

2. **Spleen Qi deficiency**: Slow onset of the disease, the patient is unable to lift the upper eyelid, the eyeball is covered by the eyelid and sight is

affected, the symptoms are better in the morning and worse in the evening, rest and relaxation can make the symptoms better while exertion makes the symptoms worse. Other symptoms are pale complexion, dizziness, loss of appetite, physical weakness, and even dysphagia, pale tongue with thin coating, weak pulse.

3. **Liver and Kidney deficiency**: Many cases start during childhood, with bilateral or unilateral ptosis, the eye cannot be opened for the whole day, the eyebrow is often lifted up, forehead wrinkles are deepened, children may have combined symptoms such as five kinds of maldevelopment and five kinds of flaccidity in infants, pale tongue, white coating, weak pulse.

Treatment
Body acupuncture

1. **Principles of treatment**

   To tonify the Kidney and strengthen the Spleen, nourish Qi and Blood for congenital deficiency and Spleen deficiency syndrome, combine acupuncture and moxibustion with the reinforcing method; dispel Wind and promote the collaterals, harmonize Qi and Blood for the syndrome of external pathogenic Wind attacking the collaterals, and apply acupuncture and moxibustion with even technique.

2. **Prescription**

   Select the points mainly from the eye region. Zanzhu (BL2), Sizhukong (TE23), Yangbai (GB14), Sanyinjiao (SP6).

3. **Explanation**

   Zanzhu (BL2), Sizhukong (TE23) and Yangbai (GB14) are located on the upper part of the eye, and can promote the meridians and collaterals, harmonize the Qi and Blood in the local area in order to lift the eyelid; Sanyinjiao (SP6) is the meeting point of the Spleen, Liver and Kidney Meridians, and it can tonify the Spleen and Kidney, nourish the Blood and tendons, harmonize the Qi and Blood.

4. **Modification**

   * *Congenital deficiency syndrome*: + Taixi (KI3), Mingmen (GV4) and Shenshu (BL23) to tonify the Kidneys.

   * *Spleen Qi deficiency syndrome*: + Zusanli (ST36) and Pishu (BL20) to strengthen the Spleen and Stomach, tonify Qi and Blood.

- *To lift up Yang Qi:* + Baihui (GV20).
- *External Wind attacking the collaterals:* + Hegu (LI4) and Fengchi (GB20) to promote the meridians and collaterals, dispel Wind and relieve the exterior syndromes.

5. **Manipulation**

   Puncture Zanzhu (BL2), Sizhukong (TE23) and Yangbai (GB14) with penetrating method or to the direction of Yuyao (EX-HN4); pay attention to the needling angle and depth when puncturing Fengchi (GB20); moxibustion is applied on Baihui (GV20).

Other therapies

1. **Cutaneous needle**

   Tap Jingming (BL1), Zanzhu (BL2), Meichong (BL3), Yangbai (GB14), Toulinqi (GB15), Muchuang (GB16), inner canthus, or from the upper eyelid to Tongziliao (GB1). Tap the points of the head moderately and the points around the eye region mildly, 15 minutes each treatment, once a day.

2. **Electrostimulation on the nerve stem**

   Select the stimulation points of the supraorbital nerve and facial nerve (the mid-point between supraauricular notch and the lateral corner of the eye). Apply electroacupuncture therapy; connect the cathode to the supraorbital nerve, anode to the facial nerve, current intensity follows patient tolerance. 20 minutes for each treatment, one treatment every other day.

Notes

1. Acupuncture has a certain degree of success in treating this disease.

2. For severe congenital cases, surgery is recommended.

4. TWITCHING OF THE EYELID

Brief introduction

Twitching of the eyelid is characterized by the involuntary tremor of the eyelid mainly due to the disharmony between Qi and Blood. Normally it happens to one side of the eye, and in the case of severe and frequent vibration, the mouth and the cheek muscles can be affected as well. Many cases are induced or aggravated by emotional tension, poor sleep, or vision fatigue, but disappear during sleep.

Aetiology and pathogenesis

Qi and Blood deficiency, poor nourishment of the tendons and muscles, and Blood deficiency producing Wind are the main etiologies and pathogenesis. It can also be due to chronic disease, fatigue, emotional injury affecting Heart and Spleen, causing both Qi and Blood deficiency, poor nourishment of the tendons and muscles; or due to prolonged Liver and Spleen Blood deficiency which produces Wind, and the internal deficient Wind causes the twitching.

Syndrome differentiation

Involuntary frequent eyelid twitching, the mouth and cheek muscles can be involved as well in severe cases. Emotional tension, fatigue, overuse of vision, symptoms are worse with poor sleep but disappear during the sleep.

1. **Heart and Spleen deficiency**: Twitching of the eyelid, sometimes better and sometimes worse, tiredness or nervousness can aggravate the symptoms, irritability, poor memory, or poor appetite and lassitude, pale tongue, thin and weak pulse.

2. **Blood deficiency producing Wind**: A longer duration of the disease, frequent eyelid twitching affecting the mouth and cheek, twitching of the eyebrow, pale complexion without lustre or sallow face, pale lips, dizziness and blurred vision, slightly red tongue, thin coating, wiry and tense pulse.

Treatment
Body acupuncture

1. **Principles of treatment**

    Tonify the Heart and Spleen, nourish the Blood and dispel the Wind, apply both acupuncture and moxibustion for the syndrome of Heart and Spleen deficiency, with reinforcing technique; apply acupuncture mainly for the syndrome of Blood deficiency producing Wind, with even method.

2. **Prescription**

Select the points mainly from the Large Intestine Meridian of Hand-Yangming and the Stomach Meridian of Foot-Yangming in the eye region. Sibai (ST2), Zanzhu (BL2), Sizhukong (TE23), Hegu (LI4), Taichong (LR3), Sanyinjiao (SP6), Zusanli (ST36).

3. **Explanation**

Sibai (ST2), Zanzhu (BL2) and Sizhukong (TE23) are the points around the eyes, and they can promote the Qi and Blood in the eye region to dispel Wind and stop spasm; Hegu (LI4) is the point from the meridian of sufficient Qi and Blood, 'Hegu (LI4) is specially used to treat face and mouth disorders', and it can promote the Qi and Blood of the face; Hegu (LI4) combined with Taichong (LR3) which is of the Liver Meridian of Foot-Jueyin are considered 'the Four Gates', and they can nourish and soothe the Liver, dispel Wind and stop spasm; Sanyinjiao (SP6) and Zusanli (ST36) are the points from the Spleen and Stomach Meridians, and they can tonify the Spleen and Stomach, produce Qi and Blood, and strengthen the acquired foundation.

4. **Modification**
   - *Both Heart and Spleen deficiency syndrome:* + Xinhua (BL15), Pishu (BL20) to strengthen the Spleen and Heart.
   - *Syndrome of Blood deficiency producing Wind:* + Xuehai (SP10) and Ganshu (BL18) to strengthen the function of stopping spasm.
   - *Upper eyelid twitching:* + Jingming (BL1) and Yuyao (EX-HN4).
   - *Lower eyelid twitching:* + Chengqi (ST1) and Quanliao (SI18).

5. **Manipulation**

Penetrating method applied on Zanzhu (BL2) and Sizhukong (BL23), or puncture these 2 points toward Yuyao (EX-HN4); puncture into the infraorbital foramen if puncturing Sibai (ST2); apply the routine acupuncture technique for the rest of the points.

Other therapies

1. **Auricular acupuncture**

   Points: Eye, Ear-Shenmen, Liver, Heart, Spleen. Choose 2–3 points each time, strong stimulation for the frequent and severe twitching of eyelid condition, retain the needles for 30 minutes; or apply embedded needling therapy, or use Vaccaria seeds.

2. **Scalp acupuncture**

   Select MS12 (Upper-Middle Line of Occiput), MS13 (Upper-Lateral Line of Occiput). Apply the routine scalp acupuncture technique.

3. **Point injection**

   Select Yifeng (TE21), Yangbai (GB14), Xiaguan (ST7), Zusanli (ST36). Inject Danshen (丹参 *Radix Salviae Miltiorrhizae*) injection or vitamin B group injection, inject 0.5–1ml in each point.

Notes

1. Acupuncture treatment is certainly effective in treating mild cases of this disease, but has poor efficacy for the chronic type.

2. If the patient has combined symptoms such as secondary facial spasm due to the cranial nerve damage, further checks should be conducted.

5. MYOPIA

Brief introduction

Myopia is referred to as 'short-sightedness', inability to see distant objects as clearly as near objects. In Western medicine, it is one of the ametropia diseases.

Aetiology and pathogenesis

This disease is normally due to congenital deficiency, acquired maldevelopment, mental stress, Heart Yang deficiency, the deficiency of Heart, Liver and Kidneys; or due to holding the reading material at an improper distance while reading, an improper writing posture, poor lighting, the stagnation of the collaterals and the poor nourishment of the eye. It mainly occurs in youth.

Syndrome differentiation

1. **Liver and Kidney deficiency**: Blurred vision, myopsis, dizziness and tinnitus, dream-disturbed sleep, soreness and weakness in the lumbar and knee joints, red tongue, less coating, thin pulse.

2. **Spleen deficiency**: Vision fatigue, preference to have the eyes closed, loss of appetite, abdominal distension and diarrhoea, limb weakness, pale tongue with white coating, weak pulse.

3. **Heart Yang deficiency**: Lassitude, chills and cold limbs, irritability, insomnia and poor memory, pale tongue with thin coating, weak pulse.

Treatment

Body acupuncture

1. **Principles of treatment**

   Tonify the Liver and Kidneys, strengthen the Spleen and nourish the Heart, nourish the Blood and brighten the eyes. Apply acupuncture and moxibustion together, with the reinforcing method.

2. **Prescription**

   Select points mainly from the local eye region and the Stomach Meridian of Foot-Yangming and the Gallbladder Meridian of Foot-Shaoyang. Jingming (BL1), Chengqi (ST1), Sibai (ST2), Taiyang (EX-HN5), Fengchi (GB20), Guangming (GB37).

3. **Explanation**

   Jingming (BL1), Taiyang (EX-HN5), Chengqi (ST1) and Sibai (ST2) are the points located in the eye region, and they are the commonly used points to treat eye diseases. They can promote the meridians and activate the collaterals, tonify Qi and brighten the eyes; Fengchi (GB20) is the meeting point of the Gallbladder Meridian of Foot-Shaoyang and the Yang Link Vessel, Guangming (GB37) is the point of the Gallbladder Meridian of Foot-Shaoyang, and the combination of these 2 points can promote the collaterals, nourish the Liver and brighten the eyes.

4. **Modification**

   - *Syndrome of deficiency of Liver and Kidney*: + Ganshu (BL18), Shenshu (KI23), Taichong (LR3), Taixi (KI3) to tonify the Liver and Kidney, nourish the Essence and brighten the eyes.

- *Spleen and Stomach deficiency syndrome:* + Pishu (BL20), Weishu (BL21), Zusanli (ST36) and Sanyinjiao (SP6) *to tonify the Qi in Middle Burner,* nourish Blood and brighten the eyes.

- *Deficiency of Heart Yang syndrome:* + Xinshu (BL15), Geshu (BL17), Neiguan (PC6) and Shenmen (HT7) to warm up the Heart Yang, calm the Mind and brighten the eyes.

5. **Manipulation**

Jingming (BL1) and Chengqi (ST1) are located in the orbit, puncture these 2 points with thin and fine needles, fix the eyeball and insert the needle gently, do not apply the thrusting and rotating method, press the needle hole for a longer time after withdrawing the needle; pay attention to the needling direction, angle and depth when puncturing Fengchi (GB20) and it is forbidden to puncture deeply and in the upward direction in order to avoid puncturing the great occipital foramen; puncture Guangming (GB37) with the tip of needle upward to lead the needling sensation to go up.

Other therapies

1. **Auricular acupuncture**

Points: Eye, Liver, Kidney, Heart, Ear-Shenmen. Select 2–3 points each time, stimulate the points moderately with filiform needles, retain the needles for 30 minutes with intermittent stimulation, once every other day; or apply the embedded needling technique, or use Vaccaria seeds.

2. **Scalp acupuncture**

Select MS13 (Upper-Lateral Line of Occiput), NS12 (Upper-Middle Line of Occiput). Apply the routine technique of scalp acupuncture. One treatment every day.

3. **Cutaneous needle**

For mild and moderate myopia, tap the points around the eyes and Fengchi (GB20). One treatment every day.

Notes

1. Acupuncture treatment is quite effective for treating mild (less than -3D) and moderate (-3D to -6D) myopia, and has a significant effect for treating pseudo myopia. The younger the patient is, the better the result of treatment

will be. Most patients without optical correction have better results from acupuncture than those with optical correction.

2. When patients get acupuncture treatment, they should also take care of the hygiene condition of the eyes. After using the eyes for a long time, patient should close their eyes for a rest or look at a distant area; keep on doing eye gymnastics regularly and do meridian and acupoint massage.

6. STRABISMUS

Brief introduction

Strabismus is a kind of eye disease in which the patient has skewed eyes while watching the target with both eyes, it is due to pathogenic factors attacking the meridians, disharmony between Qi and Blood, or flaccid and relaxed tendons and muscles because of poor nourishment. The disease is equivalent to the strabismus in Western medicine, mainly referring to paralytic strabismus.

Aetiology and pathogenesis

This disease is mainly due to pathogenic Wind attacking the eye system when the Spleen and Stomach Qi is insufficient and the collaterals are deficient; or due to Kidney Yin deficiency, internal Liver Wind stirring up; or due to trauma, Qi and Blood stagnation, flaccid muscles and tendons.

Syndrome differentiation

1. **Pathogenic Wind attacking the collaterals**: Strabismus, double vision, or combined with ptosis, sudden onset, or with eye pain, headache and fever, red tongue, wiry pulse.

2. **Internal Liver Wind stirring up**: Sudden onset of the disease, strabismus, eye movement disturbance, eye cannot move to the side of the paralyzed muscles, dizziness, tinnitus, red face, irritability, numbness and tremor of the limbs, red tongue, yellow coating, wiry pulse.

3. **Traumatic stasis**: There is a history of trauma, strabismus after head injury, or the ecchymoma of eyelid and white part of the eye, headache, distension of the eye, limitation of eye movement, double vision, or combined with other symptoms such as nausea and vomiting, red tongue, thin coating, wiry pulse.

Treatment

Body acupuncture

1. **Principles of treatment**

   Dispel Wind, calm the Liver Yang, remove the stagnation, promote the collaterals; mainly apply acupuncture therapy, with even method.

2. **Prescription**

   Select points mainly from the Gallbladder Meridian of Foot-Shaoyang. Fengchi (GB20), Hegu (LI4), Taichong (LR3), Taixi (KI3), Guangming (GB37).

3. **Explanation**

   Fengchi (GB20) and Hegu (LI4) are good at dispelling Wind and promoting the collaterals; Taichong (LR3) and Taixi (KI3) are the Yuan-Primary points from the Liver and Kidney Meridians, and can nourish Yin and suppress sthenic Yang, calm the hyperactivity of Liver and dispel the Wind; Guangming (GB37) is the Luo-Connecting point of the Gallbladder Meridian, and used together with Taichong (LR3) these are considered as the combination of the Yuan-Primary point and the Luo-Connecting point, which have the function of clearing away Heat from Liver and Gallbladder, and promoting the collaterals.

4. **Modification**

   - *Paralysis of medial rectus:* + Jingming (BL1), Zanshu (BL2) and Yintang (EX-HN3).

   - *Paralysis of lateral rectus:* + Tongziliao (GB1) and Taiyang (EX-HN5).

   - *Paralysis of inferior rectus:* + Shangming (the mid-point of the superciliary arch, the lower border of the supraorbit), and Zanzhu (BL2).

   - *Paralysis of superior oblique muscle:* + Qiuhaou (EX-HN7) and Sibai (ST2).

   - *Paralysis of the inferior oblique muscle:* + Sizhukong (TE23) and Shangming.

5. **Manipulation**

   Pay attention to the needling direction, angle and depth when needling Fengchi (GB20), it is forbidden to puncture upward deeply so as to avoid puncturing the great occipital foramen; apply very gentle technique when puncturing the points in the orbit, do not thrust or rotate the needle so as to prevent damage to the eyeball or the internal bleeding in the eye.

Other therapies

1. **Electroacupuncture**

   Select the points mainly around the eye region such as Zanzhu (BL2), Sibai (ST2), Tongziliao (GB1) and Taiyang (EX-HN5); other distal points on the limbs can be also combined such as Hegu (LI4), Taichong (LR3), Zusanli (ST36) and Guangming (GB37). After the arrival of Qi, choose disperse-dense wave or intermittent wave, and the electric current intensity follows the patient's tolerance. 20–30 minutes each time, one treatment every other day.

2. **Cutaneous needle**

   Select the acupoints around the eye region and Taiyang (EX-HN5), Fengchi (GB20), with moderate stimulation. Once a day.

Notes

1. Acupuncture is effective in treating strabismus, especially for the patient who has had a short duration of the disease. The long-term effect can be stable if the paralysis of the eye muscle is cured.

2. Many reports show that the adjacent points around the eyes have better effect.

7. COLOUR BLINDNESS

Brief introduction

Colour blindness is a kind of congenital and hereditary defect in the capacity of identifying the colour. The incidence of male patients is much higher than that of females. Colour blindness can be divided into two types: 1) Total colour blindness which is seldom seen in the clinic. 2) Partial colour blindness which is mainly seen as red and green colour blindness.

Aetiology and pathogenesis

Congenital deficiency, Liver and Kidney deficiency, disharmony of Qi and Blood in the collaterals of the eye, poor nourishment of the eye can all lead to the inability to identify the colours.

Syndrome differentiation

The patient normally has no self identified symptoms, and the inability to identify the colour is only discovered at work or in a medical examination. The patient cannot identify the red colour (red colour blindness), or cannot identify the green colour (green colour blindness), or cannot identify either red or green colours (red and green colour blindness).

Treatment

Body acupuncture

1. **Principles of treatment**

   Tonify the Liver and Kidney, regulate and nourish the Qi and Blood, apply acupuncture as the main therapy, with reinforcing technique.

2. **Prescription**

   Select the points mainly from the local eye region, the Gallbladder Meridian of Foot-Shaoyang and the Bladder Meridian of Foot-Taiyang. Jingming (BL1), Tongziliao (GB1), Fengchi (GB20), Ganshu (BL18), Guangming (GB37), Taixi (KI3).

3. **Explanation**

   Jingming (BL2), Tongziliao (GB1) and Fengchi (GB20) are the commonly used points for treating eye diseases; they can promote the collaterals of the eye, nourish the Qi and Blood; Guangming (GB37) is the Luo-Connecting point from the Gallbladder Meridian, especially used to treat eye disease; Ganshu (BL18) and Taixi (KI3) are used together to regulate and tonify the Liver and Kidneys, and produce more Essence and Blood to nourish the eyes.

4. **Modification**

   Use other points around the eye region such as Chengqi (ST1), Zanzhu (BL2), Sizhukong (TE23), Sibai (ST2) alternately with the above-mentioned points. Zusanli (ST36), Fuliu (KI7), Taichong (LR3) and Shenshu (BL23) can be also combined to strengthen the function of reinforcing the Liver and Kidneys, nourishing the eyes.

5. **Manipulation**

   Strictly comply with the procedures of puncturing the acupoints in the eye region, gentle needling technique should be applied to avoid the damage to the eyeball or internal bleeding in the orbit; pay attention to the needling direction, angle and depth when puncturing Fengchi (GB20).

Other therapies

1. **Electroacupuncture**

   Select the points around the orbital region such as Zanzhu (BL2), Sizhukong (TE23), Sibai (ST2), Tongziliao (GB1), Fengchi (GB20), Guangming (GB37), Zusanli (ST36), Taichong (LR3) and Taixi (KI3). Choose 3–5 points each time, and after the arrival of Qi, choose disperse-dense wave, the electric current intensity depends on the tolerance of the patient, 10–20 minutes each time, once every day.

2. **Cutaneous needle**

   Gently tap the points around the eye region such as Jingming (BL1), Chengqi (ST1), Yangbai (GB14), Zanzhu (BL2), Sizhukong (TE23); moderately tap the points such as Fengchi (GB20), Ganshu (BL18), Pishu (BL20), Shenshu (BL23). Once every day.

3. **Auricular acupuncture**

   Points: Anterior Inter-Tragus, Posterior Inter-Tragus, Eye, Liver. Stimulate the points with filiform needles gently; retain the needles with intermittent stimulation for 15–20 minutes. Once every second day.

4. **Point injection**

   Select Fengchi (GB20), Yifeng (TE17), Taiyang (EX-HN5), Ganshu (BL18), Zusanli (ST36). Choose 2–3 points each time, inject 0.5ml of vitamin B_1 or 5% Danggui (当归 *Radix Angelicae Sinensis*) injection, once every second day.

Notes

Experimental results show that the acupuncture points near the eye region can affect the organs sensitive to red and green light, and thus acupuncture treatment is quite effective for colour blindness.

8. GLAUCOMA

Brief introduction

Glaucoma is a syndrome of increased intraocular pressure and visual field defect due to the progressive damage to the nerve fibres. It includes primary glaucoma, secondary glaucoma and congenital glaucoma. According to the width of the camera culi angle, primary glaucoma can be divided into two types: angle-closure glaucoma and open-angle glaucoma. Secondary glaucoma is one of the complications of certain eye diseases or the eye complications of a general disease. It is mainly due to the peripheral anterior synechia causing high intraocular pressure; congenital glaucoma is hereditary eye disease mainly due to the autosomal recessive inheritance. This section mainly introduces the differentiation of syndromes and the treatment of the primary glaucoma.

This disease is equivalent to 'five Wind glaucoma' (Wind in relation to five colours; i.e., blue, green, yellow, dark and black) in Traditional Chinese Medicine. Using Wind to name the disease means that the disease starts dramatically, rapidly and changes fast; it is a very serious condition as well. Five Wind glaucoma symptoms are the symptoms showing in different stages. Blue and dark syndromes are mild cases; green and black are the urgent and severe conditions; yellow is the late stage of these five kinds of glaucoma. In the late stage, it often combines with vitreous opacity, which belongs to the category of 'Internal oculopathy'.

Aetiology and pathogenesis

Liver opens into the eyes, Liver Fire can produce Wind, Liver Yang can transform into the Wind, therefore the occurrence and development of this disease are the most closely related to the Liver. Glaucoma is the pupil system disease and pupil system belongs to the Kidney.

Internal emotional injuries, retention of Dampness and Phlegm in the collaterals, upsurge of the Wind and Fire, hyperactivity of Yang due to Yin deficiency can all lead to the disharmony of Qi and Blood, blockage of the meridians and body pores; Liver overacting on the Spleen can lead to the dysfunction of the Spleen in transporting and transforming, and result in the accumulation of liquid in eyes which is also considered a cause of this disease.

Syndrome differentiation

1. **Sudden upsurge of Liver Yang**: Sudden onset, high intraocular pressure, severe pain of the eye and head, severe ocular hyperemia, sudden decreased vision or loss of vision, hot temper, irritability, yellow urine, constipation. Red tongue, yellow coating, wiry and rapid pulse.

2. **Phlegm and Fire retention**: High intraocular pressure, severe head and eye pain, decreased vision, dizziness, chest fullness sensation, nausea, vomiting, yellow urine, constipation, red tongue, yellow sticky coating, rolling and rapid pulse.

382 of 480 TREATMENT OF DISEASES

3. **Kidney Yang deficiency**: High intraocular pressure, distension and pain of the head and eye, mydriasis, blurred vision, mental fatigue, poor appetite, chills and cold limbs, frequent urination at night, pale tongue, white coating, thin and weak pulse.

4. **Yin deficiency of the Liver and Kidney**: High intraocular pressure, distension and pain of the head and eye, mydriasis, blurred vision, dizziness and tinnitus, dry mouth and dry throat, irritability, insomnia, weakness and soreness in the lumbar and knee joints, red tongue, little coating, thin and rapid pulse.

Treatment

Body acupuncture

1. **Principles of treatment**

   To clear away Heat and reduce the Fire, remove the stagnation and promote the collaterals for the syndromes of sudden upsurge of Liver Yang and the retention of Phlegm and Fire, only use acupuncture therapy without moxibustion, and apply reducing technique; to tonify the Kidneys and Liver to brighten the eyes and stop pain for the syndromes of Kidney Yang deficiency and deficiency of Liver and Kidneys, mainly apply acupuncture therapy, with reinforcing or even method.

2. **Prescription**

   Select points mainly from the eye region. Jingming (BL1), Qiuhou (EX-HN7), Taiyang (EX-HN5), Fengchi (GB20), Taichong (LR3).

3. **Explanation**

   Jingming (BL1), Qiuhou (EX-HN7) and Taiyang (EX-HN5) are the local points in the eye region, and can promote the local Qi movement in the meridians and remove the Heat; Fengchi (GB20) is the point from Gallbladder Meridian of Foot-Shaoyang and has connections with the collaterals or the eyes, and it can reduce the Fire from the Liver and Gallbladder, clear the Mind and the eyes. Taichong (LR3) is the Yuan-Primary point of the Liver Meridian, and can regulate the Qi movement in the eye region and reduce the high intraocular pressure.

4. **Modification**

   - *Sudden upsurge of Liver Yang syndrome*: + Xingjian (LR2) and Xiaxi (GB43) to calm the Liver Yang.

- *Syndrome of retention of Phlegm and Fire:* + Fenglong (ST40) and Dadu (LR1) to resolve the Phlegm and reduce the Fire.

- *Deficiency of Kidney Yang syndrome:* + Mingmen (GV4) and Shenshu (BL23) to warm up the Kidney Yang.

- *Syndrome of Liver and Kidney Yin deficiency:* + Taixi (KI3), Ganshu (BL18) and Sanyinjiao (SP6) to nourish Yin and calm the Yang.

- *Severe pain of the head and eye:* + Yingxiang (LI20) with bleeding method to reduce the acute accumulation of Heat. It can relieve the symptoms rapidly and has very good function in protecting the vision as well.

5. **Manipulation**

Carefully puncture Jingming (BL1) and Qiuhou (EX-HN7) according to the routine needling technique for the points in the eye region, avoid damage to the eyeball and internal bleeding of the eye; pay attention to the needling direction, angle and depth when puncturing Fengchi (GB20); the bleeding technique can be applied on Taiyang (EX-HN5) and Taichong (LR3).

Other therapies

1. **Auricular acupuncture**

Points: Eye, Pressure-reducing point, Ear-Shenmen, Kidney, Adrenal Gland, Endocrine, Liver, Liver Yang 1, Liver Yang 2. Choose 3–5 points each time, stimulate the points strongly with filiform needles, and retain the needles for 4 minutes; or apply the embedded needling method or use of Vaccaria seeds.

2. **Three-edged needle**

If there is severe pain of the head and eye, bleed Yintang (EX-HN3), Neiyingxiang (EX-HN9), Ear Apex, Baihui (GV20), Zanzhu (BL2), Taiyang (EX-HN5) and Taichong (LR3) with a three-edged needle; bleed 1–2 drops of Blood for each point.

3. **Point injection**

Add 654-2 (Anisodamine) in vitamin B_{12} to inject into Ganshu (BL18), Shenshu (BL23), inject 0.5ml in each point, once every other day. It is effective in improving vision and expanding the visual field for the contraction of visual field type of condition.

Notes

1. Acupuncture is quite effective for treating glaucoma. Most of the primary glaucoma can be cured with an early diagnosis and proper treatment. There will be a risk of blindness if the treatment is improper or delayed.

2. Patients should adjust their emotions, try not to get angry and impatient, avoid over-exertion, and not eat spicy and hot food.

9. SUDDEN LOSS OF VISION

Brief introduction

Sudden loss of vision is the condition of internal oculopathy where the patient has acute decreased vision due to Qi stagnation in the collaterals of the retina and eye system (the optic nerve, internal orbital blood vessels and vision path, etc.). It is a commonly seen acute ophthalmology disease. It is equivalent to the different types of ocular fundus disease that impair vision such as central retinal artery occlusion, retinal haemorrhage and acute optic neuritis. The sudden loss of vision results from hysteria, encephalitis, sinusitis, diabetes, all kinds of poisoning, infectious diseases and vitamin deficiency. Unilateral loss of vision is more commonly seen in the clinic.

Aetiology and pathogenesis

This disease is mainly due to sudden anger and fear, and stagnation of Qi and Blood leading to the blockage of the collaterals in the eye system; or it may be due to the pathogenic Heat and hyperactivity of Liver Yang stirring up the Wind, then attacking the eye and impairing the vision; or due to prolonged Qi and Blood stagnation blocking the collaterals of the eye system, leading to deficiency of Qi and Blood, and impairment of vision.

Syndrome differentiation

Sudden loss of the vision of one eye or both eyes, which can sometimes get better and the vision be restored. It is recurrent and eventually the vision cannot be restored. The appearance of the affected eye is normal, but with very complex changes in the fundus such as arterial occlusive disease, paleness or oedema of the optic papilla, or thinning of the retinal artery.

1. **Stagnation of Qi and Blood**: The patient has a sudden loss of vision caused by abnormal emotional changes such as rage or panic, and has combined symptoms such as depressed emotion, dizziness, headache, tinnitus, hypochondriac distension, with a dark purple tongue, thin coating and thin pulse. Ocular fundus examination shows arterial occlusive changes, the optic nerve papilla gets pale and the retinal artery gets thinner.

2. **Qi and Blood deficiency**: Prolonged stagnation, loss of vision, dizziness, fatigue, pale face, or spontaneous sweating, pale tongue with thin coating, thin and weak pulse. Fundus examination shows that the colour of the optic papilla is pale and the retinal oedema is reduced.

3. **Liver-Yang transforming into Wind**: Sudden loss of vision and the vision restored again temporarily, but it is recurrent and the vision will eventually be lost. The combined symptoms include hand and foot numbness, dizziness, tinnitus, flush, irritability, hot temper, red tongue with thin coating and wiry pulse.

Treatment
Body acupuncture

1. **Principles of treatment**

   Activate Qi and Blood circulation, promote the collaterals and remove the stasis for the syndrome of Qi and Blood stagnation; calm the Liver Wind for the syndrome of Liver Yang transforming into Wind, only apply acupuncture therapy without moxibustion, with reducing technique; tonify Qi and Blood, nourish Blood and brighten the eyes for both Qi and Blood deficiency, apply both acupuncture and moxibustion, with the reinforcing method.

2. **Prescription**

   Select the points mainly from the local eye region and Gallbladder Meridian of Foot-Shaoyang. Jingming (BL1), Tongziliao (GB1), Fengchi (GB20), Taichong (LR3), Guangming (GB37).

3. **Explanation**

   Jingming (BL1) and Tongziliao (GB1) are the main points to treat eye diseases; they can activate Blood and promote the collaterals, move the Qi and brighten the eyes; Fengchi (GB20) is the appropriate point from the Gallbladder Meridian and has the function of dispelling Liver Wind, clearing Liver Heat and brightening the eyes; the Liver opens into the eyes, and

Taichong (LR3) is the Yuan-Primary point from the Liver Meridian, so it can clear away the Liver Heat, activate the Blood circulation and brighten the eyes; Guangming (GB37) is the key point of the Gallbladder Meridian of Foot-Shaoyang and is a specific point for treating eye diseases, which when combined with Taichong (LR3) is regarded as the combination of Yuan-Primary point and Luo-Connecting point.

4. **Modification**

   - *Stagnation of Qi and Blood syndrome:* + Hegu (LI4) and Geshu (BL17) to remove Qi and Blood stagnation.

   - *Syndrome of Liver Yang transforming into Wind:* + Xingjian (LR2) and Taixi (KI3) to nourish Yin and calm the hyperactivity Yang.

   - *Both Qi and Blood deficiency syndrome:* + Sanyinjiao (SP6) and Zusanli (ST36) to tonify Qi, nourish Blood and brighten the eyes.

5. **Manipulation**

   Puncture Jingming (BL1) according to the routine needling technique for the acupoints in the eye region, avoid damage to the eyeball or internal eye bleeding; pay attention to the needling direction, angle and depth when puncturing Fengchi (GB20), avoid puncturing the great occipital foramen and damaging the medullary bulb; apply the routine technique for the rest of points.

Other therapies

1. **Auricular acupuncture**

   Points: Liver, Gallbladder, Endocrine; Liver, Gallbladder, Spleen, Stomach; Liver, Ear-Apex, Ear-Shenmen, Adrenal Gland. Shallow needling technique or embedded needling therapy should be applied to one of the sets of points, or bleeding the Ear-Apex.

2. **Point injection**

   Select Tongziliao (GB1), Fengchi (GB20), Hegu (LI4), Waiguan (TE5), Guangming (GB37). Inject vitamin B_1 or B_{12} plus 0.2ml of the 0.5% Procaine Hydrochloride; inject 0.5ml in each point.

Notes

1. Acupuncture is quite effective for treating the sudden loss of vision; the sooner the treatment starts, the better the effect that can be achieved. There is a better effect for the treatment of incomplete infarction than that of the complete infarction. Western medication should be integrated in order to save the vision. Vasodilators such as amyl nitrite inhalation or sublingual nitroglycerin tablets are recommended for the sudden loss of vision due to the central retinal artery occlusion. Corticosteroids can be combined to treat the optic papilla congestion and oedema.

2. The patient should try to avoid panic and restrain anger, which may reduce the incidence of this disease.

10. OPTIC ATROPHY

Brief introduction

Optic atrophy is the extensive damage of the retinal ganglion cells axonal and the atrophic degeneration of the optic nerve. It is characterized by visual dysfunction and the pale optic papilla. It is a serious chronic ocular fundus disease which can impact upon the vision and also has a high risk of causing loss of vision. It is the final result of many internal oculopathies.

Aetiology and pathogenesis

It is mainly due to the congenital deficiency, Liver and Kidney weakness, Blood and Essence deficiency, poor nourishment of the eyes; or due to injury of the eye system that blocks the meridians and collaterals, leading to the poor nourishment of Essence and Blood in the eyes.

Syndrome differentiation

No abnormal appearance of the eyes, significant decrease of the vision or loss of vision. Simultaneous abnormal changes of visual field and vision loss, concentric visual field contraction. Red-green visual field contraction is the most significant symptom. Pupillary response gets slow or disappears due to the differing severity of the optic atrophy.

1. **Liver Qi stagnation**: Abnormal emotions, hot temper and irritability, hypochondriac distension and pain, red tongue, thin coating, wiry pulse.

2. **Qi and Blood stagnation**: There is history of head or eye trauma, headache, dizziness, poor memory, dark tongue colour or with blood spots, hesitant pulse.

3. **Liver and Kidney deficiency**: Dry eyes, dizziness, tinnitus, dry throat and the flush, seminal emission, lumbar soreness, red tongue with thin coating, thin and rapid pulse.

Treatment
Body acupuncture

1. **Principles of treatment**

    Remove the Liver Qi stagnation, activate the Blood circulation and remove the Blood stasis for the syndrome of Liver Qi stagnation and Blood stasis, only apply acupuncture therapy without moxibustion, with the reducing method; tonify the Liver and Kidneys, nourish the Essence and brighten the eyes for the Liver and Kidney deficiency syndrome, mainly apply acupuncture therapy, with reinforcing or even technique.

2. **Prescription**

    Select the points mainly from the local eye region and the Gallbladder Meridian of Foot-Shaoyang. Qiuhou (EX-HN7), Jingming (BL1), Chengqi (ST1), Fengchi (GB20), Guangming (GB37), Taichong (LR3).

3. **Explanation**

    Qiuhou (EX-HN7), Jingming (BL1), Chengqi (ST1) are the local eye points, and can promote the Qi and Blood circulation in the local area; Fengchi (GB20) can promote the collaterals and brighten the eyes; Taichong (LR3) is the Yuan-Primary point of the Liver Meridian, and is used together with Guangming (GB37) which is from the Gallbladder Meridian of Foot-Shaoyang to soothe the Liver Qi, nourish the Liver and brighten the eyes.

4. **Modification**

    *   *Liver Qi stagnation syndrome*: + Xingjian (LR2), Xiaxi (GB43) to soothe Liver Qi and remove the stagnation.
    *   *Syndrome of Qi and Blood stagnation*: + Hegu (LI4) and Geshu (BL17) to remove the stasis and promote the collaterals.
    *   *Liver and Kidney deficiency syndrome*: + Ganshu (BL18), Shenshu (BL23) and Taixi (DI3) to strengthen the Liver and Kidney, nourish the Essence and brighten the eyes.

5. **Manipulation**

Carefully puncture Jingming (BL1), Chengqi (ST1) and Qiuhou (EX-HN7) according to the routine acupuncture technique for the acupoints in the eye region, avoiding damage to the eyeball and internal bleeding of the eye; pay attention to the needling direction, angle and depth when puncturing Fengchi (GB20); the best needling sensation should be transmitted to the eyeball; apply the routine acupuncture technique for the rest of the points.

Other therapies

1. **Cutaneous needle**

Select the orbital region, both sides on T5-T12, Fengchi (GB20), Geshu (BL17), Ganshu (BL18), Danshu (BL19). Tap the eye region gently until the skin turns slightly red. Tap the other points with moderate force. Once every other day.

2. **Scalp acupuncture**

Select MS3 (Lateral Line 2 of Forehead), MS12 (Upper-Middle Line of Occiput), MS13 (Upper-Lateral Line of Occiput). After the arrival of Qi, rotate the needles rapidly with a speed of 200 times per minute, retain the needles for 3–6 hours. Electroacupuncture can be combined while the needles are retained. Once every day.

3. **Auricular acupuncture**

Points: Liver, Kidney, Subcortex, Occiput. Embedded needling technique can be applied, or use of Vaccaria seeds, pressing the points 3–5 times every day.

Notes

1. There is no satisfactory treatment for the optic atrophy. Acupuncture is quite effective for treating this disease for a short term; it can control the progression of the disease, help the recovery, improve the vision and delay the loss of vision.

2. The patient should regulate emotions, avoid anger and over-exertion.

11. PIGMENTARY DEGENERATION OF RETINA

Brief introduction

Pigmentary degeneration of retina is a group of inherited retinal diseases, which are characterized by the progressive damage of retinal photoreceptor and pigment epithelium function. It occurs usually in both eyes and men have a higher incidence than women. If it begins when the patient is young, the disease can get worse with age.

Aetiology and pathogenesis

This disease is mainly due to the congenital deficiency, declined vital Fire, Liver and Kidney deficiency and Essence and Blood deficiency. If the Spleen and Stomach are weak, the clear Yang will not be sent up normally and the vessels will not be well filled with Blood and the Blood will be stagnated. Then the eyes will lose nourishment and this will result in the loss of vision at night and the contraction of the visual field. In the late stage, the patient will lose their vision due to the blockage of the vessels and the poor nourishment of the Qi and Blood.

Syndrome differentiation

Progressive loss of vision, night blindness, visual field contraction, the fundus of pigmented retinopathy. Sometimes the central vision will be affected in the later stages.

1. **Kidney Yang deficiency**: In the early stage, there is poor vision in the darkness and the vision will be restored in the light. The disease gets worse in the long term, and the patient will have contracted visual fields or tunnel vision, and finally lose their vision. The combined symptoms are soreness and weakness of the lumbar and knee joints, pale tongue, deep pulse.

2. **Liver and Kidney Yin deficiency**: The main symptoms are the same as above-mentioned ones, combined with dry eyes, dizziness, tinnitus, insomnia or dream-disturbed sleep, red tongue with little coating, thin and rapid pulse.

3. **Spleen Qi deficiency**: The main symptoms are the same as above-mentioned ones, combined with pale face, poor appetite, lassitude, pale tongue, white coating, weak pulse.

Treatment

Body acupuncture

1. **Principles of treatment**

   Tonify the Liver and Kidney for the syndromes of Kidney Yang deficiency and Spleen Qi deficiency, acupuncture and moxibustion therapies should be combined, with reinforcing technique; nourish Yin and Blood, tonify Essence and brighten the eyes for Liver and Kidney Yin deficiency syndrome.

2. **Prescription**

   Select the points mainly from the eye region and the Gallbladder Meridian of Foot-Shaoyang. Qiuhou (EX-HN7), Jingming (BL1), Yiming (EX-HN14), Fengchi (GB20), Yanglao (SI6), Zusanli (ST36), Taichong (LR3), Guangming (GB37).

3. **Explanation**

   Qiuhou (EX-HN7) and Jingming (BL1) are the points from the eye region, and can promote the Qi and Blood in the local area and brighten the eyes; Yiming (EX-HN14) and Fengchi (GB20) can strengthen the Qi and Blood circulation in the eye region. Yanglao (SI6) is the established point for treating eye diseases. Zusanli (ST36) can activate the Qi and Blood circulation in the eye region as well as tonify the Spleen and Stomach, replenish Qi and brighten the eyes; Taichong (LR3) is the Yuan-Primary point from the Liver Meridian, combined with Guangming (GB37) which is the Luo-Connecting point from the Gallbladder Meridian of Foot-Shaoyang can nourish the Liver and brighten the eyes.

4. **Modification**

   - *Kidney Yang deficiency syndrome:* + Shenshu (BL23), Mingmen (GV4) and Guanyuan (GV4) to warm up the Kidney Yang.

   - *Liver and Kidney deficiency syndrome:* + Shenshu (BL23), Ganshu (BL18) and Taixi (KI3) to tonify the Liver and Kidney.

   - *Spleen Qi deficiency syndrome:* + Pishu (BL20) and Sanyinjiao (SP6) to tonify the Spleen Qi.

   In addition, the points around the eyes such as Zanzhu (BL2), Sizhukong (TE23), Tongziliao (GB1), Chengqi (ST1) and Sibai (ST2) can be used alternatively with the above-mentioned points.

5. **Manipulation**

Carefully puncture Jingming (BL1) and Qiuhou (EX-HN7) according to the routine technique for the acupoints in the eye region, avoiding damage to the eyeball and internal bleeding of the eye; the needling sensation of Yiming (EX-HN14) and Fengchi (GB20) should be transmitted to the eyeball; the routine acupuncture method should be applied for the rest of the points.

Other therapies

1. **Auricular acupuncture**

Points: Eye 1, Eye 2, Liver, Heart, Gallbladder, Kidney. Choose 3 points each time, puncture shallowly with filiform needles, retain the needles for 30 minutes; or apply the embedded needling method, or use of Vaccaria seeds.

2. **Point injection**

Use vitamin B_1, B_{12} or Lingzhi (灵芝 *Ganoderma Lucidum seu Japonicum*) injection, inject the both sides of Ganshu (BL18), Shenshu (BL23) alternately, 0.5ml in each point, once every other day.

Notes

1. The pigmentary degeneration of retina is a hereditary disease; there is no specific treatment for it because the aetiology and pathogenesis are not clear.

2. Genetic consultation is recommended so as to reduce the incidence of this disease.

12. OTITIS MEDIA

Brief introduction

Otitis media can be divided into two types: purulent otitis media and secretory otitis media. The purulent type is a kind of inflammatory disease in the middle ear mucosa and tympanic membrane, which is mainly due to the invasion of suppurative pathogens. It is characterized by suppuration inside the ear, belongs to the 'purulent ear' category in TCM. It can be divided into acute and chronic types according to the duration of the disease. The acute type is more commonly seen in infants and young children who are under the school age. Without immediate or proper treatment, otitis media can be recurrent and easily changes into the chronic type. Secretory otitis media, also known as 'non-suppurative otitis media' has main symptoms such as hearing loss or tinnitus, which belong to the 'the ear distension', 'the ear blockage' category in TCM. The causative factors of this disease are unclear; it occurs throughout the year and is also one of the most common causes of deafness.

Aetiology and pathogenesis

According to Traditional Chinese Medicine, acute suppurative otitis media is mainly due to exogenous pathogenic Wind Heat; or due to excessive Fire from the Liver and Gallbladder flaring up to the ear and steaming the tympanic membrane. If the treatment is improper or delayed, causing the deficiency of Zang Fu organs and the poor nourishment of the ears, then the toxic pathogens will remain in the ears and it will turn into the chronic type. Secretory otitis media is mainly due to exogenous pathogenic Wind Heat going up along the meridians and blocking the Qi in the meridians; or due to improper treatment or recurrence, the prolonged accumulation of pathogens leading to poor circulation of Qi and Blood, retention of the Phlegm and Dampness.

Syndrome differentiation

Acute suppurative otitis media is characterized by symptoms such as ear pain, pus discharge, stuffy ears or tinnitus and hearing loss. The combined general symptoms are high fever, chills, headache, fatigue, etc. Once the perforation of the tympanic membrane occurs, most of the above-mentioned symptoms will be alleviated, but the hearing ability will be reduced and can even result in deafness.

1. **Chronic suppurative otitis media**: With a history of acute disease, the duration of the disease is longer than 3 months, with ear pus discharge and hearing loss.

2. **Acute otitis media**: With a history of upper respiratory tract infection, obstruction of the ear canal, reduced hearing ability, persistent or intermittent low-frequency tinnitus.

3. **Chronic otitis media**: This is characterized by tinnitus and progressive deafness.

4. **Upsurge of Wind Heat**: A sudden onset, stuffy ears or distension and pain of the ear, tinnitus like Wind whistling, reduced hearing ability. Combined symptoms such as headache, fever, dry throat and sore throat. Red tongue, thin yellow coating, superficial and rapid pulse.

5. **Excessive Fire in the Liver and Gallbladder**: Severe drilling pain in the ear, pus discharge. Accompanied by fever, red face, irritability, hot temper, bitter taste in the mouth, dry throat, constipation, and dark yellow urine. Red tongue, thick yellow coating, rolling and rapid pulse, or wiry and rapid pulse.

6. **Accumulation of the Phlegm**: Stuffy ear, tinnitus, reduced hearing ability which gets worse gradually. Pale or purple tongue or with blood spot on it, hesitant and soft, superficial and weak pulse.

7. **Spleen deficiency and retention of Dampness**: Clear and thin pus discharge from the ear and this may last for many years. Combined symptoms are lassitude, thinness, poor appetite, loose stools, pale tongue, white or sticky coating, soft, superficial and weak pulse.

8. **Kidney Yin deficiency**: Dirty, stinking and thick pus discharge in the ear that lasts for many years. Combined symptoms are dizziness, lassitude, weakness and soreness in the lumbar and knee joints. Red or pale tongue, less or no coating, deep and thready pulse.

Treatment
Body acupuncture

1. **Principles of treatment**

   To reduce the Fire, resolve the Phlegm and remove the stagnation for syndromes of upsurge of Wind Heat and excessive Fire in the Liver and Gallbladder, only apply acupuncture therapy without moxibustion, with the reducing method; strengthen the Spleen and drain the Dampness for the syndrome of the Spleen deficiency and the retention of Dampness, apply both acupuncture and moxibustion, with the reinforcing method; nourish Yin and clear away the Heat for the Kidney Yin deficiency syndrome, only apply acupuncture therapy without moxibustion, with even method.

2. **Prescription**

   Select the points mainly from the ear region and the Triple Burner Meridian of Hand-Shaoyang. Ermen (TE21), Tinghui (GB2), Yifeng (TE17), Hegu (LI4), Waiguan (TE5).

3. **Explanation**

The Triple Burner Meridian of the Hand-Shaoyang and the Gallbladder meridian of Foot-Shaoyang run around and enter the ear. Select points around the ears from these two meridians, such as Ermen (TE21), Tinghui (GB2), Yifeng (TE17), as they can promote the Qi from the Shaoyang meridians and open the orifice; Waiguan (TE5) is the Luo-Connecting point from the Triple Burner Meridian of Hand-Shaoyang, and it can harmonize the Shaoyang, reduce the Heat and promote the Qi from Shaoyang meridians; combining with Hegu (LI4) from the Large Intestine Meridian of Hand-Yangming strengthens the function of reducing Heat and removing the toxic material. All the points are used together to activate the Qi movement, clear away the Heat and remove the stagnation.

4. **Modification**

- *Wind and Heat syndrome:* + Dazhui (GV14), Fengchi (GB20) to dispel the Wind and clear away the Heat.

- *Syndrome of excessive Heat in the Liver and Gallbladder:* + Xingjian (LR2) and Xiaxi (GB43) to sooth the Liver and Gallbladder.

- *Phlegm retention syndrome:* + Sanyinjiao (SP6) and Fenglong (ST40) to resolve the Phlegm and remove the stagnation.

- *Syndrome of Spleen deficiency and the retention of Dampness:* + Sanyinjiao (SP6) and Yinlingquan (SP9) to strengthen the Spleen and drain the Dampness.

- *Kidney Yin deficiency syndrome:* + Taixi (KI3) and Shenshu (BL23) to tonify the Kidney and fill the Essence.

- *Headache:* + Taiyang (EX-HN5).

- *To promote the collaterals and relieve the pain:* + Shangxing (GV23).

5. **Manipulation**

Pay attention to the needling angle and direction for the acupoints around the ears, and avoid damage to the tympanic membrane; select the thin needle to puncture Yifeng (TE17) and only apply the rotating technique but not thrusting, in order to avoid damage to the facial nerve; the needling sensation should be transmitted to the bottom of the ear; apply the routine needling technique for the rest of the points. The moxibustion method can be also applied; clean the external auditory canal discharge before applying the moxibustion, and apply moderate moxibustion with moxa stick over the ear points until the local skin turns slightly red and gets warm, 15 minutes each time.

Other therapies

1. **Auricular acupuncture**

   Points: Ear-Apex, Ear-Shenmen, Adrenal Gland, Kidney, Internal Ear, Liver, Gallbladder, External Ear, Endocrine. Select 3–5 points each time, apply acupuncture and retain the needles for 20 minutes.

2. **Point injection**

   Use complex Danshen (丹参 *Radix Salviae Miltiorrhizae*) injection, Danggui (当归 *Radix Angelicae Sinensis*) injection or vitamin B_1, B_{12} injection, select 2–4 points each time, inject 1–2ml in each point, once every other day.

Notes

1. Acupuncture treatment is effective in treating different types of otitis media, particularly in the acute stage. Acupuncture has a very obvious effect in dispelling the Wind, clearing away the Heat, removing the toxic materials and relieving the pain. Acupuncture treatment can promote the absorption and recovery of the perforation due to the suppuration. Try to clear the pus or empyema, and keep the ear drainage canal opened.

2. Physical exercises are recommended for the patient to enhance physical fitness. Prevent and properly treat common cold and chronic diseases of the nose and nasopharynx to avoid acute middle ear disease. During the illness, try to avoid the improper blowing of the nose, so as to avoid water and tears flowing into the ear.

3. Observe the change in the conditions for acute suppurative otitis media and avoid the dangerous development of the disease.

13. TINNITUS, DEAFNESS

Brief introduction

Tinnitus and deafness are auditory disturbances. Tinnitus is characterized by a ringing sound in the ears; the sound is like a cicada or wave, which disturbs the hearing ability. Deafness refers to different degrees of decreased hearing ability or hearing loss. Although these two diseases are different, they occur mainly at the same time. The deafness develops from the tinnitus. Similar treatment can be recommended for a small number of the conditions caused by the maldevelopement of the auditory organs such as congenital deafness, otitis media, auditory nerve disease, deafness induced by high blood pressure and certain forms of drug poisoning.

Aetiology and pathogenesis

Ears are located in an area connected to the Gallbladder Meridian. Abnormal emotional changes can lead to Qi stagnation and transform into the Fire; fury can injure the Liver and make Qi rebel along the meridian and disturb the clear orifices; or an improper diet, retention of Dampness, accumulation of Phlegm transforming into Fire and disturbing the clear orifices can all result in this disease. The constitutional deficiency or Essence deficiency after illness, or excessive sexual activity consuming the Kidney Qi can empty the sea of the marrow and result in deafness; or improper diet and over exertion can injure the Spleen and Stomach, so that there is a lack of the source for producing Qi and Blood, and the deficiency of the meridians, which are unable to nourish the ears, can lead to the occurrence of this disease.

Syndrome differentiation

Tinnitus is manifested as ear ringing with different tones such as a cicada singing, Wind whistling, thunder, waves, car horn or a whistling sound. Many patients with tinnitus also suffer from hearing loss.

The term deafness covers different degrees of decreased hearing ability, or complete hearing loss. Some patients have combined symptoms such as tinnitus, and ear canal obstruction.

1. **External pathogenic Wind**: Starts with cold symptoms which is followed by sudden tinnitus, deafness and the ear distension. Combined with headache, aversion to Wind, fever, dry mouth; red tongue, thin yellow or thin white coating, superficial and rapid pulse.

2. **Liver and Gallbladder Fire**: Sudden onset of tinnitus and deafness and worsened by anger, distension and pain of the ear, red face, bitter taste in mouth and dry throat, irritability, hot temper, constipation; red tongue, yellow coating, wiry and rapid pulse.

3. **Accumulation of Phlegm and Fire**: Ears ringing like a cicada singing, ear obstruction and hearing loss. Combined with dizziness, blurred vision, fullness of the chest, a lot of sputum. Red tongue with yellow sticky coating, rolling and wiry pulse.

4. **Kidney Essence deficiency**: Progressive hearing loss, tinnitus is worse at night. Combined with insomnia, dizziness, soreness and weakness in the lumbar and knee joints, red tongue, less or no coating, wiry and thin or thin and weak pulse.

5. **Spleen and Stomach deficiency**: Tinnitus and deafness aggravated by exertion and alleviated by rest. Combined with lassitude, abdominal

distension, small appetite and loose stools; pale tongue, thin white coating or slightly sticky coating, thin and weak pulse.

Treatment
Body acupuncture

1. **Principles of treatment**

   To dispel Wind and reduce Fire, resolve Phlegm, open the orifices for syndromes of external pathogenic Wind and excessive Fire in the Liver and Gallbladder, only apply acupuncture therapy without moxibustion, with the reducing method; strengthen the Spleen and tonify Qi, tonify the Kidneys and fill the Essence for syndromes of Spleen and Stomach deficiency and Kidney Essence deficiency, apply both acupuncture and moxibustion for Spleen and Stomach deficiency syndrome, with reinforcing technique; apply acupuncture mainly for Kidney Essence deficiency syndrome with even method.

2. **Prescription**

   Select the points mainly from the ear area and the Triple Burner Meridian of Hand-Shaoyang and the Gallbladder Meridian of Foot-Shaoyang. Ermen (TE21), Tinggong (SI19), Tinghui (GB2), Yifeng (TE17), Zhongzhu (TE3), Xiaxi (GB43).

3. **Explanation**

   The Triple Burner Meridian of Hand-Shaoyang and the Gallbladder Meridian of Foot-Shaoyang run through the anterior and posterior areas of the ear. Choose Ermen (TE21) and Tinggong (SI19) to dispel Wind Heat, and clear the stuffy feeling of the ears; they are the key points for treating ear disorders; Yifeng (TE17) and Tinghui (GB2) to soothe the Qi in the Shaoyang meridians; Xiaxi (GB43) to reduce the Fire from the Liver and Gallbladder; Zhongzhu (TE3) to reduce the Fire from the Triple Burner and clear the orifices. All the points are used together to connect the upper and lower part of the body, promote the meridians and collaterals.

4. **Modification**

   - *External pathogenic Wind*: + Fengchi (GB20), Waiguan (TE5) and Hegu (LI4) to dispel Wind and clear away the Heat.
   - *Syndrome of excessive Fire in Liver and Gallbladder*: + Xingjian (LR2), Qiuxu (GB40) and Zulinqi (GB41) to clear away the Fire from the Liver and Gallbladder.

- *Accumulation of Phlegm and Fire syndrome:* + Fenglong (ST40), Neiting (ST44) to break the Phlegm and reduce the Fire.

- *Kidney Essence deficiency syndrome:* + Shenshu (BL23), Taixi (KI3), Guanyuan (CV4) to tonify the Kidney and fill the Essence, nourish the ears.

- *Spleen and Stomach deficiency syndrome:* + Qihai (CV6), Zusanli (ST36) and Pishu (BL20) to tonify the Spleen and Stomach, nourish the ear.

5. **Manipulation**

The needling sensation of the points around the ear should be transmitted to the ear scapha; apply the routine acupuncture technique for the rest of the points; moxibustion or warming needling technique can be added on Qihai (CV6), Zusanli (ST36) and Pishu (BL18). Once every day.

Other therapies

1. **Auricular acupuncture**

Points: Kidney, Liver, Gallbladder, Triple Burner, Internal Ear, External Ear, Subcortex. Choose 3–5 points each time, puncture the points shallowly with filiform needles, retain the needles for 30 minutes; or the use of Vaccaria seeds.

2. **Scalp acupuncture**

Select MS11 (Posterior Temporal Line) bilaterally. Insert filiform needle rapidly to a certain depth and rotate the needle rapidly for about one minute, retain the needles for 30 minutes. Once every other day.

3. **Point injection**

Select Yifeng (TE17), Wangu (GB12), Shenshu (BL23) and Yanglingquan (GB34). Use Danshen (丹参 *Radix Salviae Miltiorrhizae*) injection or vitamin B_{12} injection, inject 0.5–1ml in each point.

Notes

1. Acupuncture treatment is quite effective for treating tinnitus and deafness except in cases of complete deafness caused by the tympanic membrane damage.

2. The causes of tinnitus and deafness are very complicated; a clear diagnosis should be made so as to cooperate with the primary disease treatment.

3. Patients should regulate their life rhythm and their emotions so as to assist the treatment. They should try to avoid over exertion and excessive sexual activity, and keep the ear canal clean.

14. RHINITIS

Brief introduction

Rhinitis refers to the inflammation of the nasal mucous membranes and it is classified into acute, chronic and allergic types. Acute rhinitis is the acute infectious inflammation of the nasal mucous membranes. Chronic rhinitis is the chronic inflammation of the nasal mucous membranes or submucous layers. Allergic rhinitis is the allergic reaction of nasal mucous membranes caused by various specific sensitizers.

Aetiology and pathogenesis

Acute rhinitis may occur in invasion by pathogenic Wind or common cold in TCM. Invasion of external Wind Cold leads to dysfunction of Lung Qi in dispersing, or upward invasion of Wind Heat leads to the dysfunction of the Lungs in clearing and descending. Either of these results in the accumulation of toxic pathogens in the nose. Chronic rhinitis is caused by: 1) obstruction of pathogenic factors, which is due to Qi deficiency of the Lungs and Spleen, or 2) Qi and Blood stagnation obstructing the nose, which is due to long-term presence of toxic pathogens. Allergic rhinitis is because pathogenic Wind Cold invades the nose under conditions of Lung Qi deficiency or disturbance of Lung Qi due to deficiency of the Spleen or Kidneys, which causes obstruction of Body Fluid in the nose.

Syndrome differentiation

The main symptoms of acute rhinitis may include nasal obstruction, nasal discharge, sneezing and hyposmia accompanied by general discomfort. Symptoms of chronic simple rhinitis include intermittent or alternate nasal obstruction, which becomes better in the daytime and worse at night, usually profuse mucous nasal discharge or sometime purulent nasal discharge. While symptoms of chronic hypertrophic rhinitis include continuous nasal obstruction, a small amount of purulent nasal discharge that it is difficult to discharge, pain of the head, low mood and distinct hyposmia. While in chronic atrophic rhinitis, besides nasal obstruction, there is dry nose and throat, epistaxis, dysosmia and a fetid smell in the nose. Symptoms of allergic rhinitis may include paroxysmal itching of the nose, clear nasal discharge, sneezing, and a history of other allergic diseases.

1. **Invasion of external pathogenic Wind**:

   - *Wind Cold*: Severe nasal obstruction, frequent sneezing, profuse and clear nasal discharge, hard and dull nasal voice, accompanied by pain of the head and body, anhidrosis, chills, pale tongue with thin white coating, superficial tense pulse.

   - *Wind Heat*: Paroxysmal Dryness and obstruction of the nose, or itching and Heat sensation of the nose, pain of the head and throat, thirst with desire to drink water, red tongue with white or yellow coating, superficial rapid pulse.

2. **Stagnation of Qi and Blood**: Continuous nasal obstruction, profuse and viscous nasal discharge of white or yellow colour, red tongue or tongue with ecchymosis, wiry, thready and hesitant pulse.

3. **Stagnation of pathogens due to Qi deficiency**: Paroxysmal nasal obstruction, which is better in the day and worse at night; viscous and clear nasal discharge aggravated by cold, dizziness, heaviness of the head, red tongue with thin white coating, retarded pulse.

   - *Lung Qi deficiency*, in addition, itching and distension of the nose, frequent sneezing, nasal obstruction, clear nasal discharge, spontaneous sweating.

   - *Spleen Qi deficiency*, in addition, short breath, low voice, lassitude, disliking to speak, anorexia, abdominal distension, loose stools.

   - *Kidney Qi deficiency*, in addition, cold limbs, soreness and weakness of the lumbar region and knee joint, pale tongue with thin white coating, weak pulse.

Treatment
Body acupuncture

1. **Principles of treatment**

   - *Invasion of Wind Heat*: To eliminate Wind, relieve exterior symptoms, disperse and improve circulation in the nose with acupuncture alone and the reducing method.

   - *Invasion of Wind Cold*: Wind Cold syndrome is treated by acupuncture combined with moxibustion, the reducing method.

   - *Stagnation of Qi and Blood*: To promote flow of Qi, activate Blood circulation, relieve stagnation, and remove obstruction of the nose with acupuncture and the reducing method.

- *Stagnation of pathogens due to Qi deficiency*: To reinforce the Lungs, strengthen the Spleen, benefit the Kidneys, with acupuncture and moxibustion, reinforcing or even method.

2. **Prescription**

Select local points of the nose and points of the Large Intestine Meridian of Hang-Yangming as main points, Yingxiangg (LI20), Bitong (Extra), Yintang (EX-HN3), Hegu (LI4).

3. **Explanation**

Yingxiangg (LI20), located at both sides of the nose, has the effect of improving circulation in the nose and treats various diseases of the nose. Bitong (Extra), located at the root of nose, and Yintang (EX-HN3), superior to the nose, are two important points for rhinitis. Hegu (LI4), the Yuan-Primary point of the Large Intestine Meridian of Hand-Yangming, is effective for various diseases of the head and face.

4. **Modification**
   - *External Wind Cold*: + Lieque (LU7) and Fengchi (GB20) to eliminate Wind and dispel Cold.
   - *External Wind Heat*: + Quchi (LI11) and Waiguan (SJ5) to eliminate Wind and clear Heat.
   - *Stagnation of Qi and Blood*: + Geshu (BL17) and Tongtian (BL7) to activate Blood circulation and remove obstruction of the nose.
   - *Stagnation of pathogens due to Qi deficiency*: + Baihui (DU20) and Feishu (BL13) to reinforce Qi and expel pathogenic factors.
   - *Lung Qi deficiency*: + Feishu (BL13) and Taiyuan (LU9) to reinforce the Lung Qi.
   - *Deficiency of the Spleen Qi*: + Pishu (BL20) and Zusanli (ST36) to strengthen the Middle Burner and reinforce Qi.
   - *Deficiency of the Kidney Qi*: + Mingmen (DU4) and Shenshu (BL23) to reinforce the Kidneys and assist the Lungs.

5. **Manipulation**

Puncture from Yingxiangg (LI20) obliquely and upward toward Bitong (Extra). Apply routine needling techniques to other points. Add moxibustion if it is due to external Wind Cold, or deficiency of the Lungs, Spleen or Kidneys.

Other therapies

1. **Auricular acupuncture**

   Points: External Nose, Internal Nose, Adrenal Gland, Forehead, Lung, Large Intestine, Spleen, Kidney. Choose 3–5 points each time, puncture with fili-form needles and retain for 20–30 minutes. Needle-embedding or Vaccaria seeds may also be applied to the points.

2. **Point injection**

   Apply to Hegu (LI4) and Yingxiangg (LI20) with injections of vitamin B complex, Danshen (丹参 *Radix Salviae Miltiorrhizae*), and Danggui (当归 *Radix Angelicae Sinensis*). Inject 0.2–0.5ml into each point every second day.

3. **Point application**

   Apply to Dazhui (GV14), Feishu (BL13), Gaohuang (BL43), Shenshu (BL23) and Danzhong (CV17). Combine 30g Baijiezi (白芥子 *Semen Sinapis Albae*), 10g Yanhusuo (延胡索 *Rhizoma Corydalis Yanhusuo*), 10g Gansui (甘遂 *Radix Kansui*), 10g Xixin (细辛 *Herba Asari*), 10g Dingxiang (丁香 *Flos Caryophylli*), 10g Baizhi (白芷 *Radix Angelicae Dahuricae*), grind them into powder, mix the powder with pepper water and make it into a paste, spread in a piece of gauze, sprinkle some Rougui powder (肉桂 *Cortex Cinnamomi*), apply to the points and retain for more than 4 hours. Apply once every week for 3 consecutive weeks.

Notes

1. Acupuncture is quite effective for this disease. As for acute rhinitis, there is a marked effect usually after 2 or 3 treatments with especially quick improve-ment to the ventilation of the nose. A longer course is needed for patients with chronic types and the curative effect for chronic simple rhinitis is better than that for chronic hypertrophic rhinitis.

2. Patients in the acute stage should ensure they get proper rest, eat food that is easily digested and rich in nutrition, and drink more boiled warm water to nourish unblocked defecation.

3. In patients with allergic rhinitis, the sensitinogen should be found and contact avoided.

4. Patients should take regular exercise, especially appropriate outdoor exer-cise, which is good for improving resistance.

5. Treat diseases of the upper respiratory tract if there are any.

15. EPISTAXIS

Brief introduction

Epistaxis, or bleeding of the nose, may be seen in many diseases. Local causes include trauma of the nose, inflammation and tumour of the nasal cavity, deflection of the nasal septum, and complications caused by a foreign body in the nasal cavity of children. General causes in the body include hypertension, arteriosclerosis, blood diseases, influenza, haemorrhagic fever, cirrhosis, uraemia, vicarious menstruation, heavy metal or drug poisoning, vitamin deficiency, and malnutrition. In TCM, a small quantity of nosebleed is regarded as epistaxis. Nosebleed during menstruation is called retrograde menstruation.

Aetiology and pathogenesis

Extravasation of Blood due to

1. Lung Heat, Stomach Fire or Liver Fire which impairs the collaterals of the nose to cause extravasation,

2. Qi deficiency which cannot restrict Blood to circulating in the vessels, or

3. Deficiency of Yin causing hyperactivity of Fire which impairs the vessels in the nose.

Syndrome differentiation

Epistaxis usually occurs unilaterally or flows from one side of the nasal cavity to the other side via the nasopharynx. In the case of a small nosebleed, there is just some blood in the nasal discharge, while in a large nosebleed, blood gushes from the nostrils. In patients with considerable blood loss, there is shock in different degrees, such as a pale face, lowering of blood pressure or a feeble pulse.

1. **Stagnation of Heat in the Lung Meridian**: Sudden onset, drop-by-drop nosebleed of a large amount of Blood of red colour, dry nasopharynx, accompanied by cough, yellow sputum, dry mouth and Heat sensation of the body, red tongue, thin white and dry coating, rapid pulse.

2. **Hyperactivity of Fire in the Stomach**: Nosebleed with a large amount of Blood of deep red colour, accompanied by thirst with desire to drink water, redness, swelling or even bleeding of the gingival, constipation, yellow and scanty urine, red tongue, yellow coating, rolling and rapid pulse.

3. **Flare-up of the Liver Fire**: Sudden onset, nosebleed with a large amount of deep red coloured Blood, accompanied by irritability, restlessness,

headache, dizziness, tinnitus, bitter taste in the mouth, pain in the chest and hypochondrium, red face and eyes, red tongue, yellow coating, wiry and rapid pulse.

4. **Hyperactivity of Fire due to Yin deficiency**: Paroxysmal nosebleed in red colour without a large amount of Blood, dry mouth with no desire to drink water, tinnitus, blurred vision, feverish sensation in the chest, palms and soles, deep red tongue, scanty coating, thready and rapid pulse.

5. **Spleen Qi deficiency**: Oozing and dribbling nosebleed of red colour, lustreless face, lassitude, disliking of speaking, dizziness, anorexia, loose stools, pale tongue, thin coating, retard and weak pulse.

Treatment
Body acupuncture

1. **Principles of treatment**

   - *Stagnation of Heat in the Lung Meridian, Hyperactivity of Fire in the Stomach and Flare-up of the Liver Fire*: Clear Heat, purge Fire, cool Blood, stop bleeding with acupuncture alone and the reducing method.

   - *Spleen Qi deficiency*: With both acupuncture and moxibustion, the reinforcing method.

   - *Hyperactivity of Fire due to Yin deficiency*: With acupuncture alone and even method.

2. **Prescription**

   Select local points of the nose and points of the Large Intestine Meridian of Hand-Yangming as main points. Yingxiangg (LI20), Yintang (EX-HN3), Shangxing (GV23), Hegu (LI4).

3. **Explanation**

   Yingxiangg (LI20), located on both sides of the nose, has the effect of improving circulation in the nose and treats various diseases of the nose. Shangxing (GV23) Ashi point in the Governor Vessel and Yintang (EX-HN3) is also along the running course of the Governor Vessel, which descends to pass the nose. Both of these points may clear the Heat in all the Yang meridians and purge the Fire in the nose. Hegu (LI4), Yuan-Primary point of the Large Intestine Meridian of Hand-Yangming, is effective in reducing the Heat of the head and face to stop a nosebleed.

4. **Modification**

- *Stagnation of Heat in the Lung Meridian*: + Shaoshang (LU11) and Chize (LU5) to clear the Heat in the Lungs.

- *Hyperactivity of Fire in the Stomach*: + Neiting (ST44) and Lidui (ST45) to clear Heat and purge Fire.

- *Flare-up of the Liver Fire*: + Taichong (LR3) and Xingjian (LR2) to purge Liver Fire.

- *Hyperactivity of Fire due to Yin Deficiency*: + Taixi (KI3) and Taichong (LR3) to tonify Yin and clear Heat.

- *Spleen Qi deficiency*: + Zusanli (ST36) and Sanyinjiao (SP6) to strengthen the Spleen, benefit Qi and control Blood.

5. **Manipulation**

Puncture from Yingxiang (LI20) toward Bitong (Extra). If there is extreme Fire or Heat, prick Yintang (EX-HN3), Shangxing (GV23) and Lidui (ST45) with a three-edged needle to cause bleeding. Apply routine puncture techniques to other acupoints.

Other therapies

1. **Finger pressure**

Apply finger pressure to Bailao for 2–5 minutes. As for patients with continuous epistaxis due to certain causes such as trauma, nip bilateral Kunlun (BL60) and Taixi (KI3) with thumb and index fingers of both hands together, which is usually effective.

2. **Cutaneous needle**

Select Baihui (GV20), Fengchi (GB20), Yingxiangg (LI20), Neiguan (PC6), nasal area, Jiaji points of C1 to C4 and T3–T10. Tap nasal area, Baihui (GV20), and Yingxiangg (LI20) with gentle pressure, and other points with medium pressure.

3. **Auricular acupuncture**

Points: External Nose, Internal Nose, Adrenal Gland, Ear-Shenmen and Forehead. Puncture with filiform needles and retain for 20–30 minutes, or apply Vaccaria seeds.

Notes

1. Acupuncture and moxibustion have a marked effect on simple epistaxis. After the nosebleed has stopped, primary causes should be explored and treated actively.

2. If there is a large amount of blood during the nosebleed, local haemostasis with packs should be combined with the treatment to avoid ill effects due to a serious haemorrhage.

3. Epistaxis due to blood diseases is contraindicated for acupuncture. Moxibustion or topical application of drug may be applied.

4. The patient should not eat food with pungent, spicy or dry properties.

16. TOOTHACHE

Brief introduction

Toothache refers to the pain of the teeth caused by certain reasons and it is one of the most common symptoms in diseases of the oral cavity. It occurs or worsens as a result of cold, Heat, sour or sweet stimulation. Toothache in this section includes dental caries, pulpitis, apicitis, periodontitis and dental hypersensitivity. It occurs at any age and in any season.

Aetiology and pathogenesis

Causative factors are Stomach Fire, Wind Fire and Kidney Yin deficiency. The Large Intestine Meridian of Hand-Yangming and Stomach Meridian of Foot-Yangming enter the lower and upper teeth respectively, so the accumulated Fire of the Stomach and intestines, overeating of pungent and spicy food, or invasion of external pathogenic Wind Heat may cause Stomach Fire to flare up along the meridian and affect the gingiva and collaterals. The Kidneys dominate the bones. Teeth are the tips of the bones. A weak body due to congenital deficiency or senile feebleness causes Yin deficiency of the Kidneys. In such cases Fire of the deficiency type flares up to the gingiva. Insufficiency of bone marrow results in a lack of nourishment to the teeth, which become loose and painful.

Syndrome differentiation

Toothache occurs or is aggravated by cold, Heat, sour or sweet stimulation, together with swelling, haemorrhage and atrophy of gingiva, loose teeth, dysmasesia, or dental caries.

1. **Invasion of external Wind Fire**: Acute onset, sharp toothache, redness and swelling of gingiva, preferring cold to Heat, fever, thirst, red tongue with thin yellow coating, superficial and rapid pulse;

2. **Hyperactivity of Fire in the Stomach**: Sharp toothache, redness and swelling of gingiva or even pus and blood, pain referred to the cheek, dysmasesia, foul breath, constipation, red tongue with dry yellow coating, surging and rapid pulse;

3. **Flare-up of deficiency Fire**: Intermittent dull toothache that is aggravated in the afternoon or at night, gradually loosening and weak teeth, soreness and weakness in the lumbar region and knees, Heat sensation in the palms, soles and the Heart, red tongue with scanty coating, thready and rapid pulse.

Treatment
Body acupuncture

1. **Principles of treatment**

   - *Invasion of external Wind Fire and hyperactivity of Fire in the Stomach*: To clear Heat, purge Fire, reduce swelling and relieve pain with acupuncture alone and the reducing method.

   - *Flare-up of deficiency Fire*: To nourish Yin, clear Heat, purge Fire and relieve pain with acupuncture alone and even method.

2. **Prescription**

   Select mainly acupoints in the cheek, the Large Intestine Meridian of Hand-Yangming, and the Stomach Meridian of Foot-Yangming. Jiache (ST6), Xiaguan (ST7), Hegu (LI4), Erjian (LI2), Neiting (ST44).

3. **Explanation**

   The Large Intestine Meridian of Hand-Yangming and the Stomach Meridian of Foot-Yangming enter the lower and upper teeth. Stagnation of Heat in Yangming flares up along the meridians and cause toothache. Jiache (ST6), Xiaguan (ST7) may promote flow of Qi in the Large Intestine and Stomach Meridians and relieve pain. Hegu (LI4), Erjian (LI2) and Neiting (ST44) may clear the Fire and Heat in Yangming. These points together may clear Heat, purge Fire, circulate the collaterals and relieve pain.

4. **Modification**

   - *Invasion of external Wind Fire:* + Yifeng (SJ17) and Fengchi (GB20) to disperse Wind and clear Heat.

   - *Hyperactivity of Fire in the Stomach:* + Lidui (ST45) and Quchi (LI11) to purge Fire and relieve pain.

   - *Flare-up of deficiency Fire:* + Taixi (KI3) and Zhaohai (KI6) to nourish Kidney Yin, purge Fire and relieve pain.

   - *Upper toothache:* + Taiyang (EX-HN5), Quanliao (SI18).

   - *Lower toothache:* + Daying (ST5), Chengjiang (CV24).

5. **Manipulation**

   First puncture the local points and then the distal points with strong stimulation and the reducing method. Prick Erjian (LI2) and Neiting (ST44) to cause bleeding. Treat patients who have sharp pain twice per day.

Other therapies

1. **Point application**

   Pound garlic into pulp, apply to bilateral Yangxi (LI5) and remove after a blister appears. This is for toothache due to dental caries.

2. **Auricular acupuncture**

   Points: Mouth, Triple Burner, Maxilla or Mandible, Teeth, Ear-Shenmen, Ear Apex, Stomach, Large Intestine, and Kidney. Choose 3–5 points each time, puncture shallowly with filiform needles and retain for 30 minutes. Prick Ear Apex to cause bleeding. Needle-embedding or Vaccaria seeds may be also applied to these points.

3. **Electroacupuncture**

   Select Jiache (ST6) and Xiaguan (ST7), Hegu (LI4) or Erjian (LI2). After achieving the needling sensation by acupuncture, connect pulse current and stimulate with dense wave for 20–30 minutes.

4. **Point injection**

   Select Jiache (ST6), Xiaguan (ST7), Hegu (LI4) and Yifeng (SJ17). Choose 1–2 points each time and inject 0.5–1ml Antodine into each point.

Notes

1. Acupuncture and moxibustion have marked curative effects on toothache. The pain is alleviated or treated usually after a single treatment, although pain due to dental caries can only be alleviated temporarily.

2. There are many causes of toothache. Treatment should be given according to the different primary causes.

3. The patient should pay attention to hygiene in the oral cavity, and avoid over chewing of hard matter and stimulation of cold, Heat, sour or sweet substances.

4. Be sure to distinguish the toothache from trigeminal neuralgia.

17. SORE THROAT

Brief introduction

Sore throat is characterized by redness, swelling and pain of the throat with discomfort in swallowing. It is seen in acute pharyngitis, tonsillitis, peritonsillar abscess, retropharyngeal abscess, parapharyngeal abscess, and acute laryngitis in the sense of Western medicine.

Aetiology and pathogenesis

Causative factors:

1. Stagnation of pathogenic Wind or Heat, which is due to invasion of external Wind Heat or flaring up of the accumulated Heat of the Lung Meridian and the Stomach Meridian.

2. Flare-up of deficiency Fire to the throat, which is due to deficiency of the Lungs and Kidneys in people with a weak constitution, tiredness or prolonged diseases.

It may be induced by invasion of External Wind Heat or by eating food with pungent, spicy and dry properties. Location of this syndrome is in the throat but the Lungs, Stomach, Liver and Kidneys are also related.

Syndrome differentiation

Main symptoms include acute onset, redness, swelling and pain of the throat with discomfort in swallowing, which is accompanied by symptoms of upper respiratory tract infection such as fever and cough, and general symptoms such as anorexia.

1. **Stagnation of Wind Heat in the Lung**: Redness, swelling and pain in the throat with dry and hot sensation, accompanied by fever, sweating, headache, cough with sputum, and yellow urine, red tongue with thin coating that is white or slightly yellow, superficial rapid pulse.

2. **Hyperactivity of Fire in the Stomach**: Redness, and pain of the throat with a sensation of Heat and obstruction, high fever, thirst with a desire to drink water, headache, yellow and viscous sputum, constipation, yellow and scanty urine, red tongue with yellow coating, rapid forceful pulse.

3. **Hyperactivity of Fire due to Yin deficiency**: Swelling of the throat with pain, the sensation of a foreign object and Dryness, hoarse voice, no desire to drink water, sensation of Heat in the palms, soles and the Heart that is aggravated at night, red tongue with scanty coating, thready rapid pulse.

Treatment

Body acupuncture

1. **Principles of treatment**

   • *Stagnation of Wind Heat in the Lungs and hyperactivity of Fire in the Stomach*: To clear Heat, purge Fire, reduce swelling and relieve pain with acupuncture alone and the reducing method.

   • *Hyperactivity of Fire due to Yin deficiency*: To nourish Yin, suppress hyperactivity of Yang, descend Fire with acupuncture alone and even method.

2. **Prescription**

   Tianrong (SI17), Lieque (LU7), Zhaohai (KI6), Hegu (LI4).

3. **Explanation**

   Tianrong (SI17), in the Small Intestine Meridian of Hand-Taiyang, is located near the throat with marked efficacy in clearing Heat and circulation of the throat. Lieque (LU7), in the Lung Meridian of Hand-Taiyin, is a commonly used point to treat diseases of the Lung system. And Zhaohai (KI6) is in the Kidney Meridian of Foot-Shaoyin. These 2 points form one of the pairs of Eight Confluent Points, which are specially used to treat diseases of the throat. Hegu (LI4), the Yuan-Primary point of the Large Intestine Meridian of Hand-Yangming, is used to clear Heat in the Lungs and Stomach.

4. **Modification**

- *Stagnation of Wind Heat in the Lungs*: + Chize (LU5), Waiguan (TE5) and Shaoshang (LU11) to disperse Wind and clear Heat.

- *Hyperactivity of Fire in the Stomach*: + Neiting (ST44) and Quchi (LI11) to clear pathogenic Heat.

- *Hyperactivity of Fire due to Yin deficiency*: + Taixi (KI3), Yongquan (KI1) and Sanyinjiao (SP6) to nourish Yin and reduce Fire.

- *Severe swelling and pain of the throat*: + Tiantu (CV22) and Ashi points near the laryngeal prominence to reduce swelling and relieve pain.

- *Hoarseness of voice*: + Fuliu (KI7) and Futu (LI18) to nourish throat and promote voice.

- *Constipation*: + Quchi (LI11) and Zhigou (TE6) to clear Heat and promote defecation.

5. **Manipulation**

Apply routine needling techniques to all the points. Tell patients to keep swallowing while manipulating Lieque (LU7) and Zhaohai (KI6). Prick Shaoshang (LU11) to cause bleeding. The treatment is given 1–2 times per day initially, and later once every day or every other day.

Other therapies

1. **Cutaneous needle**

   Select Hegu (LI4), Dazhui (GV14), in the posterior part of the neck, inferior part of the chin, and inferior part of the auricular lobule. If there is fever, add the cubital fossa, hyperthenar and hypothenar eminences. If there is a cough, add bilateral sides of the trachea and Taiyuan (LU9). Use medium or strong stimulation and treat 1–2 times every day.

2. **Three-edged needle**

   Prick Shaoshang (LU11), Shangyang (LI1) and the vein in dorsum of the ear to cause bleeding. The treatment is given once per day.

3. **Burning rush moxibustion**

   Select Quchi (LI11), Hegu (LI4), Chize (LU5), Fengchi (GB20) and Neiting (ST44). Use a piece of Taichong (LR3), immerse it in balm, and clean the balm on the surface of the Taichong (LR3), ignite one end and apply quickly 1–2 times to the points. The treatment is given once per day.

4. **Auricular acupuncture**

- Select Throat, Lung, Neck, Trachea, Kidney, Large Intestine, Helix 1–6. Choose 2–3 points each time, puncture shallowly and retain the needles for 30 minutes. Or apply Vaccaria seeds.

- Select the vein in dorsum of the ear and ear apex, or Helix 3, 4 and 6. Prick to cause bleeding.

- Select Tonsil and Throat. Inject 0.1ml distilled water into each point.

5. **Point injection**

Select Hegu (LI4), Quchi (LI11) and Kongzui (LU6). Choose these points on one side each time and inject 1–2ml of 10% Glucose or injection of Banlangen (板蓝根 *Radix Isatidis*), Yuxingcao (鱼腥草 *Herba Houttuyniae*) and Chaihu (柴胡 *Radix Bupleuri*) into each point. Use the points on bilateral sides alternately and treat once every day.

Notes

1. Acupuncture and moxibustion have a good effect on sore throat. But attention should be paid to treating primary causes in the meantime.

2. Patients should avoid stimulation of harmful gas and eating of spicy and stimulating food. They should try to abstain from smoking and drinking alcohol.

3. Patients should ensure they get enough rest and should reduce or avoid excessive speaking and should be careful not to strain the voice.

4. Patients are advised to do more body exercise in order to strengthen their bodily constitution and to improve the resistance of the body.

18. CHRONIC PHARYNGITIS AND LARYNGITIS

Brief introduction

Chronic pharyngitis refers to chronic diffuse inflammation of the mucous membrane, submucous tissues and lymphatic tissues in the throat with discomfort in the throat as a main symptom. *Chronic laryngitis* refers to chronic inflammation caused by germs in the mucous membrane of the larynx with hoarseness of voice as a main symptom, which is caused by repeated attack of acute pharyngitis or laryngitis after improper treatment, or the chronic inflammation of adjacent tissues.

Aetiology and pathogenesis

Causative factors:

1. Constitutional Yin deficiency of the Lungs and Kidneys causes the flare-up of deficiency Fire, which consumes Yin and Body Fluid.

2. Repeated attack of pharyngitis caused by Wind Heat resulting in stagnation of the remaining pathogens, which consumes Body Fluid and causes malnutrition of the throat.

3. Improper use of the throat in speaking such as shouting, which consumes Qi and Yin, and impairs the collaterals of the throat.

4. Stagnation of Qi, Blood and Phlegm.

Location of this disease is in the throat with the Lung and Kidney involved.

Syndrome differentiation

Chronic pharyngitis and laryngitis are classified into simple, hypertrophic and atrophic types according to degrees of the disease. The main symptom of chronic pharyngitis is discomfort in the throat. There is usually the sensation of a foreign body or a dry sensation in the throat, itching of the throat which induces coughing, viscous sputum that is difficult to expectorate and causes nausea, sometimes mild pain of the throat that is better in the morning and worse at night.

The main symptom of chronic laryngitis is hoarseness of the voice, which is intermittent in the beginning, gradually becoming constant and is worse after much speaking. There is discomfort and a little sticky secretion in the throat.

1. **Lung Yin deficiency**: Dryness and mild pain with an unproductive cough or with little and sticky sputum, flushed cheeks in the afternoon, lassitude, hot palms and soles, irritability, shortness of breath, weakness, red tongue with dry scanty coating, thready rapid pulse.

2. **Kidney Yin deficiency**: Discomfort, Dryness and mild pain in the throat, no desire to drink much water, soreness and weakness in the lumbar region and knee joint, irritability, insomnia, dizziness, blurred vision, red and delicate tongue, thready rapid pulse.

3. **Stagnation of Phlegm and Blood**: Discomfort in the throat, yellow sputum that is difficult to expectorate, nausea, desire to vomit, pain in the throat as if blocked, red tongue or with ecchymosis, yellow thick or sticky coating, thready rolling or thready hesitant pulse.

Treatment

Body acupuncture

1. **Principles of treatment**

   Nourish Yin to reduce Fire, unblock the throat, with acupuncture alone, and even method.

2. **Prescription**

   Select mainly acupoints from the Lung Meridian of Hand-Taiyin, and the Kidney Meridian of Foot-Shaoyin. Tiantu (CV22) Lieque (LU7) Zhaohai (KI7) Yuji (LU10) Tailunxi (KI3).

3. **Explanation**

   Tiantu (CV22) is located near the throat and is effective in unblocking the throat. Lieque (LU7) belongs to the Lung Meridian of Hand-Taiyin, and is a commonly used point to treat diseases of the Lung. Zhaohai (KI7) belongs to the Kidney Meridian of Foot-Shaoyin. In combination these 2 points are one of the pairs of Eight Confluent Points to nourish Yin, moisten the Lungs and unblock the throat. Yuji (LU10) is Ying-Spring point of the Lung Meridian of Hand-Taiyin and clears Lung Heat and unblocks the throat. Taixi (KI3), Yuan-Primary point of the Kidney Meridian of Foot-Shaoyin, nourishes Kidney Yin and reduces deficiency Fire.

4. **Modification**

   - *Lung Yin deficiency*: + Feishu (BL13) to nourish Yin and moisten the Lung.

   - *Kidney Yin deficiency*: + Taiyuan (LU9) to relieve convulsions so that Metal promotes Water to clear deficiency Heat.

   - *Stagnation of Phlegm and Blood*: + Fenglong (ST40), Taichong (LR3) and Sanyinjiao (SP6) to relieve stagnation, resolve Phlegm, and unblock the throat.

5. **Manipulation**

   For Tiantu (CV22), first puncture perpendicularly 0.2–0.3 cun, then erect the handle of needle and insert 1–1.5 cun along the posterior aspect of the sternum. It is not advised to puncture too deeply or obliquely toward the lateral side. Apply routine needling techniques to all the other points. Retain the needles for 20 minutes and tell patient to keep swallowing while the needles are being manipulated.

Other therapies

1. **Cutaneous needle**

   Select the posterior of the neck, inferior of the mandible, Yifeng (TE17), Hegu (LI4) and Dazhui (GV14). Tap with medium pressure 1–2 times every day.

2. **Medicinal moxibustion**

   Select Tiantu (CV22), Shuitu (ST10), Quchi (LI11), Hegu (LI4) and Fengchi (GB20). Ignite the thread, blow out the flame, and press it quickly on the points. Apply once every day on each point.

3. **Auricular acupuncture**

   Points: Throat, Lung, Neck, Trachea, Kidney, Large Intestine, Helix 1–6. Choose 2–3 points each time, puncture shallowly with filiform needles and retain for 30 minutes. Vaccaria seeds may also be applied.

4. **Point injection**

   Select Tiantu (CV22) and Quchi (LI11). Mix 2ml injection of Danggui (当归 *Radix Angelicae Sinensis*) and vitamin B_{12} injection. Inject 0.5–1ml into each point.

Notes

1. Acupuncture and moxibustion are certainly effective in treating the symptoms of this disease, but it is rather difficult to cure it. Patients need to persevere in the treatment.

2. Pay attention to treating the chronic diseases of the throat and its adjacent tissues.

3. During the treatment, tell patients not to eat food of spicy or dry properties and to abstain from smoking and alcohol.

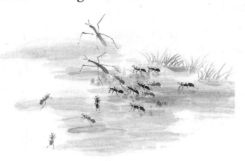

VIII. ACUTE DISEASES

1. HIGH FEVER

Brief introduction

When the temperature in the oral cavity is above 39°C, it is diagnosed as high fever. It is one of the commonly seen acute symptoms in clinic. High fever occurs in many diseases, and is especially common in acute infectious diseases, rheumatism, collagen diseases, some malignant tumours, severe moxibustion, sunstroke and atropine poisoning.

Aetiology and pathogenesis

High fever is seen in febrile diseases of TCM. The six exogenous factors are the main causes, among which Wind Cold, Wind Heat, warm and Heat pathogen, and pestilence are more commonly seen. Endogenous factors may also cause high fever.

Syndrome differentiation

A main symptom is an oral temperature above 39°C, axillary temperature above 39.5°C or temperature above 38.5°C. There is acute onset, short duration, thirst, yellow urine, red tongue, yellow coating, and surging rapid pulse.

1. **Invasion of Wind Cold**: Chills, fever, no sweating, headache, general aching, nasal obstruction with clear nasal discharge, thin white tongue coating, superficial and tense pulse.

2. **Accumulation of Wind Heat**: Fever, sweating, chills and aversion to Wind, headache, nasal obstruction, sore throat, cough with sticky sputum, thirst with preference for cold drinks, deep yellow urine, red tongue with superficial and rapid pulse.

3. **Invasion of Heat to Qi stage**: High fever, sweating, thirst with a desire to drink, deep yellow urine, constipation, abdominal pain which is worse on pressure, red tongue, yellow coating, and surging rapid pulse.

4. **Invasion of Heat to Ying-nutrient and Blood stages**: Fever which is worse at night, mental restlessness, insomnia; in severe cases mental confusion, delirium, faint skin rashes, haematemesis, haematochezia, dry red tongue, and thready rapid pulse.

5. **Severe pestilence**: High fever, irritability, redness, swelling, Heat and pain of the head and face, sore throat which may even have erosion, scarlet skin eruption, red tongue, yellow coating, and rapid pulse.

Treatment

Body acupuncture

1. **Principles of treatment**

   To clear Heat and purge Fire. *Invasion of Heat to Ying-nutrient and Blood stages:* Clear Heat and cool Blood. *Severe pestilence:* Purge Fire and expel toxic material. To apply acupuncture alone with the reducing method.

2. **Prescription**

   Dazhui (GV14), Quchi (LI11), Hegu (LI4), Waiguan (TE5).

3. **Explanation**

   Dazhui (GV14), a point in the Governor Vessel, is a meeting point of various kinds of Yang and is able to dispel the Yang and Heat of the whole body. The Lungs and Large Intestine are externally and internally related, so Quchi (LI11), a point in the Large Intestine Meridian of Hand-Yangming, combines with Hegu (LI4) to disperse Lung Qi, relieve exterior syndrome and clear excess Heat. Waiguan (TE5), a Luo-Connecting point of the Triple Burner Meridian of Hand-Shaoyang and confluent point of the Yin Link Vessel, disperses Qi in the Triple Burner and dispels Wind Heat.

4. **Modification**
   - *Wind Cold:* + Fengchi (GB20) and Fengmen (BL12) to dispel Cold and relieve exterior syndrome.
   - *Wind Heat:* + Chize (LU5), Yuji (LU10) and Shaoshang (LU11) clear Heat, disperse Lung Qi and unblocks the throat.
   - *Heat in Qi stage:* + Neiting (ST44), twelve Jing-Well points and Zhigou (TE6) to promote defecation and reduce Heat.
   - *Heat to Ying-nutrient and Blood stages:* + Quze (PC3), Weizhong (BL40), Shenmen (HT7) and Zhongchong (PC9) clear Heat in Ying-nutrient and cool Blood.
   - *Mental confusion, delirium:* + Shuigou (GV26), Suliao (GV25) and Shixuan (EX-UE11) to wake up Mind and reduce Heat.
   - *Scarlet skin eruption:* + Xuehai (SP10), Geshu (BL17) and Weizhong (BL40) to clear Heat, expel toxic material, cool Blood and stop bleeding.

5. **Manipulation**

   Apply routine needling techniques to all the points with the reducing method and retain the needles for one hour. Manipulate the needles intermittently. Prick Dazhui (GV14), Chize (LU5), Quze (PC3), twelve Jing-Well points,

Weizhong (BL40), Shixuan (EX-UE11) to cause bleeding. Add moxibustion to Fengmen (BL12), Fengchi (GB20), Dazhui (GV14) for Wind Cold. Treat 2–3 times every day.

Other therapies

1. **Auricular acupuncture**

   Points: Ear Apex, Ear-Shenmen, the vein in dorsum of the ear and Adrenal Gland. Prick ear apex and the vein in dorsum of the ear with a three-edged needle to cause bleeding. Puncture the other points shallowly with filiform needles and strong stimulation. Retain for 15–30 minutes.

2. **Point injection**

   Select Quchi (LI11), Fengmen (BL12) and Zusanli (ST36). Each time inject 1–2ml into each point with an injection of Chaihu (柴胡 *Radix Bupleuri*), Yinhuang Zhusheye, Yuxingcao (鱼腥草 *Herba Houttuyniae*), or 5%–10% Glucose. Or inject 0.3–0.5ml vitamin B$_1$ into bilateral Fengchi (GB20). Note: Yinhuang Zhusheye is an injection made from Jinyinhua (金银花 *Flos Lonicerae*) and Huangqin (黄芩 *Radix Scutellarie*).

Notes

1. Acupuncture and moxibustion have quite a good effect in abating fever and can be applied as one of the measures for high fever. But the aetiology should be established so as to give the right treatment based on the aetiology. If the effect of acupuncture and moxibustion is not marked, other methods of treatment should be combined.

2. Patients with high fever and considerable sweating should drink more sugar and salt water, eat easily digested food, and avoid greasy or spicy food, fish and shrimp.

2. SUNSTROKE

Brief introduction

Sunstroke is an acute exogenous febrile disease that may occur in places with high temperatures in the Heat of summer. The main symptoms are high fever, sweating, palpitations, dizziness, irritability, and even coma and convulsions.

Aetiology and pathogenesis

The causative factor is the invasion of summer Heat and Damp in conditions of extreme fatigue from prolonged working or walking under Heat Yang; old and weak people are vulnerable in places without enough ventilation, or if they have had insufficient sleep or food intake. In mild cases, there is a stagnation of pathogens in the body surface, which obstructs Qi. In severe cases, the hyperactivity of summer Heat invades the Pericardium to obstruct the Mind, or consumes Qi and Body Fluid to cause collapse of Qi and Yin.

Syndrome differentiation

There is sudden onset in the Heat of summer or in places with high temperatures, with high fever, hidrosis or anhidrosis, dizziness, irritability, or even coma and convulsions.

1. **Mild type**: Yang syndrome with dizziness, headache, oppressive feeling in the chest, nausea, thirst, hot body, hidrosis, lassitude, weakness, red face and tongue, yellow coating with little moisture, and surging pulse; Yin syndrome with cold body, anhidrosis, lassitude, oppressive feeling in the chest, shortness of breath, anorexia, loose stools, nausea and vomiting, thirst without the desire to drink, pale tongue, thin white coating, surging and retarded pulse.

2. **Severe type**: High fever with hidrosis or anhidrosis, oppressive feeling in the chest, vomiting, dry mouth and lips, or even sudden collapse, loss of consciousness, convulsions of the four limbs, red tongue with little moisture, surging and rapid pulse or superficial and feeble pulse; or hyperactivity of Heat consuming Qi and Yin with pale face, irritability, cold sweating in drops, loss of consciousness, red tongue, scanty coating, thready and feeble pulse.

Treatment

Body acupuncture

1. **Principles of treatment**

   To clear summer Heat, tranquillize the Heart and Mind with mainly acupuncture and the reducing method; Baihui (GV20), Dazhui (GV14), Hegu (LI4), Neiguan (PC6), Quze (PC3).

2. **Prescription**

   Baihui (GV20), Dazhui (GV14), Hegu (LI4), Neiguan (PC6), Quze (PC3).

3. **Explanation**

Baihui (GV20) and Dazhui (GV14) are points in the Governor Vessel, which is a meeting vessel of all Yang, and are used to unblock Yang and clear Heat. Yangming dominates the body surface. Hegu (LI4), the Yuan-Primary point of the Large Intestine Meridian of Hand-Yangming, clears summer Heat and stops convulsions. Neiguan (PC6), the Luo-Connecting point of the Pericardium Meridian of Hand-Jueyin and Confluent point of the Yin Link Vessel, clears the Heart, unblocks the chest, regulates Qi, and harmonizes the Stomach to stop vomiting. Quze (PC3), the He-Sea point of the Pericardium Meridian of Hand-Jueyin, clears Heat in the Ying-nutrient and Blood.

4. **Modification**

- *Dizziness and headache*: + Taiyang (EX-HN5), Touwei (ST8) and Yintang (EX-HN3) to cleat Heat and relieve pain.

- *Vomiting*: + Zhongwan (CV12) and Gongsun (SP4) to harmonizes the Stomach and stop vomiting.

- *Yin syndrome of sunstroke*: + Zusanli (ST36), Guanyuan (CV4) and Qihai (CV6) to harmonizes the Middle Burner and eliminate Damp.

- *Yang syndrome of sunstroke*: + Neiting (ST44) and Xiagu (ST43) to clear Heat in Yangming.

- *Loss of consciousness*: + Renzhong (GV26) and Shixuan (EX-UE11) to clear Heat and wake up the Mind.

- *Convulsions of the four limbs*: + Yanglingquan (GB34) and Taichong (LR3) to eliminate Wind and relieve convulsions.

- *Cold limbs after sweating and feeble pulse*: + Guanyuan (CV4), Qihai (CV6) and Taiyuan (LU9) to benefit Qi, preserve Yin and save Yang from collapse.

5. **Manipulation**

Prick Baihui (GV20), Dazhui (GV14), Taiyang (EX-HN5), Yintang (EX-HN3), Shixuan (EX-UE11), Quze (PC3) and Weizhong (BL40) with a three-edged needle to cause bleeding. Apply routine needling techniques to the other points with the reducing method. For the Yin syndrome of sunstroke, add Zusanli (ST36), Guanyuan (CV4), Qihai (CV6) and Baihui (GV20) with moxibustion or warming needle moxibustion.

Other therapies

1. **Warm compress**

   Choose moderately warm articles such as heated towels, hot water bottles, heated soil or fried salt wrapped in cloth bags. Apply them on the abdomen or Guanyuan (CV4) and Shenque (CV8) for the Yin syndrome of sunstroke in the case of sudden coma.

2. **Auricular acupuncture**

   Points: Ear Apex, Ear-Shenmen, Adrenal Gland, Subcortex, Heart, and Occiput. Puncture shallowly with filiform needle and strong stimulation. Retain for 20 minutes. Prick ear apex to cause bleeding.

Notes

1. Sunstroke is characterized by sudden onset and rapid change. Timely emergency treatment is necessary. First shift the patient from the hot place to a cool place with good ventilation, then give emergency treatment.

2. Acupuncture and moxibustion have a confirmed effect on sunstroke and are convenient. They may be applied as an initial measure for First Aid. In cases where sunstroke seems severe, observe the changes in the patient's state carefully in order to adopt comprehensive measures.

3. To avoid sunstroke, individuals should avoid high temperatures in summer and prepare drinks with cool properties. Keep rooms ventilated and take proper rests alongside work.

3. CONVULSIONS

Brief introduction

Convulsions refers to involuntary muscular contractions. It is seen in Western medicine in high fever, acute intracranial infection, hypertensive encephalopathy, epilepsy, gestational epilepsy, tetanus, intracranial space with occupying lesions, craniocerebral trauma and hyperia.

Aetiology and pathogenesis

This disease relates to the Heart, Liver and Kidneys, and especially to the Liver, which controls the tendons. Extreme Heat stirring up Wind, internal disturbance of Liver Wind or Blood deficiency causing Wind may lead to contraction of the tendons. In addition, invasion of toxic Wind to the interior, incisions, insect or animal stings and bites, insufficiency of Yin and Blood are also important causes of convulsions.

Syndrome differentiation

The main symptoms include involuntary contraction of the four limbs, stiffness and rigidity of the neck, clenched jaws, and opisthotonus. In severe cases there is coma. If it is caused by exogenous toxic Heat, there is sudden onset and short duration. If it is caused by insufficiency of Yin and Blood in prolonged diseases, there is slow onset and long duration.

1. **Extreme Heat stirring up Wind**: Stiffness and rigidity of the neck, or even opisthotonus, high fever, headache, hidrosis, thirst with desire for cold drinks, loss of consciousness, red tongue, yellow coating, surging and rapid pulse.

2. **Internal disturbance of deficiency Wind**: Mild convulsions, low fever, mental restlessness, dry mouth and tongue, lassitude, deep red tongue, scanty coating, thready and rapid pulse. In cases of consumption of Qi and Blood, these symptoms are accompanied by dizziness, blurred vision, sweating, shortness of breath, lassitude weakness, pale tongue, weak pulse. In case of Yin deficiency of the Liver and Kidneys, symptoms are accompanied by soreness and weakness of the lumbar region and knee joints, burning pain in the hypochondrium, low fever in the afternoon, deep red tongue, thready and rapid pulse.

Treatment
Body acupuncture

1. **Principles of treatment**

   To eliminate Wind and relieve convulsions with acupuncture alone, the reducing method for excess and even method for deficiency.

2. **Prescription**

   Mainly select points in the Governor Vessel. Shuiguo (GV26), Dazhui (GV14), Jinsuo (GV8) Hegu (LI4), Taichong (LR3), Yanglingquan (GB34).

3. **Explanation**

The Governor Vessel governs all Yang. Shuiguo (GV26), Dazhui (GV14) and Jinsuo (GV8) are used to eliminate Wind, unblock the collaterals and relieve convulsions. Hegu (LI4), the Yuan-Primary point of the Large Intestine Meridian of Hand-Yangming, dispels Wind. The Liver controls the tendons. Taichong (LR3), the Yuan-Primary point of the Liver Meridian, subdues the Liver, eliminates Wind and stops convulsions. The combination of bilateral Taichong (LR3) and Hegu (LI4) are called 'the Four Gates' points, and are an important pair to relieve convulsions, tranquillize the Mind, subdue the Liver and eliminate Wind. Yanglingquan (GB34), the He-Sea point of the Gallbladder Meridian and Confluent Point of Tendon, subdues the Liver, eliminates Wind and stops convulsions.

4. **Modification**

- *Accumulation of toxic Heat*: + Laogong (PC8), Quchi (LI11) and Zhongchong (PC9) to clear Heat and relieve convulsions.
- *Hyperactivity of pathogenic Wind*: + Fengfu (GV16) and Fengmen (BL12) to dispel Wind and relieve convulsions.
- *Deficiency of Qi and Blood*: + Geshu (BL17), Zusanli (ST36) and Qihai (CV6) to tonify Qi and Blood.
- *Yin deficiency of the Liver and Kidneys*: + Shenshu (BL23), Ganshu (BL18), Sanyinjiao (SP6) and Taixi (KI3) to tonify the Liver and Kidneys.
- *Loss of consciousness*: + Baihui (GV20) and Yongquan (KI1) to wake up the Mind and regain consciousness.

5. **Manipulation**

Apply strong stimulation and the reducing method to extreme Heat stirring up Wind. Prick Zhongchong (PC9) to cause bleeding. Do not puncture Fengfu (GV16) and Fengmen (BL12) deeply so as to avoid injuring the spinal cord and apex of the Lung. Apply medium stimulation and even method to internal disturbance of deficiency Wind. For patients with frequent convulsions, treat 2–3 times every day.

Other therapies

1. **Auricular acupuncture**

Points: Liver, Kidney, Subcortex, Ear-Shenmen, and Brain Stem. Apply strong stimulation with filiform needle and retain for 30–60 minutes. Or apply needle-embedding for several hours.

2. **Electroacupuncture**

Select Hegu (LI4), Taichong (LR3) and Yanglingquan (GB34). When there is the arrival of Qi, connect the points to electroacupuncture stimulator with continuous wave and quick frequency for 20–30 minutes.

3. **Point injection**

Select Hegu (LI4), Taichong (LR3), Taiyang (EX-HN5) Yanglingquan (GB34), Quchi (LI11) and Sanyinjiao (SP6). Choose 2–3 points each time and inject 0.5–1ml into each point with injection of Dilong (地龙 *Pheretima*).

Notes

1. For patients who appear to be about to have a convulsion, timely treatment should be given. Acupuncture is very effective for this condition. But after the convulsions have stopped, treatment should be given aimed at the aetiology.

2. When puncturing during convulsions or if there is attack of convulsions during puncturing, pay attention to the prevention of stuck, bent or broken needles.

4. SYNCOPE
Brief introduction

The main symptoms of syncope include sudden loss of consciousness, pale face, sweating and cold limbs. In mild cases, it is of short duration with no sequela after patients regain consciousness. In severe cases, it is of long duration and death may even occur after syncope. It corresponds to fainting, shock, sunstroke, hypoglycaemia, hysteria, etc. in Western medicine.

Aetiology and pathogenesis

The aetiology includes external pathogenic Cold or summer Heat, pestilence, emotional factors, food intake, overstrain and stress. The pathogenesis includes imbalance of Yin-Yang, and the adverse flow of Qi and Blood. The affected part is the brain with all the Zang Fu organs involved, and it is especially closely related to the Liver.

Syndrome differentiation

The main symptoms include sudden loss of consciousness and cold limbs, accompanied by coarse breathing, rattling, trismus, pale face, spontaneous sweating. There is sudden onset and it has a short duration.

1. **Qi syncope**: Manifestations of the excess syndrome are onset after sudden anger, sudden loss of consciousness, clenched jaws and fists, coarse breathing, cold limbs, superficial pulse or deep and string-taut pulse. Manifestations of the deficiency syndrome are weak body, loss of consciousness after tiredness, fear or fright, dizziness, pale face, feeble breathing, sweating, cold limbs, pale tongue, deep and feeble pulse.

2. **Blood syncope**: Manifestations of the excess syndrome are onset after sudden anger, sudden loss of consciousness, trismus, red face, purple lips, red tongue, deep and string-taut pulse. Manifestations of the deficiency syndrome are sudden loss of consciousness after much blood loss, pale face, lustreless lips, tremor of the four limbs, mouth agape, spontaneous sweating, cold skin, feeble breathing, pale tongue, thready and weak pulse.

3. **Phlegm syncope**: Constitutional Phlegm and Damp, sudden syncope after anger, rattling in the throat or vomiting of foams, coarse breathing, white sticky coating, deep and rolling pulse.

4. **Cold syncope**: Direct invasion of pathogenic Cold to the interior caused by insufficiency of congenital Yang with cold body and limbs, mental confusion, diarrhoea with undigested food in the stools, scanty urine or enuresis, pale tongue, white coating; deep and thready pulse.

5. **Heat syncope**: Initially there is feverishness of the body, headache, a burning sensation in the chest and abdomen, thirst with the desire to drink water, constipation with offensive smelling stools, irritability. Then there is loss of consciousness, cold extremities, and rapid pulse.

Treatment
Body acupuncture

1. **Principles of treatment**

   To wake up the Mind and regain consciousness, with acupuncture alone and the reducing method for excess syndrome, with acupuncture and more moxibustion, the reinforcing method for deficiency syndrome.

2. **Prescription**

   Mainly select points in the Governor Vessel, Shuigou (GV26), Baihui (GV20), Neiguan (PC6).

3. **Explanation**

   The location of this disease is in the brain. The Governor Vessel connects the brain and governs all Yang. Shuigou (GV26) and Baihui (GV20), points in the Governor Vessel, wake up the Mind and regain consciousness. Neiguan (PC6), the Luo-Connecting point of the Pericardium Meridian, wakes up the Mind.

4. **Modification**

   - *Excess syndrome in Qi syncope:* + Taichong (LR3) and Xingjian (LR2) to disperse the Liver Qi.

   - *Deficiency syndrome in Qi syncope:* + Zusanli (ST36) and Qihai (CV6) to benefit Qi and ascend Yang.

   - *Excess syndrome in Blood syncope:* + Xingjian (LR2) to descend Liver Fire or Yongquan (KI1) to descend Blood.

   - *Deficiency syndrome in Blood syncope:* + Guanyuan (CV4), Geshu (BL17) and Zusanli (ST36) to benefit Yin and save collapse.

   - *Phlegm syncope:* + Zhongwan (CV12), Fenglong (ST40) to wake up the Mind and resolve Phlegm.

   - *Heat syncope:* + Dazhui (GV14), Zhongchong (PC9) to reduce Heat.

   - *Cold syncope:* + Moxibustion on Shenque (CV8), Guanyuan (CV4) to warm Yang and dispel Cold trismus: Jiache (ST6), Xiaguan (ST7) and Hegu (LI4).

5. **Manipulation**

   - *Excess or Heat syndrome:* Apply strong stimulation and the reducing method to all the points. Prick Baihui (GV20) to cause bleeding. Puncture from Hegu (LI4) toward Houxi (SI3) and Taichong (LR3) toward Yongquan (KI1), or puncture Baihui (GV20), bilateral Laogong (PC8) and Yongquan (KI1) together.

   - *Deficiency or Cold syndrome:* Apply acupuncture and more moxibustion, the reinforcing method. Apply indirect-moxibustion with salt insulation on Shenque (CV8) and Guanyuan (CV4), or on Baihui (GV20), bilateral Laogong (PC8) and Yongquan (KI1).

Other therapies

1. **Finger pressure**

   Nip Shuigou (GV26), Hegu (LI4) and Neiguan (PC6) with the thumb with heavy pressure until the patient appears to react to the pain or regains consciousness.

2. **Three-edged needle**

   For excess syndrome, select Dazhui (GV14), Baihui (GV20), Taiyang (EX-HN5), Weizhong (BL40) and Shixuan (EX-UE11). Prick these points to cause bleeding.

3. **Auricular acupuncture**

   Points: Heart, Brain, Ear-Shenmen, Inferior Apex of Tragus, Inferior Foot of Helix. Choose 2–3 points each time. Apply strong stimulation for the excess syndrome and weak stimulation for the deficiency syndrome. Retain the needles for 30 minutes. Rotate and twirl once every 5 minutes.

4. **Electroacupuncture**

   For the excess syndrome, connect the points to electroacupuncture stimulator after the needling sensation has been achieved with continuous wave until the patients regain consciousness.

Notes

1. Syncope is a common severe disease in clinic and timely treatment should be given. Acupuncture and moxibustion have an immediate effect in some cases of syncope. But afterward the immediate attack, treatment should be given to the primary causes.

2. Syncope and collapse can be converted into each other. Syncope is usually the forerunner of collapse and collapse is the further development of syncope. During treatment, attention should be paid to preventing a sudden change of the state.

5. COLLAPSE

Brief introduction

Collapse is a common severe disease in clinic. The main symptoms include pale face, dribbling of cold sweat, cold limbs, irritability or coma, incontinence of urine and stools, feeble pulse. It usually corresponds to shock from various causes in Western medicine.

Aetiology and pathogenesis

It is classified into collapse of Yin or Yang in TCM, which indicates severe consumption of Yin, Yang, Qi and Blood, and anti-pathogenic Qi.

The pathogenesis is that Yin fails to preserve Yang and Yang fails to consolidate Yin, leading to separation of Yin and Yang.

Syndrome differentiation

There is a pale face, cold limbs, dribbling of sweat, incontinence of urine and stools or scanty urine, irritability or even coma, decreasing blood pressure, feeble pulse or disorder of pulse.

1. **Collapse of Yin**: Accompanied by fever, irritability, palpitations, hidrosis, thirst with desire to drink, scanty and yellow urine, Dryness and redness of the lips and tongue, no coating, thready and rapid or deep and feeble pulse.

2. **Collapse of Yang**: Feeble breathing, dark face, cyanosis of mouth and lips, scanty urine or incontinence of urine, diarrhoea with undigested food in the stools, pale tongue, white coating, feeble pulse.

3. **Collapse of Yin and Yang**: A severe case of collapse with loss of consciousness, eyes open, mouth agape, platycoria, rattling in the throat, shallow breathing, hidrosis, relaxed hands, cold body, incontinence of urine and stools, feeble pulse.

Treatment
Body acupuncture

1. **Principles of treatment**

   To save Yang from collapse, regulate Yin and Yang, with acupuncture and more moxibustion, the reinforcing method.

2. **Prescription**

   Select points in the Conception Vessel and the Governor Vessel. Shenque (CV8), Guanyuan (CV4) Suliao (GV25), Baihui (GV20).

3. **Explanation**

The Conception Vessel controls Yin of the whole body and the Governor Vessel governs Yang of the whole body. Selection of points in these two vessels may regulate Yin and Yang to prevent their separation from each other. Shenque (CV8) and Guanyuan (CV4) are related to primary Qi. Moxibustion may save Yang from collapse. Suliao (GV25) wakes up the Mind and excites Yang Qi. Moxibustion on Baihui (GV20), a meeting point of all Yang, tonifies and ascends Yang Qi to prevent collapse.

4. **Modification**

- *Collapse of Yin*: + Taixi (KI3) and Yongquan (KI1) to nourish Yin and save collapse.

- *Collapse of Yang*: + Qihai (CV6) and Zusanli (ST36) to benefit Qi and save collapse.

- *Hidrosis*: + Hegu (LI4) and Fuliu (KI7) to arrest sweating and save collapse.

- *Cold limbs after sweating*: + Dazhui (GV14), Mingmen (GV4) and Sanyinjiao (SP6) to warm Yang.

- *Incontinence of urine and stools*: + Huiyin (CV1) and Shenshu (BL23) to strengthen the Kidneys and arrest the discharges.

5. **Manipulation**

Apply strong stimulation and the reducing method to Suliao (GV25). Mainly apply moxibustion to Guanyuan (CV4), Qihai (CV6), Dazhui (GV14) and Baihui (GV20). Use indirect moxibustion with salt insulation on Shenque (CV8). Apply the reinforcing method or warming needle moxibustion on the other points.

Other therapies

1. **Finger pressure**

Select Suliao (GV25), Neiguan (PC6) and Shenmen (HT7). Press with thumb for 1–3 minutes.

2. **Moxibustion**

Select Shenque (CV8), Guanyuan (CV4), Zusanli (ST36) and Baihui (GV20). Use a moxa stick above the points for 30–60 minutes. Or apply more moxibustion to Baihui (GV20), bilateral Laogong (PC8) and Yongquan (KI1) until the patient regains consciousness.

3. **Auricular acupuncture**

   Select Adrenal Gland, Heart, Ear-Shenmen (HT7), Subcortex, Occiput. Apply gentle stimulation and retain the needles for 1–2 hours.

4. **Point injection**

   Select Guanyuan (CV4) and Zusanli (ST36). Inject 1ml of Shenmai Zhusheye or Shenfu Zhusheye into each point. Note: Shenmai Zhusheye is an injection made from Ginseng and *Radix Ophiopagonis*. Shenfu Zhusheye is made from Ginseng and prepared Aconite.

Notes

1. Collapse is a severe disease. Timely emergency treatment should be given. Acupuncture and moxibustion, especially moxibustion, are quite effective in treating this disease. But treatment should be given to the primary diseases combined with First Aid in Western medicine if necessary.

2. Intensive care should be given to patients with severe collapse. Observe carefully changes in their condition and record pulse, body temperature, respiration, blood pressure.

6. ANGINA PECTORIS

Brief introduction

Angina Pectoris is a major clinical manifestation of coronary heart disease. Main symptoms include severe pain in the precordial region of the left chest, palpitations, oppressive feeling in the chest and shortness of breath. It is a comprehensive syndrome caused by severe and temporary ischaemia and anoxia of the cardiac muscle as a result of insufficient blood supply from the coronary artery. It usually occurs in males over 40 years old. Common inducing factors are fatigue, emotional stimulation, overeating, invasion of external Cold, cloudy or rainy weather, acute circulation failure.

Aetiology and pathogenesis

Causative factors:

1. Deficiency of anti-pathogenic Qi and invasion of external Cold causing obstruction of Yang in the chest.

2. Liver Qi stagnation causing stagnation of Qi and Blood.

3. Irregular food intake causing Phlegm, which obstructs the Heart, resulting in pain.

4. Lack of physical exercise, overstrain, or Kidney deficiency in senile people consuming Ying-nutrient and Blood, in which case obstruction of Heart Yang fails to nourish the vessels of the Heart.

The location of the disease is in the Heart with the Liver, Spleen and Kidneys involved. The basic pathogenesis is imbalance of Qi and Blood, and obstruction of the vessels in the Heart.

Syndrome differentiation

Main symptoms include sudden oppressive feeling in the chest, severe pain in the precordial region of the left chest, palpitations, shortness of breath, referred pain to the back. It occurs after exposure to cold, food intake, tiredness or emotional disturbance with duration of 1–5 minutes and refers to the left neck, shoulder and arm. Accompanying symptoms are hidrosis, oppressive and suffocating feeling in the chest, fear, dyspnoea, pale face, and cold limbs with dark purple tongue, string-taut and hesitant pulse.

1. **Stagnation of Qi and Blood**: Stabbing pain in the chest with fixed location, asthmatic breathing, discomfort lying down, palpitations, hidrosis, dark face, cyanosis of lips and nails, dark purple tongue or tongue with ecchymosis, hesitant, knotted or intermittent pulse.

2. **Stagnation of pathogenic Cold**: Chest pain radiating to the back, asthmatic breathing and discomfort lying down that becomes worse when cold and better when warm, pale face, cold limbs, slightly red tongue, thin white coating, string-taut and tense or deep and slow pulse.

3. **Obstruction of Phlegm and Damp**: Oppressive feeling and stuffiness in the chest, or chest pain radiating to the back, asthmatic breathing, discomfort lying down, rattling in the throat, being overweight, heaviness of the body, sticky and tasteless mouth, sticky tongue coating, deep and rolling pulse.

4. **Declining of Yang Qi**: Oppressive feeling in the chest, shortness of breath, or even chest pain radiating to the back, palpitations, hidrosis, discomfort lying down, soreness and weakness of lumbar region, insomnia, pale face, cyanosis or pale colour of lips and nails, slightly red tongue with teeth mark, thin moistened or white glossy coating, deep thready or deep feeble pulse.

Treatment

Body acupuncture

1. **Principles of treatment**

   To promote flow of Qi, unblock Yang and relieve pain, with acupuncture and moxibustion, the reducing method; the reinforcing method for deficiency.

2. **Prescription**

   To select mainly points in the Pericardium Meridian of Hand-Jueyin and related Front-Mu points; Neiguan (PC6) Ximen (PC4) Yinxi (HT6) Juque (CV14) Danzhong (CV17).

3. **Explanation**

   Neiguan (PC6), a point in the Pericardium Meridian of Hand-Jueyin and Confluent Point of the Yin Link Vessel, unblocks the chest, regulates Qi, activates Blood and unblocks the collaterals. Ximen (PC4) and Yinxi (HT6) are respectively Xi-Cleft points of the Pericardium Meridian of Hand-Jueyin and the Heart Meridian of Hand-Shaoyin. They promote the flow of Qi, unblock the collaterals, relieve stagnation and relieve pain. Juque (CV14) and Danzhong (CV17) are respectively Front-Mu points of the Heart and Pericardium. They activate Blood, relieve stagnation, and tranquillize the Heart and Mind. Besides, Danzhong (CV17), an Influential point of Qi, promotes the flow of Qi, unblocks Yang, relieves stagnation and alleviates pain.

4. **Modification**

   - *Stagnation of Qi and Blood*: + Taichong (LR3) and Geshu (BL17) to promote flow of Qi and relieve stagnation.

   - *Stagnation of pathogenic Cold*: + Moxibustion on Shenque (CV8) and Guanyuan (CV4) to dispel Cold and relieve pain.

   - *Obstruction of Phlegm and Damp*: + Zhongwan (CV12) and Fenglong (ST40) to resolve Phlegm and eliminate Damp.

   - *Yang deficiency of the Heart and Kidney*: + Xinshu (BL15), Jueyinshu (BL14) and Shenshu (BL23) to warm and reinforce the Heart and Kidneys.

   - *Tachypnoea*: + Tiantu (CV22) and Kongzui (LU6) to regulate Qi and relieve pain.

5. **Manipulation**

   Pay attention to the direction, angle and depth of Juque (CV14) and Back-Shu points. Usually the reducing method is applied. For patients with deficiency, apply the reinforcing method, or more moxibustion to warm and unblock collaterals.

Treat twice every day if it is during an attack, or once every 2 days if during intermission.

Other therapies

1. **Finger pressure**

   Select Xinshu (BL15), Jueyinshu (BL14), Geshu (BL17), Neiguan (PC6), Jianshi (PC5), Sanyinjiao (SP6), Ashi points in the precordial region. Choose 3–4 points each time and press with the thumb for 3–5 minutes on each point.

2. **Point application**

   Take some Qili San (Anti-bruise Powder) and spread it on Shexiang (麝香 *Moschus*) Hugu (虎骨 *Os Tigris*), Gao to apply on Tanzhong (CV17), Juque (CV14), Xinshu (BL15), and Jueyinshu (BL14). This treatment is given once every 2 days.

3. **Auricular acupuncture**

   Points: Heart, Ear-Shenmen, Sympathetic Nerve, Subcortex, and Endocrine. Choose 3–4 points each time with strong stimulation and retain for 30–60 minutes.

4. **Electroacupuncture**

   Select Yinxi (HT6), Ximen (PC4), Tanzhong (CV17) and Juque (CV14). Stimulate with continuous wave and quick frequency for 20–30 minutes.

5. **Point injection**

   Select Ximen (PC4), Xinshu (BL15), Jueyinshu (BL14), Zusanli (ST36). Choose 2 points each time. Inject 2ml Fufang Danshen Zhusheye or Chuanxiongqin Zhusheye into each point. The treatment is given once every day.

Notes

1. Angina pectoris is a severe disease. Timely and careful treatment should be given. Acupuncture and moxibustion have a confirmed effect on alleviating angina pectoris or arrythmia, and are quite effective for myocardial infarction.

2. Continuation of treatment during intermission helps to reduce attacks of angina pectoris, alleviate symptoms and improve electrocardiogram results.

3. Tell patients to pay attention to diet and lifestyle. They should follow a light diet without greasy food, and abstain from smoking and alcohol.

4. Patients should keep in a good mood. They should not become too joyful, sad or excited, but be tranquil and happy.

7. GASTROINTESTINAL SPASM

Brief introduction

Gastrointestinal spasm refers to severe gastric and abdominal pain caused by sudden, fitful, intense contraction of the gastrointestinal smooth muscles. It is a common symptom in clinical settings. Gastric spasm is seen in Western medicine in acute gastritis, gastric ulcer, or neurosis amongst other conditions. Intestinal spasm usually occurs in children with a history of repeated attacks.

Aetiology and pathogenesis

It is usually caused by food retention or accumulation of Cold in gastrointestine. The location of this disease is in the Stomach and intestine with a nature of deficiency or a complicated condition of deficiency and excess.

Syndrome differentiation

It is characterized by sudden paroxysmal gastric and abdominal pain. Inducing factors are local exposure to Cold, irregular food intake, and intense exercise after meals.

1. **Food retention**: Severe epigastric pain that is worse on pressure, nausea, vomiting, belching with a fetid odour, pale face, cold limbs after sweating, white sticky tongue coating, string-taut and tense pulse.

2. **Accumulation of Cold in gastrointestine**: Severe and stabbing pain in the epigastrium, contracture of skin in the abdomen (all of which become better on warmth and pressure), pale face, cold limbs after sweating, white coating, and tense pulse.

Treatment

Body acupuncture

1. **Principles of treatment**

   To improve digestion, relieve retained food, unblock the Qi of the Fu organs, warm the Middle Burner, dispel Cold, and relieve pain with mainly acupuncture and the reducing method.

2. **Prescription**

   Mainly select acupoints in the Stomach Meridian of Foot-Yangming and related Front-Mu and Xi-Cleft points. Zhongwan (CV12), Tianshu (ST25), Liangqiu (ST34), Zusanli (ST36).

3. **Explanation**

   Zhongwan (CV12) unblocks Qi of the Fu organs, regulates Stomach Qi and relieves pain. Tianshu (ST25), the Front-Mu point of the Large Intestine, combines with Zhongwan (CV12) to strengthen the effect of unblocking the Qi of the Fu organs, stopping convulsions and relieving pain. Liangqiu (ST34) is especially effective in acute paroxysmal pain syndrome. Zusanli (ST36), is the Lower He-Sea point of the Stomach that is effective for the symptoms of Fu organs. It is also one of the Four General Points to be used for symptoms of the abdomen.

4. **Modification**

   - *Food retention*: + Jianli (CV11) and Gongsun (SP4) to improve digestion and regulate Stomach Qi.

   - *Accumulation of Cold in gastrointestine*: + moxibustion on Shenque (CV8) and Guanyuan (CV4) to warm and dispel Cold, relieve pain.

   - *Gastric spasm*: + Neiguan (PC6) and Liangmen (ST21) to regulate Stomach Qi and relieve convulsions.

   - *Intestinal spasm*: + Shangjuxu (ST37) and Xiajuxu (ST39) to regulate the intestine and relieve convulsions.

   - *Nausea and vomiting*: + Neiguan (PC6) and Geshu (BL17) to unblock the chest and regulate Stomach Qi.

   - *Contracture of skin in the abdomen*: + Jinsuo (GV8) and Yanglingquan (GB34) to relieve convulsions and relieve pain.

5. **Manipulation**

Apply routine needling techniques to all the points with strong stimulation and the reducing method. Retain needles for 20–30 minutes. Add moxibustion or warming needle moxibustion.

Other therapies

1. **Finger pressure**

Select Zhiyang (GV9) or tender points in the back. Press and pluck with the thumb for 3–5 minutes, and repeat once after a 5 minute interval.

2. **Heat compress**

Fry salt and Wuzhuyu (吴茱萸 *Fructus Evodiae*) until they become warm, then enclose in a hop-pocket, and apply this to the epigastrium until the pain disappears. This method is particularly applicable for children.

3. **Topical application of drug**

Grind equivalent dosages of Wuzhuyu (吴茱萸 *Fructus Evodiae*), Dingxiang (丁香 *Flos Caryophylli*), dried ginger, Aiye (艾叶 *Folium Artemisiae Argyi*), and white pepper into powder. Take 2g powder and enclose into a fine gauze bag of 2cm × 3cm. Then apply it on the umbilicus and fix with adhesive plasters.

4. **Auricular acupuncture**

Points: Stomach, Large Intestine, Small Intestines, Ear-Shenmen, Sympathetic Nerve, Abdomen, and Subcortex. Choose 4–5 points each time. Puncture with filiform needles, apply strong stimulation, and retain for 20–30 minutes.

5. **Electroacupuncture**

When there is the arrival of Qi by the use of the puncturing needles, connect the points in the abdomen and distal points to the electroacupuncture stimulator. Stimulate with continuous wave, quick frequency and strong stimulation for 20–30 minutes.

6. **Point injection**

Select Zhongwan (CV12), Tianshu (ST25), Zusanli (ST36), Weishu (BL21), Dachangshu (BL25), Xiaochangshu (BL27), Neiguan (PC6). Choose 1–3 points each time, and inject 0.5–1ml of Atropine or 2% Lidocaine into each point.

Notes

1. Acupuncture and moxibustion have quite a good effect on analgesia for this disease. If the pain is not alleviated after this treatment, the causes should be found so as to give treatment based on the aetiology.

2. Tell patients to form good habits of eating with regular food intake and to avoid overeating and overdrinking. They should also eat more food rich in fibre and less food that may produce gas. They should abstain from cold drinks, and should not do intensive exercise immediately after heavy meals.

8. GALLBLADDER COLIC

Brief introduction

Gallbladder colic is a common acute syndrome in the abdomen. It is characterized by colic pain in the hypochondrium of the right upper abdomen. The pain is paroxysmally worse or continuous. It is included in hypochondriac pain in TCM and seen in Western medicine in various diseases of the biliary duct such as cholecystitis, inflammation of the biliary duct, Gallbladder calculi, and ascariasis. It occurs more often in females than in males.

Aetiology and pathogenesis

1. Emotional factors cause Qi stagnation of the Liver and Gallbladder.

2. Irregular food intake impairs the Spleen and Stomach to cause an accumulation of Phlegm and Damp, which transforms into Heat or calculi.

3. Ascariasis moves into the biliary duct.

The location of this disease is in the Liver and Gallbladder with the Spleen, Stomach and intestines involved.

Syndrome differentiation

Main symptoms include sudden severe and continuous colic pain in the right upper abdomen, which is paroxysmally worse. The pain is also worse on pressure with tenderness or pounding pain, and radiates to the right shoulder in the back. Inducing factors are melancholy, over-thinking, anger, overeating of greasy food, being too hungry and exposure to cold or heat.

1. **Qi stagnation of the Liver and Gallbladder**: Onset of colic pain induced by emotional turbulence, oppressive feeling in the chest, belching, nausea, vomiting, anorexia, irritability, hot temper, thin white tongue coating, string-taut tense pulse.

2. **Damp Heat in the Liver and Gallbladder**: Colic pain in the right upper abdomen, chills, fever, bitter taste in the mouth, dry throat, nausea, vomiting, or even yellow eyes, body and urine, constipation, dribbling of cold sweat, yellow sticky tongue coating, string-taut and rapid pulse.

3. **Moving of ascariasis into the biliary duct**: Severe pain in the right upper abdomen and inferior of the sternocostal angle that is worse on pressure, insomnia, chills, fever, nausea, vomiting, or vomiting of ascariasis, anorexia, thin white tongue coating, string-taut and tense pulse.

Treatment
Body acupuncture

1. **Principles of treatment**

   To pacify the Liver and Gallbladder, promote flow of Qi and relieve pain, with mainly acupuncture and the reducing method.

2. **Prescription**

   Mainly select points in the Gallbladder Meridian of Foot-Shaoyang, related Front-Mu and Back-Shu points. Zhongwan (CV12), Riyue (GB24), Danshu (BL20), Yanglingquan (GB34), Dannang (EX-LE6).

3. **Explanation**

   Zhongwan (CV12), the Influential point of Fu organs, unblocks and regulates the Qi of the Fu organs. Riyue (GB24), the Front-Mu point of the Gallbladder, and Danshu (BL20), Back-Shu point of the Gallbladder, may together pacify and regulate the Qi of the Liver and Gallbladder. Yanglingquan (GB34), the Lower He-Sea point of the Gallbladder, is the first choice for disorders of the Gallbladder. Dannang (EX-LE6) is an established point for disorders of the Gallbladder.

4. **Modification**

   - *Qi stagnation of the Liver and Gallbladder*: + Taichong (LR3) and Ligou (LR5) to strengthen the effect of pacifying the Liver and Gallbladder.

   - *Damp Heat in the Liver and Gallbladder*: + Sanyinjiao (SP6) and Yinlingquan (SP9) to clear Damp Heat.

- *Moving of ascariasis*: + Baichongwo and penetrating from Yingxiang (LI20) toward Sibai (ST2) to expel ascariasis.

- *Fever and chills*: + Quchi (LI11), Zhigou (TE6) and Waiguan (TE5) to harmonize Shaoyang.

- *Nausea and vomiting*: + Neiguan (PC6) and Zusanli (ST36) to harmonize the Middle Burner and stop vomiting.

- *Jaundice caused by Damp Heat*: + Zhiyang (GV9), Ganshu (BL18) and Yinlingquan (SP9) to clear Damp Heat and relieve jaundice.

5. **Manipulation**

   Riyue (GB24) is punctured obliquely and laterally along the intercostal space. Danshu (BL20) is punctured downward or obliquely toward the spinal column without deep insertion to avoid injuring the internal organs. Ganshu (BL18) and Danshu (BL20) may be applied with big moxibustion cones to cause a burning sensation in the skin or blisters. Apply routine needling techniques to the rest of the points with strong stimulation and longer retention, for 1–2 hours. Manipulate the needles intermittently to maintain the strong needling sensation. The treatment is given twice every day.

Other therapies

1. **Finger pressure**

   Select Danshu (BL20) or its adjacent tender spots. Press with the thumb strongly for 10–20 minutes.

2. **Auricular acupuncture**

   Points: Liver, Gallbladder, lower portion of Rectum, Abdomen, Chest, Ear-Shenmen, Sympathetic Nerve, Stomach, and Spleen. Choose 3–4 points each time. Puncture with filiform needles and use strong stimulation. Retain for 30 minutes and treat once every day.

3. **Electroacupuncture**

   Connect points in the abdomen and lower limbs to an eletroacupuncture stimulator, and stimulate with continuous wave and quick frequency for 30–60 minutes. Apply 1–2 times every day.

4. **Point injection**

   Select tender points in the right upper abdomen, Riyue (GB24), Qimen (LR14), Yanglingquan (GB34), Dannang (EX-LE6). Inject 0.5–1ml of 654-2 (Anisodamine) injection into each point. Treat once every day.

Notes

1. Acupuncture and moxibustion have quite a good effect on Gallbladder colic and are especially effective in cases with acute onset, short duration, and no severe complications. But during the treatment, the aetiology should be found and a combination of treatment aimed at the aetiology will increase the effect.

2. Tell patients to follow a light diet rather than one containing greasy food and keep warm.

9. URINARY COLIC

Brief introduction

Urinary colic refers to the severe pain caused by urinary calculus. It is characterized by paroxysmal colic in the lower back or sides of the abdomen that radiates downward or upward along the urethra, urodynia, and haematuria. It is seen in lower back pain and dysuria in TCM.

Aetiology and pathogenesis

Fundamental causes of this disease include irregular food intake, Damp-Heat in the Lower Burner, and Kidney Yang deficiency. The direct cause of the colic pain is the stimulating of the Zang Fu organs and tissues during discharge of calculi. A main factor for haematuria is that the calculi injure the mucous membranes and vessels in the Zang Fu organs and tissues. The location of this disease is in the Kidneys and Bladder and it is closely related with the Liver and Spleen.

Syndrome differentiation

According to the location of the calculi, there can be a calculus in the Kidneys, ureter, Bladder, and urethra. But all these are accompanied by sudden severe colic in the lower back with a dragging pain in the lower abdomen, which also radiates to the anterior of the pudendum, perineum and medial of the thigh. Or there is a sudden interruption of the urine stream, severe stabbing pain in the urethra, haematuria, and percussive pain in the Kidney area. Patients with longstanding pain experience a pale face, nausea, vomiting, dribbling of cold sweat, or even syncope.

1. **Damp Heat in the Lower Burner**: Dark yellow and turbid urine, haematuria or presence of calculi in the urine, dribbling of urine, red tongue,

yellow or yellow sticky coating, string-taut and tense or string-taut and rapid pulse.

2. **Kidney Qi deficiency**: Acraturesis with dribbling of urine, lassitude, pale tongue, thin white or thin yellow coating, string-taut and tense pulse.

Treatment

Body acupuncture

1. **Principles of treatment**

   - *Damp Heat in the Lower Burner*: To clear Heat, eliminate Damp, restore free urination and relieve pain with acupuncture alone and the reducing method.

   - *Kidney Qi deficiency*: To reinforce Kidney Yang, promote diuresis, discharge calculi with mainly acupuncture or moxibustion according to some conditions, reinforcing or even method.

2. **Prescription**

   To mainly select the Back-Shu and Front-Mu points of the Kidneys and Bladder. Zhongji (CV3), Jingmen (GB25), Shenshu (BL23), Pangguangshu (BL28), Sanyinjiao (SP6).

3. **Explanation**

   The location of this disease is in the Kidneys and Bladder. Zhongji (CV3) and Jingmen (GB25) are respectively the Front-Mu points of the Bladder and the Kidneys. Shenshu (BL23) and Pangguangshu (BL28) are respectively Back-Shu points of the Kidneys and Bladder. The combination of the Front-Mu and Back-Shu points may promote the Qi activity of the Bladder, clear Damp Heat in the Lower Burner, unblock Qi in the Kidneys and Bladder and relieve pain. Sanyinjiao (SP6), a meeting point of the Spleen, Kidney and Liver Meridians, invigorates Kidney Qi, promotes diuresis, restores free urination, and strengthens the function of Zhongji (CV3) in clearing Damp Heat in the Lower Burner.

4. **Modification**

   - *Damp Heat*: + Qugu (CV2) and Yinlingquan (SP9)to clear Damp-Heat.

   - *Kidney Qi deficiency*: + Mingmen (GV4), Qihai (CV6) and Guanyuan (CV4) to warm and reinforce Kidney Qi.

   - *Nausea and vomiting*: + Neiguan (PC6) and Zusanli (ST36) to harmonize the Middle Burner.

- *Dribbling of urine*: + Shuifen (CV9), Shuidao (ST28), Weiyang (BL39) and Sanjiaoshu (BL22) to promote diuresis and restore free urination.

- *Calculi in the urine*: + Weiyang (BL39), Ciliao (BL32), Rangu (KI2) and Zhibian (BL54) to discharge calculi and relieve pain.

- *Haematuria*: + Geshu (BL17) and Xuehai (SP10) to clear Heat and cool Blood.

5. **Manipulation**

Zhongji (CV3) and Jingmen (GB25) must not be punctured deeply or perpendicularly in order to avoid injuring the internal organs. Apply routine needling techniques to the other points. Apply strong stimulation and retain the needles for 30–60 minutes. Treat twice every day.

Other therapies

1. **Wrist-ankle acupuncture**

Select 4 points located 3-finger breadth superior to the medial leg, midline in the lateral side, tip of the medial and external malleolus. Puncture obliquely upward 1.5 cun and retain for 30 minutes. Treat once every day.

2. **Auricular acupuncture**

Points: Kidney, Bladder, Urethra, Ear-Shenmen, Sympathetic Nerve, Subcortex, Triple Burner and Brain. Choose 3–4 points each time, puncture with filiform needles and strong stimulation, and retain for 30–60 minutes. Treat once every day.

3. **Cupping**

Select Shenshu (BL23) and Ashi points. Apply cupping and retain for 5–10 minutes. This is used during an attack of the pain.

4. **Electroacupuncture**

After inserting the needles, choose 2 pairs of points and stimulate with continuous wave and quick frequency for 30–60 minutes until the pain is relieved.

5. **Point injection**

Select tender points in the lumbus, Shenshu (BL23), Jingmen (GB25), Zhongji (CV3), Guanyuan (CV4), Sanyinjiao (SP6), and Yinlingquan (SP9). Choose 3–4 points each time, inject 3–5ml of 5%–10% Glucose, 2% Lidocaine, physiology saline, or injection of Danggui (当归 *Radix Angelicae Sinensis*) into each time point. Treat once every day.

Notes

1. Acupuncture, especially electroacupuncture, has a confirmed effect on urinary colic in terms of relieving pain and discharging calculi. To strengthen the effect, tell patients to drink a lot of water, and do more running and jumping.

2. For patients with constant colic that is not relieved, the aetiology should be established to adopt a comprehensive treatment. If surgery is really necessary, tell patients to undergo the surgery as soon as possible.

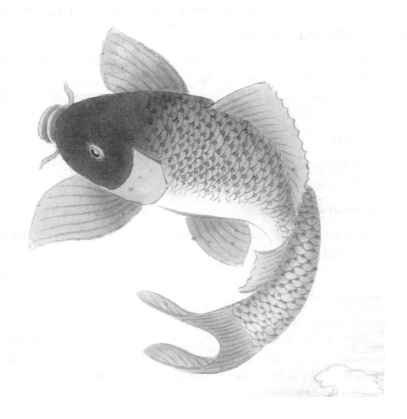

IX. OTHER DISEASES

1(A). WITHDRAWAL SYNDROME DURING ABSTINENCE FROM SMOKING

Brief introduction

Smoking injures the respiratory, cardiovascular, and nervous systems of the human body to different extents. It is one of the important causes for the increase in the occurrence and death rates of cancer, chronic bronchitis, cor pulmonale, gastric and duodenal ulcers, and cirrhosis. Withdrawal syndrome during abstinence from smoking refers to general weakness, irritability, yawning, lack of taste in the mouth and tongue, and even mental dullness, oppressive feeling in the chest, anxiety, and dysaesthesia.

Aetiology and pathogenesis

This condition is named in TCM, but there are similar manifestations in cough, depression, somnolence, and epilepsy. TCM holds that the inhalation of the harmful materials in tobacco over a long period of time will cause an imbalance between Yin and Yang, and disharmony of Qi and Blood in the Zang Fu organs, meridians and collaterals. Puncturing related points may regulate Qi and Blood in the Zang Fu organs, meridians and collaterals, and balance Yin–Yang in order to remove the addiction caused by smoking.

Syndrome differentiation

There is a long-term history of smoking, with 10–20 or over 20 cigarettes every day. Once people stop smoking, there is strong desire to smoke. If this cannot be met, symptoms include lassitude, anxiety, yawning, lacrimation, hypersalivation, lack of taste in the mouth, discomfort in the throat, or oppressive feeling in the chest, nausea, vomiting, and even trembling of the muscles and dysaesthesia.

Treatment

Body acupuncture

1. **Principles of treatment**

   To disperse Lung Qi, resolve Phlegm, and tranquillize the Heart and Mind with mainly acupuncture, the reducing method or even method.

2. **Prescription**

   Chize (LU5), Fenglong (ST40), Hegu (LI4), Shenmen (HT7), Hegu (LI4), Jieyan Xue (quitting smoking point). Note: Jieyan Xue is in the middle between the line joining Lieque (LU7) and Yangxi (LI5).

3. **Explanation**

   Chize (LU5), Hegu (LI4) and Fenglong (ST40) may disperse Lung Qi, resolve Phlegm, and regulate Qi and Blood in the meridians and collaterals passing the neck. Shenmen (HT7) calms the Heart and Mind. Jieyan Xue is an effective point for abstinence from smoking, as it can lead to a bitter taste in the mouth, dry throat, nausea and vomiting during smoking, and cause an aversion to cigarettes to support abstinence from smoking.

4. **Modification**

   * *Oppressing feeling in the chest, asthmatic breathing, and profuse sputum:* + Neiguan (PC6) and Danzhong (CV17) to unblock the chest, regulate and promote Qi, and resolve Phlegm.

   * *Discomfort in the throat:* + Tiantu (CV22), Lieque (LU7) and Zhaohai (KI6) to resolve Phlegm and unblock the throat.

   * *Irritability:* + Shuigou (GV26), Shenmen (HT7) and Neiguan (PC6) tranqulize the Heart and Mind.

   * *Mental dullness:* + Pishu (SP20) and Zusanli (ST36).

   * *Trembling of the muscles:* + Shuigou (GV26) and Taichong (LR3) to relieve convulsions and tranquillize the Mind.

5. **Manipulation**

   Puncture Jieyan Xue perpendicularly 0.3 cun. Apply the reducing method by rotating and twirling on Jieyan Xue, Lieque (LU7), Fenglong (ST40), Hegu (LI). Retain for 30 minutes each time and treat once or twice every day.

Other therapies

1. **Auricular acupuncture**

   Points: Lung, Mouth, Internal Nose, Subcortex, Sympathetic Nerve, and Ear-Shenmen. Puncture with filiform needles and apply strong stimulation. Retain for 15 minutes and treat once every day. The two ears may be used alternately. Needle-embedding or Vaccaria seeds may also be applied. Tell patients to press 3–5 times every day, especially when they have the desire to smoke. This may inhibit their desire to smoke.

2. **Electroacupuncture**

When there is arrival of Qi, connect the points to an electroacupuncture stimulator and stimulate with a disperse and dense wave, strong stimulation for 20–30 minutes. Treat once every day.

Notes

1. Acupuncture, especially auricular acupuncture, has quite good effect on abstinence from smoking. For most people who voluntarily receive treatment for abstinence from smoking, the expected effect is reached. The effect is not so good on people with a long history of smoking, especially of smoking many cigarettes every day, or whose smoking habits are related to their occupation or environment. The long-term follow-up result is not so good as the short-term result.

2. When applying Vaccaria seeds or needle-embedding, tell people to press the auricular points for stronger stimulation after meals or when the desire to smoke becomes the strongest during mental work. The purpose of this is to stop the addiction to cigarettes. Select related points according to the symptoms during abstinence from smoking. The effect is consolidated only when these symptoms are relieved.

1(B). WITHDRAWAL SYNDROME DURING ABSTINENCE FROM ALCOHOL

Brief introduction

This occurs in people with a long history of drinking too much alcohol when they abstain from alcohol. The symptoms include general lassitude, weakness, yawning, lacrimation, nasal discharge, anorexia, nausea, vomiting, irritability and depression.

Treatment

Body acupuncture

1. **Principles of treatment**

To regulate Qi and Blood, and tranquillize the Heart and Mind using mainly acupuncture and with the even method.

2. **Prescription**

Baihui (GV20), Shenmen (HT7), Pishu (BL20), Weishu (BL21), Zusanli (ST36), Sanyinjiao (SP6).

3. **Explanation**

Baihui (GV20), located in the head, is a point in the Governor Vessel. It connects with the brain and may tranquillize the Mind. Shenmen (HT7) tranquilizes the Heart and Mind. Pishu (SP20), Weishu (BL21), Zusanli (ST36) and Sanyinjiao (SP6) may strengthen the Spleen, regulate Stomach Qi, and regulate Qi and Blood.

4. **Modification**

- *Irritability and depression*: + Shuigou (GV26), Xinshu (BL15) and Neiguan (PC6) to calm the Heart and Mind.

- *Dizziness, soreness and weakness in the lumbar region and knees*: + Ganshu (BL18) and Shenshu (BL23) to reinforce the Liver and Kidneys.

- *Nausea and vomiting*: + Neiguan (PC6) and Zhongwan (CV12) to descend the abnormal rising of Stomach Qi.

- *Abdominal pain and diarrhoea*: + Tianshu (ST25) and Shangjuxu (ST37) to regulate the intestines.

5. **Manipulation**

Apply routine needling techniques to all the points. Retain for 30–60 minutes to maintain a stronger needling sensation. Treat once or twice every day.

Other therapies

1. **Auricular acupuncture**

Points: Stomach, Mouth, Endocrine, Subcortex, Ear-Shenmen, Throat, and Liver. Puncture shallowly with filiform needles and retain for 30 minutes. Treat once every day. Or apply Vaccaria seeds, and tell people to press 3–5 times every day or at any time when the desire for alcohol appears.

2. **Electroacupuncture**

When there is arrival of Qi, connect the points to an electroacupuncture stimulator and stimulate with continuous wave, strong stimulation for 40–60 minutes. Treat once every day.

Notes

1. Acupuncture has an obvious effect on abstinence from alcohol. For most people who voluntarily receive treatment for abstinence from alcohol, the expected effect is reached. The effect is not so good for people with a long history of drinking alcohol, drinking too much alcohol, or with habits of drinking alcohol related to their occupation and environment.

2. When applying Vaccaria seeds, tell people to press the auricular points for stronger stimulation when the desire to drink alcohol occurs until the desire disappears. Select related points according to the symptoms during the abstinence from drinking alcohol to consolidate the effect.

1(C). WITHDRAWAL SYNDROME DURING ABSTINENCE FROM DRUGS

Brief introduction

In patients who have taken or injected opium drugs more than 2–3 times, withdrawal syndrome usually occurs within 4–16 hours of stopping the medicine and reaches a peak in 36–72 hours. Early manifestations include yawning, lacrimation, nasal discharge, and hidrosis, symptoms which are similar to the common cold. Then the withdrawal syndrome occurs, and symptoms include sneezing, chills, goose flesh, anorexia, nausea, vomiting, abdominal colic, diarrhoea, spasms of the whole body, weakness, insomnia or waking up easily at night, tachycardia, raised blood pressure, hot temper, irritability or depression, and even aggressive behaviour. These are accompanied by strong psychological desire for the drug. Most of the symptoms disappear within 7–10 days.

Syndrome differentiation

1. **Internal disturbance of Liver Wind**: Hot temper, irritability, convulsions, aggressive behaviour such as smashing things, insomnia for the whole night, red eyes, bitter taste in the mouth, lacrimation and nasal discharge, abdominal pain, diarrhoea, red tongue, yellow coating, string-taut rolling and rapid pulse.

2. **Deficiency of the Spleen and Kidney**: Lassitude, mental depression, hypersalivation, anorexia, dizziness, insomnia, palpitations, shortness of breath, abdominal pain, diarrhoea, hidrosis, lacrimation, tremor of muscles, collapse, lying on the bed, incontinence of urine and stools, pale tongue, white coating, deep thready and weak pulse.

3. **Disharmony between the Heart and Kidneys**: Trance, mental restlessness, waking up easily, dizziness, palpitations, lack of taste in the mouth, anorexia, weakness of the four limbs, red tongue, white coating, string-taut and thready pulse.

Treatment
Body acupuncture

1. **Principles of treatment**

   - *Internal disturbance of Liver Wind*: To clear Liver Fire, eliminate Wind and resolve Phlegm, with acupuncture alone and the reducing method.

   - *Deficiency of the Spleen and Kidney, and disharmony between the Heart and Kidneys*: Strengthen the Spleen and Kidneys, harmonize the Heart and Kidneys, use both acupuncture and moxibustion, the reinforcing method or even method.

2. **Prescription**

   Shuigou (GV26), Fengchi (GB20), Neiguan (PC6), Hegu (LI4), Laogong (PC8), Fenglong (ST40).

3. **Explanation**

   Shuigou (GV26) and Fengchi (GB20) may wake up the Mind. Neiguan (PC6) and Laogong (PC8) may tranquillize the Heart and Mind, and clear Heart Fire. Hegu (LI4) circulates Qi and Blood, relieves pain and calms the Mind. Fenglong (ST40) strengthens the Spleen, resolves Phlegm, and eliminates Wind.

4. **Modification**

   - *Internal disturbance of Liver Wind*: + Taichong (LR3), Xingjian (LR2) and Xiaxi (GB43) to clear Fire in the Liver and Gallbladder.

   - *Deficiency of the Spleen and Kidneys*: + Pishu (SP20), Shenshu (BL23) and Sanyinjiao (SP6) to strengthen the Spleen and Kidneys, and regulate Qi and Blood.

   - *Disharmony between the Heart and Kidneys*: + Xinshu (BL15), Shenshu (BL23) and Taixi (KI3) to harmonize the Heart and Kidneys, and regulate Yin–Yang.

   - *Abdominal pain and diarrhoea*: + Tianshu (ST25) and Sahngjuxu (ST37) to regulate Qi in the Stomach and intestines.

   - *Irritability*: + Zhongchong (PC9), Yongquan (KI1) to calm the Mind.

- *Occurrence of desire for the drug*: + Hegu (LI4) and Taichong (LR3).
- *Convulsions*: + Yanglingquan (GB34).

5. **Manipulation**

Puncture from Shuigou (GV26) toward the nasal septum with strong stimulation. Be careful with the direction, angle and depth of Fengchi (GB20) to avoid injuring the medullary bulb. Apply routine needling techniques to the other points and retain for 60 minutes Treat 1–2 times every day.

Other therapies

1. **Bleeding and cupping**

Tap the Governor Vessel, Jiaji points and Back-Shu points in the Bladder Meridian with cutaneous needles and heavy pressure. Then add cupping or moving cupping.

2. **Auricular acupuncture**

Points: Lung, Mouth, Endocrine, Adrenal Gland, Subcortex and Ear-Shenmen.

- *Hyperactivity of Fire in the Liver and Gallbladder*: Ear Apex, Liver Yang, and Liver.
- *Deficiency of the Spleen and Kidneys*: Spleen, Kidney, Lumbosacral.
- *Disharmony between the Heart and Kidneys*: Heart, Kidney and Sympathetic Nerve.
- *Convulsions*: Knee.
- *Abdominal pain and diarrhoea*: Sympathetic Nerve, Abdomen, Stomach, Large Intestine.

Choose 3–5 points each time, puncture shallowly with filiform needles, and retain for 30–60 minutes. Treat 1–2 times every day. Or apply Vaccaria seeds, and change to the other ear every 2–3 days.

3. **Electroacupuncture**

When there is arrival of Qi, connect the points to an electroacupuncture stimulator and stimulate with disperse and dense wave, strong stimulation for 40–60 minutes. Treat once every day.

Notes

1. Acupuncture has quite good effects on abstinence from drugs. As long as patients are determined to do it, it usually succeeds.

2. Make detailed inquiries of the reasons for the drug addiction and the patients' situation. Give the same treatment to patients taking drugs because of diseases such as tumours, respiratory system conditions, digestive system conditions and neuralgia so as to avoid accidents.

3. Assistance from the family and society is an essential factor in consolidating the effect of the treatment and to help the patient to avoid taking drugs again.

4. Adopt timely comprehensive measures for patients with syncope or collapse.

2. CHRONIC FATIGUE SYNDROME

Brief introduction

Chronic Fatigue syndrome (CFS) is a group of symptoms associated with more than half a year of chronic and recurrent fatigue, of which the causes remain unknown and for which there are no organic problems discovered as a result of appropriate Western examinations. It is seen in TCM in headache, insomnia, palpitations, depression and dizziness.

Aetiology and pathogenesis

This disease is related to the Liver, Spleen and Kidneys. Overstrain, emotional factors or invasion of exogenous pathogens causes dysfunction of the Liver, Spleen and Kidneys. The Liver maintains the free flow of Qi, which influences the emotions and mental activities. The Liver controls the tendons and stores Blood, which is related to movement and tiredness. Dysfunction of Liver in maintaining the free flow of Qi, storing Blood and controlling the tendons may cause symptoms in the nervous, cardiovascular, and motor systems. The Spleen is the acquired foundation of the body, and governs transportation and transformation, and dominates the muscles. Spleen Qi deficiency results in failure to transport and transform Water and food Essence, which leads to tiredness and weakness of the limbs and muscles. The Kidneys are the congenital foundation of the body, they store Essence, dominate the bones, and produce marrow. Insufficiency of Kidney Essence causes weakness of bones.

Syndrome differentiation

More than half a year of fatigue in the nervous, cardiovascular, and motor systems. Rule out tumour, immune diseases, local infection, chronic mental disorders, nervous and muscular diseases, and endocrine diseases. There may be mild fever, dizziness, weakness or pain of muscles, pain and discomfort of the throat, pain of lymph nodes in the anterior or posterior of the neck, isthmus of fauces, insomnia, poor memory, depression, anxiety, unstable emotions and lack of attention, which are not alleviated after bed rest and influence the patient's daily life and work.

Treatment

Body acupuncture

1. **Principles of treatment**

   To pacify the Liver and regulate Qi, reinforce the Heart and Kidneys, nourish the Mind, and relieve fatigue, with acupuncture and moxibustion, the reinforcing method.

2. **Prescription**

   Baihui (GV20), Yintang (EX-HN3), Shenmen (HT7), Taixi (KI3), Taichong (LR3), Sanyinjiao (SP6), Zusanli (ST36).

3. **Explanation**

   Baihui (GV20) and Yintang (EX-HN3), located in the Governor Vessel, unblock the head and nourish the Mind. Shenmen (HT7) and Taixi (KI3), Yuan-Primary points of the Heart and Kidney Meridians, may harmonize the Heart and Kidneys. Taichong (LR3), Sanyinjiao (SP6) and Zusanli (ST36) pacify the Liver and regulate Qi.

4. **Modification**

   - *Insomnia, dream-disturbed sleep, easily waking up:* + Anmian (halfway between Yifeng (TE17) and Fengchi (GB20)) and Neiguan (PC6) to nourish the Heart and Mind.

   - *Palpitations and anxiety:* + Neiguan (PC6) and Xinshu (BL15).

   - *Dizziness and lack of attention:* + Sishencong (EX-HN1), Xuanzhong (GB39).

5. **Manipulation**

   Apply routine needling techniques to all the points. Treat 2–3 times every week.

Other therapies

1. **Auricular acupuncture**

   Points: Heart, Kidney, Liver, Spleen, Brain, Subcortex, Ear-Shenmen, and Sympathetic Nerve. Choose 3–5 points each time, apply Vaccaria seeds to the two ears alternately and change every 2–3 days.

2. **Electroacupuncture**

   When there is arrival of Qi, connect the points to an electroacupuncture stimulator and stimulate with disperse and dense wave, weak stimulation for 20–30 minutes.

3. **Cutaneous needle**

   Tap the Governor Vessel, Jiaji points and Back-Shu points gently for 15–20 minutes each time. Treat once every day.

Notes

1. Acupuncture has quite good effect in relieving the symptom of fatigue in the body, regulating the emotions and sleep, and improving the weak body constitution of the patient.

2. Besides acupuncture treatment, diet therapy should be combined with more vitamins and minerals. Advise patients to take Chinese herbal drugs and antidepressant, and immunopotentiator (drug to strengthen immunity) in Western medicine.

3. Tell patients to be optimistic and avoid emotional stimulation, adopt a regular lifestyle and avoid overstrain. Appropriate physical exercise and other entertainments are good to aid recovery from this disease.

3. COMPETITION STRESS SYNDROME

Brief introduction

Competition Stress syndrome includes that arising from games or exams. It refers to a series of symptoms in the nervous, digestive and cardiovascular systems caused by mental tension before or during competitions. It often occurs in athletes and students.

Aetiology and pathogenesis

It is caused by emotional factors. Too much joy, anger or over-thinking leads to dysfunction of the Zang Fu organs.

Symptoms include headache, dizziness, palpitations, insomnia or somnolence, anorexia, abdominal pain, diarrhoea, cold sweating, irritability, tremor of hands and muscles, lassitude, weakness, and lack of attention. Athletes may suffer from hypertension and syncope during games. Students may suffer from poor memory, difficulty in writing, blurred vision, frequent and urgent urination, and syncope.

Treatment

Body acupuncture

1. **Principles of treatment**

   To reinforce the Heart and Spleen, pacify the Liver and regulate Qi, and tranquillize the Mind with mainly acupuncture, and even method.

2. **Prescription**

   Baihui (GV20), Sishencong (EX-HN1), Shenmen (HT7), Neiguan (PC6), Sanyinjiao (SP6).

3. **Explanation**

   Baihui (GV20) and Sishencong (EX-HN1) may strengthen the brain and tranquillize the Mind. Shenmen (HT7) and Neiguan (PC6) can reinforce Heart Blood, and tranquillize the Mind. Sanyinjiao (SP6) strengthens the Spleen, benefit the Kidneys, and pacify the Liver.

4. **Modification**

   - *Headache and dizziness*: + Yintang (EX-HN3), Taiyang (EX-HN5).
   - *Irritability and tremor of hands*: + Shuigou (GV26), Hegu (LI4).
   - *Tremor of muscles*: + Taichong (LR3), Yanglingquan (GB34).
   - *Difficulty in writing and blurred vision*: + Fengchi (GB20), moxibustion on Baihui (GV20).
   - *Raised blood pressure*: + Dazhui (GV14), Renying (ST9).
   - *Syncope*: + Suliao (GV25), Shuigou (GV26).

5. **Manipulation**

   Puncture subcutaneously from Baihui (GV20) toward Sishencong (EX-HN1). Or puncture subcutaneously from Sishencong (EX-HN1) toward Baihui (GV20). After puncturing Neiguan (PC6), carry out slight rotating and twirling without a strong needling sensation. Apply strong stimulation to Shuigou (GV26) without retaining the needle. Renying (ST9) is punctured perpendicularly, avoiding the arteria carotis, with a slight lifting and thrusting, no retaining. Puncture Fengchi (GB20) 1 cun towards the tip of the nose. Add moxibustion to Baihui (GV20) and Zusanli (ST36) after acupuncture.

Other therapies

1. **Auricular acupuncture**

   Points: Ear-Shenmen, Heart, Subcortex, Sympathetic Nerve, Occiput, Brain, Spleen, and Liver. Choose 2–3 points each time and apply medium stimulation with filiform needles or electroacupuncture. Vaccaria seeds may also be applied.

2. **Electroacupuncture**

   When there is arrival of Qi, connect the points to an electroacupuncture stimulator and stimulate with disperse and dense wave, weak stimulation for 15–20 minutes. Treat 1–2 times every day.

3. **Scalp acupuncture**

   Select the middle line of the forehead, lateral line 2 of the forehead, the posterior temporal line. Apply routine needling techniques and retain for 30 minutes. Rotate and twirl quickly every 5 minutes. Or connect to an electroacupuncture stimulator for 30 minutes.

4. **Cutaneous needle**

   Tap Baihui (GV20), Sishencong (EX-HN1) and Fengchi (GB20) for 2–3 minutes on each point. The treatment is given once every day.

Notes

1. Acupuncture and moxibustion have a confirmed effect on competition stress syndrome without side effects and will not influence the result of drug tests.

2. Vaccaria seeds may be applied before the competition. When the patients feel stressed during games or exams, they may press the auricular points by themselves to tranquillize the Mind.

3. Competition stress syndrome is caused by mental tension. So besides the above-mentioned treatment, psychological assistance may be combined.

4(A). COSMETIC TREATMENT: FRECKLES

Brief introduction

Freckles refers to black or light yellow spots on the skin after exposure to the sun. It does not differ according to sex. It usually appears at around the age of 5 and the amount increases with the gaining of age.

Aetiology and pathogenesis

Invasion of external pathogenic Wind and stagnation of Fire in the Blood stage of the minute collaterals, attacks the face along the meridians.

Syndrome differentiation

It mostly occurs in the face, especially around the nose and sides of the als nasi. Occurrence changes with the seasons. In summer, the amount of freckles increases, the colour deepens and the area of lesion becomes bigger. In winter, the amount decreases, the colour lightens and the area of lesion becomes smaller. There are no other subjective symptoms.

Treatment

Body acupuncture

1. **Principles of treatment**

   To disperse Wind, clear Heat, cool Blood and dissipate rash with mainly acupuncture and even method.

2. **Prescription**

   Select mainly points in the cheek, the Large Intestine Meridian of Hand-Yangming, and the Spleen Meridian of Foot-Taiyin; Yingxiang (LI20), Sibai (ST2), Yintang (EX-HN3), Quanliao (SI18), Hegu (LI4), Xuehai (SP10), Sanyinjiao (SP6).

3. **Explanation**

   Yingxiang (LI20), Sibai (ST2), Yintang (EX-HN3) and Quanliao (SI18) are all located in the cheek. They unblock Qi of the local meridians and collaterals, activate Blood circulation and dissipate rashes. Hegu (LI4), the Yuan-Primary point of the Large Intestine Meridian of Hand-Yangming, is effective in various diseases of the face, and clears Wind Fire in Yangming, cool Blood and dissipate rash. Xuehai (SP10) and Sanyinjiao (SP6) are located in the Spleen Meridian of Foot-Taiyin. The Spleen dominates the muscles and its Divergent Meridian reaches the face. So these 2 points may tonify the Blood, nourish Yin, and harmonize Qi and Blood.

4. **Manipulation**

Apply routine needling techniques to the points.

Other therapies

1. **Fire needling**

Do routine sterilization in the area with freckles. Burn the Fire needle to red, and do spot burning accurately and quickly on the freckles without puncturing too deeply. After the treatment, keep the surface of wound clean to prevent infection. Treat once every 3–4 days.

2. **Auricular acupuncture**

Points: Lung, Heart, Stomach, Large Intestine, Endocrine, and Ear-Shenmen. Choose 2–4 points each time, stimulate with filiform needles and medium pressure, and retain for 20–30 minutes. Or apply Vaccaria seeds.

3. **Cutaneous needle**

Tap the freckle on the face gently, Fengchi (GB20), and Feishu (BL13) until the skin becomes slightly red. Treat once every day.

4. **Electroacupuncture**

When there is arrival of Qi, connect the points to an electroacupuncture stimulator and stimulate with disperse and dense wave, medium stimulation for 20–30 minutes. Treat once every day.

5. **Point injection**

Select Zusanli (ST36), Xuehai (SP10), Feishu (BL13) and Geshu (BL17). Choose 2 points each time. Inject 1–2ml of injection of Danggui (当归 *Radix Angelicae Sinensis*) or Danshen (丹参 *Radix Salviae Miltiorrhizae*) into each point.

Notes

1. Acupuncture is quite effective in treating this disease.

2. Carry out strict sterilization in Fire needling. Manipulate accurately and quickly. Do not apply in too big an area each time and treat different areas

alternately. After the treatment, keep the surface of the wound clean to prevent infection.

3. During the treatment, advise patients to avoid exposure to sun as much as possible so as to avoid influencing the effect.

4(B). COSMETIC TREATMENTS: CHLOASMA

Brief introduction

Chloasma refers to symmetrically patchy brown skin of the face. It is seen in women in pregnancy, and after abortion or miscarriage. It is related to disorders of oestrogen metabolism and the vegetative (autonomic) nervous system. Other related factors include exposure to sun, using certain cosmetic products for a long time, contraception pills, irregular menstruation, inflammation in the pelvis, Liver disease, chronic alcohol poisoning, tuberculosis and tumour.

Aetiology and pathogenesis

This disease is closely related to the Liver, Spleen and Kidneys. Pathogenesis is that Qi and Blood cannot ascend to nourish the face. Low mood or sudden anger impairing the Liver, worry impairing the Spleen, fright and fear impairing the Kidneys, all cause adverse flow of Qi. Then Qi and Blood cannot ascend to nourish the face.

Syndrome differentiation

The colour of chloasma in the face is yellow brown, light brown or dark brown. Initially, spots appear in different areas and gradually fuse into patches symmetrically in the face. It is more obvious in the malar, forehead and two cheeks. The form is sometimes like the wings of butterfly with clear or diffused borders. There is no inflammation or scales on the face.

1. **Stagnation of Qi and Blood**: Dark face, deep colour of the rashes, dark red mouth and lips, abdominal pain before menstruation, distending pain in the chest and hypochondrium, hot temper, sighing, dark red tongue with ecchymosis, string-taut and hesitant pulse.

2. **Yin deficiency of the Liver and Kidneys**: Dark brown rash, feverish sensation in the palms and soles, insomnia, dream-disturbed sleep, soreness and weakness in the lumbar regions and knees, delicate and red tongue, scanty coating, thready and rapid pulse.

3. **Spleen deficiency causing Damp**: White bright face, rash of light colour, overweight, lassitude, weakness, swollen tongue with teethmarks, soft and thready pulse.

Treatment

Body acupuncture

1. **Principles of treatment**

   To harmonize Qi and Blood, relieve stagnation and dissipate the rash with acupuncture and moxibustion, even method.

2. **Prescription**

   Select mainly points in the cheek, the Large Intestine Meridian of Hand-Yangming, and the Spleen Meridian of Foot-Taiyin. Yingxiang (LI20), Quanliao (SI18), Hegu (LI4), Xuehai (SP10), Sanyinjiao (SP6).

3. **Explanation**

   Yingxiangg (LI20) and Quanliao (SI18), as local points, may unblock Qi of the local meridians and collaterals, relive stagnation and dissipate the rash. Hegu (LI4), Xuehai (SP10) and Sanyinjiao (SP6) reinforce the Spleen and Stomach, and regulate Qi and Blood, to ascend Essence and Blood in the Zang Fu organs to the face to dissipate the rash.

4. **Modification**

   - *Stagnation of Qi and Blood*: + Taichong (LR3) and Geshu (BL17) to pacify the Liver, regulate Qi, activate Blood circulation and relieve stagnation.

   - *Yin deficiency of the Liver and Kidneys*: + Ganshu (BL18), Shenshu (BL23) and Taixi (KI3) to nourish Yin, clear Heat, and reinforce the Liver and Kidneys.

   - *Spleen deficiency causing Damp*: + Pishu (SP20) and Yinlingquan (SP9) to reinforce the Spleen, benefit Qi, promote diuresis and eliminate Damp.

   - *Areas with chloasma*: + Ashi points to unblock the collaterals and dissipate the rash.

5. **Manipulation**

   Apply routine needling techniques to the points. Be careful with the angle, direction and depth of the Back-Shu points. Moxibustion may be added to Pishu (BL20).

Other therapies

1. **Auricular acupuncture**

   Points: Lung, Liver, Kidney, Heart, Endocrine, Subcortex, Internal Genitals, and Cheek. Choose 2–4 points each time. Puncture with filiform needles and medium stimulation or apply electroacupuncture. Vaccaria seeds may also be applied. Or select Ear Apex, Lung, Large Intestine, Cheek, and Endocrine. Choose 2–4 points each time, and prick with a three-edged needle to cause bleeding. There may be bleeding in the ear apex with 5–8 drops.

2. **Electroacupuncture**

   When there is arrival of Qi, connect the points to an electroacupuncture stimulator and stimulate with disperse and dense wave, medium stimulation for 20–30 minutes. Treat once every other day.

3. **Point injection**

   Select Feishu (BL13), Weishu (BL21), Zusanli (ST36), and Xuehai (SP10). Choose 2 points each time. Inject 1–2ml of injection of Danggui (当归 *Radix Angelicae Sinensis*) or Danshen (丹参 *Radix Salviae Miltiorrhizae*) into each point. Treat once every the other day.

Notes

1. Acupuncture is quite effective for treating chloasma, but it may need longer courses of treatment.

2. Occurrence of chloasma can be influenced by various factors and active treatment should be given to the primary diseases. If it is caused by certain medicines or cosmetic products, the patient should stop using them.

3. During the treatment, tell the patient to avoid exposure to the sun as much as possible.

5. ANTI-AGING

Brief introduction

Aging is the result of a series of physiological and pathological processes. Along with the gaining of age, the immunity of the body gradually decreases to cause aging. Through peroxidation of the lipids, the free radicals in the human body can lead to impairment of the tissues and retrograde changes of organs, and thus accelerate the process of aging. Besides, functional decline of the nerves and endocrine system, disorders of lipid metabolism, and obstacles to Blood circulation are also closely related to aging.

Aetiology and pathogenesis

The root cause is that Kidney Qi deficiency fails to consolidate Kidney Essence. The Essence that the Kidneys store is the foundation of the Yin–Yang balance, and Qi and Blood of the whole body, and determines growth, development and aging. Along with the declining of Kidney Qi, the functions of the Zang Fu organs, meridians and collaterals, Qi and Blood also gradually decline, causing an imbalance of Yin–Yang, and aging occurs.

Syndrome differentiation

Main symptoms include slow thinking, indifference of expression, slow reactions, and poor memory. Senile symptoms are difficult to control and the coordination of muscular motion, slowing action, lassitude, weakness, aversion to cold, cold limbs, soreness and weakness in the lumbar region and knee joints, dizziness, tinnitus, insomnia, poor memory, hair loss and loose teeth are all aging symptoms. Because of decreasing bodily resistance, it is easy for older people to suffer from various senile diseases.

Treatment
Body acupuncture

1. **Principles of treatment**

   To reinforce the Kidneys, fill up Essence, regulate Qi and Blood and benefit the Zang Fu organs for the purposes of anti-aging, use acupuncture and moxibustion, and the reinforcing method.

2. **Prescription**

   Zusanli (ST36), Sanyinjiao (SP6), Shenshu (BL23), Guanyuan (CV4), Baihui (GV20).

3. **Explanation**

   Zusanli (ST36), the Lower He-Sea point of the Stomach, benefits the Spleen, nourishes the Stomach, reinforces Qi and Blood, and improves immunity. Thus it is a commonly used acupoint to prevent diseases, preserve health and prolong life. Sanyinjiao (SP6), a meeting point of the three Yin meridians of the foot (the Liver, Spleen and Kidney Meridians), strengthens the Spleen and Stomach, reinforces the Liver and Kidneys, nourishes Blood and fills up Essence. Guanyuan (CV4), a meeting point of the Conception Vessel and the three Yin meridians of the foot, benefits the Zang Fu organs, reinforces the Kidneys and fills up Essence to reinforce the congenital foundation. Baihui (GV20), an important point in the Governor Vessel, supplements the brain for anti-aging.

4. **Modification**

   - *Heart and Lung Qi deficiency*: + Xinshu (BL13) and Feishu (BL13) to reinforce the Heart and Lungs.

   - *Spleen Qi deficiency*: + Pishu (BL20) and Weishu (BL21) to reinforce the Middle Burner and benefit Qi.

   - *Insufficiency of Liver and Kidneys*: + Ganshu (BL18), Mingmen (GV4) Qihai (CV6) and Taixi (KI3) to benefit the Liver and Kidneys.

5. **Manipulation**

   Apply routine needling techniques to all the points. Setting mountain on Fire, a reinforcing method, may be applied to Zusanli (ST36), Sanyinjiao (SP6), Qihai (CV6), Guanyuan (CV4), Shenshu (BL23) and Mingmen (GV4). Or apply various methods of moxibustion.

Other therapies

1. **Indirect Moxibustion**

   Select Pishu (BL20), Shenshu (BL23), Guanyuan (CV4), Qihai (CV6) and Zusanli (ST36). Choose 2–4 points each time and apply indirect moxibustion with Fuzi (附子 *Radix Aconiti Lateralis Preparata*) insulation. The treatment is given once every 2 days.

2. **Auricular acupuncture**

   Points: Subcortex, Endocrine, Kidney, Heart, Brain, Ermigen (Vagus Root). Choose 2–4 points each time. Apply Vaccaria seeds once every week.

3. **Cutaneous needle**

   Tap gently the head, the Governor Vessel and the Bladder Meridian in the back to make these parts slightly red. Apply once every 2 days.

4. **Point injection**

   Select Qihai (CV6), Guanyuan (CV4), Sanyinjiao (SP6), Pishu (BL20), Shenshu (BL23). Choose 2 points each time. Inject 1–2ml into each point with a mixture of human placenta tissue fluid, injection of Lurong extract

(鹿茸 *Cornu Cervi Pantotrichum*), Huangqi (黄芪 *Radix Astragali seu Hedysari*) and Danggui (当归 *Radix Angelicae Sinensis*). This method is applied twice every week.

Notes

1. Acupuncture and moxibustion have quite a good effect for anti-aging. Moxibustion should be applied the most frequently. However it is crucial to persevere.

2. Besides acupuncture and moxibustion, other methods should be combined including massage, Qigong, physical exercise, entertainment and diet to preserve health.

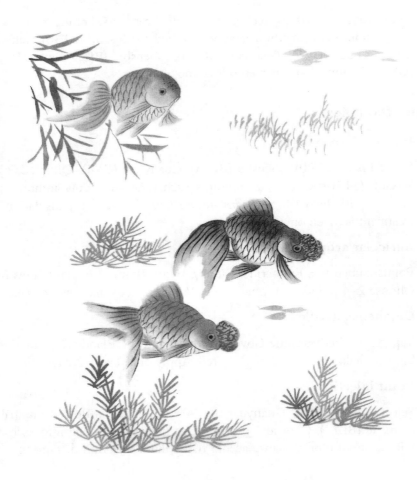

GLOSSARY

Acra Pertaining to a limb or other extremity.

Ablactation Weaning.

Adenomyoisis See *Endometriosis*.

Als nasi Either of the two rounded sections on the outside of the nose.

Analgesia Pain relief.

Anhidrosis The absence of perspiration where it should have been triggered.

Anoxia A condition in which the tissues of the body receive inadequate amounts of oxygen.

Anterior synechia An adhesion between the iris and the cornea.

Aponeurosis plantaris The thick connective tissue that supports the arch of the foot.

Arteriosclerosis A general term to refer to any of several conditions affecting the arteries.

Ascariasis A genus of parasitic nematode worms.

Asthenospermia See *Oligospermia*.

Ataxia The shaky movements that result from the brain's failure to regulate the body's posture, and strength and direction of limb movements.

Athetosis A writhing involuntary movement especially affecting the hands, face and tongue.

Atrial fibrillation Chaotic electrical and mechanical activity of the upper chambers of the heart, resulting in rapid and irregular pulse rate.

Atrioventricular block   The impairment of the conduction between the atria and ventricles of the heart.

Autonomic nervous system   The part of the peripheral nervous system responsible for the control of involuntary muscles.

Autosomal recessive inheritance   Two copies of an abnormal gene must be present in order for a particular trait, disorder or disease to be passed through a family this way.

Bell's palsy   Paralysis of the facial nerve causing weakness of the muscles in one side of the face and an inability to close the eye.

Biliary   Pertaining to the bile duct.

Biliary ascariasis   The infestation of biliary channels by an ascaris lumbricoides worm.

Bradycardia   An abnormally low heart rate.

Bradykinesia   Difficulty in initiating and executing movements. A symptom of Parkinson's.

Bronchiectasis   Widening of the bronchi or their branches.

Bruxism   A habit in which an individual grinds their teeth.

Calcaneus   The heel bone.

Canthus   Corner of the eye.

Caput radii   The cylindrical head of the radius.

Carcinoma   Cancer that arises in the epithelium, the tissue that lines the skin and internal organs of the body.

Cervical spondylosis   Degenerative osteoarthritis of the vertebrae of the neck.

Cholecystitis   The inflammation of the gall bladder.

Cholelithiasis   Gallstones.

Choreiform movement   Involuntary movements associated with the movement disorder choreia.

Chyluria   The presence of chyle (milky bodily fluid consisting of lymph and emulsified fats) in the urine.

Cirrhosis A consequence of chronic liver disease characterized by replacement of liver tissue by fibrosis, scar tissue and regenerative nodules (lumps that occur as a result of a process in which damaged tissue is regenerated), leading to loss of liver function.

Claudication Limping.

Cor pulmonale Enlargement of the right ventricle of the heart due to excessive pressure loading that results from diseases of the lungs or pulmonary arteries. Also known as pulmonary heart disease.

Cun A Chinese unit of length. Traditionally equal to the width of a person's thumb at the knuckle, it has now been standardized to 3.33cm.

Cyanic Blue in colour.

Cystitis Inflammation of the urinary bladder, often caused by infection.

Desquamation The process in which the outer layer of the epidermis of the skin is removed by scaling.

Detrusor The muscle of the urinary bladder wall.

Diabrosis Perforation, especially by ulcer.

Diuresis Increased secretion of urine by the kidneys.

Dysacusis A hearing impairment characterized by difficulty in processing details of sound due to distortion in frequency or intensity.

Dysaudia Difficulty in hearing.

Dyscrasia An abnormal state of the body or part of the body, especially one due to abnormal development or metabolism.

Dysaesthesia The abnormal, usually unpleasant, sensations felt by a patient with partial damage to sensory nerve fibres when skin is stimulated.

Dysgenesis Faulty development.

Dysmasesia Difficulty in chewing.

Dysphonia Difficulty in voice production.

Dysphoria An unpleasant or uncomfortable mood.

Dyspnoea Difficulty breathing.

Dysuria Difficult or painful urination.

Ecchymoma A slight haematoma following a bruise.

Ecchymosis   A bruise.

Eclampsia   A complication of pregnancy characterised by seizures and coma that are not caused by existing or organic brain disorders.

Encephalitis   Acute inflammation of the brain.

Endometriosis   The presence of endometrial tissue (the inner lining of the uterus) at sites in the pelvis outside of the uterus.

Epicondyle   A rounded projection at the end of a bone, located on or above a condyle (a rounded projection that forms an articulation with another bone).

Erythema   Flushing of the skin due to dilatation of the blood capillaries in the dermis.

Exophthalmos   Protrusion of the eyeballs in their sockets.

Extrapyramidal   Relating to the extrapyramidal system of nerve tracts and pathways, which is concerned with the regulation of stereotyped reflexor muscle movements.

Flexor digitorum brevis   The muscle in the middle of the sole of the foot, which flexes the toes.

Foot drop   An inability or difficulty in moving the ankle and toes upwards.

Gallbladder calculi   A hard, pebble-like mass formed within the gallbladder. Also known as gallstones.

Gastrectasia   Dilatation of the stomach.

Gastric mucosa   The layer of the stomach which contains the glands and the gastric pits.

Gastroptosis   A condition in which the stomach hangs low in the abdomen.

Gestational epilepsy   The occurrence of seizures exclusively during (usually the first) pregnancy or in the postpartum period.

Glycosuria   The presence of Glucose in the urine in abnormally large amounts.

Haematemesis   The vomiting of blood.

Haematochezia   The passing of bright red, bloody stools.

Haematoma   An extravasation of blood outside the blood vessels, generally the result of haemorrhage.

Haematuria   The passing of blood in the urine.

Haemoptysis   The coughing up of blood from the trachea, larynx, bronchi or lungs.

Haemorrhage   The escape of blood from a ruptured blood vessel, externally or internally.

Hemiplegia   Paralysis of one side of the body.

Hepato-   Relating to the liver.

Heteroptics   Incorrect or perverted perception of what is seen.

Hidrosis   Sweating.

Humeral epicondylitis   Inflammation of several structures of the elbow. Also known as tennis elbow.

Hyperia   Laboured breathing.

Hyperaesthesia   Excessive sensibility, especially of the skin.

Hyperosmotic non-ketotic coma   A type of diabetic coma; a state of extreme hyperglycaemia (high blood sugar) seen in type 2 diabetes.

Hypersomnia   Sleep lasting for exceptionally long periods, occurs in some cases of brain inflammation.

Hypertension   High blood pressure; a chronic medical condition in which the systemic arterial blood pressure is elevated.

Hypertensive encephalopathy   A neurological dysfunction induced by malignant hypertension (organ damage resulting from hypertension).

Hyperthyroidism   Overactivity of the thyroid gland.

Hypoaesthesia   Diminished sense of touch.

Hypophrenia   Deficiency of the mind.

Hyposmia   A reduced ability to detect odours, often caused by allergies or viral infection.

Hypotension   Abnormally low blood pressure, most commonly experienced when rising from a sitting or lying position.

Hypothenar eminence   A group of three muscles of the palm that control the motion of the little finger.

Indigitation   The telescoping of one part of the bowel into another.

Ischaemia   Inadequate flow of blood to a part of the body.

Isthmus of fauces   The passage from the mouth to the oropharynx, between the soft palate and the root of the tongue.

Ketoacidosis   A type of metabolic acidosis (increased acidity in the blood) associated with high levels of ketone bodies (normal by-products of fat metabolism, which are oxidized to produce energy) in the body tissues.

Leucorrhoea   A discharge of mucus from the vagina.

Ligamentum plantarae longum   A long ligament on the underside of the foot that connects the heel bone with the second to fifth metatarsals.

Lingua   The tongue.

Lochiorrhoea   The excessive discharge of blood, mucous and cell material through the vagina for an unusually long period of time after labour.

Lumbus   Lower back.

Lymphangitis   Inflammation of the lymphatic vessels.

M. sternocleidomastoideus   A paired muscle in the superficial layers of the anterior portion of the neck, which acts to flex and rotate the head.

Medulla   The inner region of any organ or tissue when it is distinguishable from the outer region.

Meniere's syndrome   A disease of the inner ear characterized by episodes of deafness, buzzing in the ears and vertigo.

Meningitis   Inflammation of the protective membranes covering the brain and spinal cord, known collectively as the meninges, due to infection by viruses, bacteria or fungi.

Micrographia   Abnormally small, cramped handwriting. A symptom of Parkinson's.

Muscular fasciitis   Painful inflammation of the muscles.

Myasthenia gravis   A chronic disease marked by muscle weakness and fatiguability.

Mydriasis   Widening of the pupil, which occurs normally in dim light.

Myocardial infarction   Death of a segment of heart muscle, which follows the interruption of its blood supply.

Myoma   A benign tumour of muscle.

Myotonia   A disorder of the muscle fibres that results in prolonged contractions.

Necrosis   The death of some or all of the cells in an organ or tissue.

Nephritis   Inflammation of the kidney.

Neurothlipsis   Pressure on one or more nerves.

Oedema   Excessive accumulation of fluid in the body tissues.

Oligospermia   Reduced sperm motility.

Oliguria   The production of an abnormally small volume of urine.

Opisthotonus   A state of severe hyperextension and spasticity in which an individual's head, neck and spinal column enter into a complete 'bridging' or 'arching' position.

Orthopnoea   Shortness of breath which occurs when lying flat.

Orthostatic   Relating to the upright position of the body.

Pancreatitis   Inflammation of the pancrease.

Paralysis agitans   Parkinson's disease.

Parotid   One of a pair of salivary glands situated in front of each ear.

Paroxysmal   Short, frequent and stereotyped symptoms that can be observed in various clinical conditions.

Petechia   Small round flat dark red spots caused by bleeding into the skin or beneath the mucous membrane.

Phlebitis   Inflammation of the wall of a vein, which is most commonly seen in the legs as a complication of varicose veins.

Phrenospasm   Spasm of the diagram, as when hiccupping.

Plantar fascia   The thick connective tissue that supports the arch of the foot.

Plasmodia   The malaria parasite.

Platycoria   A dilated condition of the pupil of the eye.

Polydipsia   Abnormally intense thirst, leading to the drinking of large quantities of water.

Polyphagia   Excessive eating.

Polyuria   The production of large volumes of urine.

Prostatitis   Inflammation of the prostate gland.

Ptosis   The drooping of a body part.

Pubic symphysis   Joint uniting the left and right pubic bones.

Pulmonary emphysema   A long-term, progressive disease of the lung that primarily causes shortness of breath

Purpura   A skin rash resulting from bleeding into the skin from small blood vessels.

Pylorospasm   Closure of the outlet of the stomach due to muscle spasm, leading to delay in the passage of stomach contents to the duodenum and vomiting.

Pyopoiesis   The formation or discharge of pus.

Quadrantus plantae   A muscle in the foot that aids flexing of the second to fifth toes.

Retinal ganglion cells   A type of neuron located near the inner surface (the ganglion cell layer) of the retina of the eye.

Rheumatic cardiomyopathy   The deterioration of the function of the heart muscle as a result of rheumatic fever.

Scapha   The hollow at the end of the helix of the ear.

Sclera   The white fibrous outer layer of the eyeball.

Seborrhoea   Excessive secretion of sebum by the sebaceous glands (glands of the skin).

Splenomegaly   Enlargement of the spleen.

Strephexopodia   Ankle sprain.

Strephenopodia   Ankle sprain.

Subluxation   The presence of an incomplete or partial dislocation of a joint or organ.

Syringomyelia   A disorder in which a cyst or cavity forms within the spinal cord.

Tachycardia   An abnormally high heart rate.

Tenesmus   Straining, especially ineffective and painful straining, during a bowel movement or urination.

Thenar eminence   The group of muscles on the palm of the hand at the base of the thumb.

Trigeminal neuralgia   A severe burning or stabbing pain following the course of the trigeminal nerve in the face.

Trismus   A spasm in the jaw muscles preventing the mouth from opening.

Tubercle   A small rounded protuberance on a bone.

Uraemia   The presence of excessive amounts of urea and other nitrogenous waste compounds in the blood.

Urethra   The tube that conducts urine from the bladder to the exterior.

Urinary calculus   A hard mass of mineral salts in the urinary tract.

Urodynia   Pain on urination.

Urticaria   A skin rash notable for dark red, raised, itchy bumps. Also known as hives.

Vaccaria seeds   Seeds from the Vaccaria plant, which are used to stimulate ear acupuncture points.

Vasoneurosis   Any disorder primarily affecting the blood vessels.

Vasospasm   Refers to a condition in which blood vessels are unduly reactive and enter spasm, leading to vasoconstriction.

Vertebro-basilar artery   The two vertebral arteries and the basilar artery.

Volvulus   Twisting of part of the digestive tract, usually leading to partial or complete obstruction.

Whitlow   An inflamed swelling of the nail folds (the folds of skin that lie above the roots).

BIBLIOGRAPHY

Huang Di Nei Jing Su Wen (1979) 'Plain Questions.' *The Yellow Emperor's Classic of Internal Medicine.* Beijing: People's Health Publishing House.

Huang Di Nei Jing Ling Shu (1979) 'Miraculous Pivot.' *The Yellow Emperor's Classic of Internal Medicine.* Beijing: People's Health Publishing House.

Huang-fu Mi (1979) *Systematic Classic of Acupuncture and Moxibustion.* Bejing: People's Press.

Zhang Zhong Jing (2007) *Treatise on Febrile Diseases.* Translated by Luo Xiwen. Canada: Redwing Book Company.